THE
ENCYCLOPEDIA
OF
OBESITY
AND
EATING DISORDERS

THE ENCYCLOPEDIA OF OBESITY AND EATING DISORDERS

Dana K. Cassell

with

Félix E. F. Larocca, M.D., F.A.P.A.

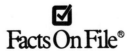

Facts On File®

AN INFOBASE HOLDINGS COMPANY

The Encyclopedia of Obesity and Eating Disorders

Copyright © 1994 by Dana K. Cassell
Foreword copyright © 1994 by Félix E. F. Larocca, M.D.

Facts On File, Inc.
460 Park Avenue South
New York, NY 10016

Library of Congress Cataloging-in-Publication Data
Cassell, Dana K.
  Encyclopedia of obesity and eating disorders / Dana K. Cassell.
    p. cm.
  Includes bibliographical references and index.
  ISBN 0-8160-1985-1
  1. Eating disorders—Encyclopedias. 2. Obesity—Encyclopedias.
I. Title.
  [DNLM: 1. Eating Disorders—encyclopedias. 2. Obesity—encyclopedias.
WD 210 C344e]
RC552.E18C37   1993
616.85'26'003—dc20   92-18289

A British CIP catalogue record for this book is available from the British Library.

Facts On File books are available at special discounts when purchased in bulk
quantities for businesses, associations, institutions or sales promotions. Please call
our Special Sales Department in New York at 212/683-2244 or 800/322-8755.

Composition by the Maple-Vail Book Manufacturing Group
Manufactured by Book Press
Printed in the United States of America

10 9 8 7 6 5 4 3 2 1

This book is printed on acid-free paper.

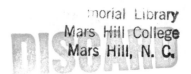

CONTENTS

ACKNOWLEDGMENTS

First, thanks to Kate Kelly, the editor whose idea this book was, and to Meg Ruley, the agent who brought us together. Several other editors at Facts On File worked on the project, but none more than Drew Silver, who edited the entire manuscript and contributed greatly to the work.

In preparing this volume we have reviewed books, journal and mass media articles, monographs and studies by the score to distill current opinion and research findings, and we have carefully tried to give full attribution to authors and researchers whose work we have consulted. Among those who have been especially helpful in sending material, or who have contributed significantly to the literature—and thus indirectly to the success of this book—are Paul E. Garfinkel, M.D.; David M. Garner, Ph.D.; Paul Ernsberger, Ph.D.; George A. Bray, M.D.; D. A. Booth, Ph.D.; Kelly D. Brownell, Ph.D.; Maria P. P. Root, Ph.D.; Patricia Fallon, Ph.D.; William N. Friedrich, Ph.D.; Patricia A. Neuman, Ed.S.; Patricia A. Halvorson, Ph.D.; Janet Polivy, Ph.D.; W. J. Kenneth Rockwell, M.D.; Gerald F. M. Russell, M.D.; the BASH Treatment and Research Center; the Renfrew Centers; and the National Association to Aid Fat Americans, Inc. (NAAFA). We owe much to the helpful staffs at the National Medical Library in Bethesda, Maryland and the Louis Calder Memorial Library, University of Miami Medical School/Jackson Memorial Medical Center in Miami. Special thanks to Frank DeLalla II for his computer expertise and to Vicki DeLalla for her research and assistance.

Given the unexpected length of time this project has taken, we fear there are some whose contributions we have failed to acknowledge. We hope they will forgive us; we are grateful to them all.

Dana K. Cassell
Félix E. F. Larocca, M.D., F.A.P.A.

FOREWORD

Never before the waning years of our century has so much attention been paid to what we might call the unwelcome side effects of eating: obesity, anorexia nervosa, bulimia nervosa, radical dieting and other disordered behaviors.

A great industry has arisen to take advantage of the yearning for thinness that has spread through developed nations. No-calorie or low-calorie foods and drinks, sugarless sweeteners, and pills sold as appetite suppressants pour onto the market. Writers make fortunes propagating new diets and *cuisine minceur* recipes. "Health clubs" and the makers of exercise machines sell people the presumed benefits of a "workout."

At the same time, obesity flourishes and hospital units fill with people, mostly women, mostly young, to whom eating has become an implacable and powerful enemy. Some are driven straight to the grave in an unequal contest with appetite. Many smoke cigarettes to take their minds off food, thus compounding the damage inflicted on their bodies by disordered eating habits.

The oldest eating disorder is anorexia nervosa of the restrictive type—that is, unremitting self-starvation in the pursuit of thinness. Cases began to appear around 1870, a decade after publication of the world's first book on how to lose weight.

Some writers have wanted to diagnose anorexia in fasters of various kinds, mostly medieval. The conduct usually described by the word *fasting,* however, has deep roots in ancient Judeo-Christian religious practices. It was inspired by a wish to show mortification of the flesh, contempt for the material world, closeness to God and a miraculous ability to sustain life without food.

The difference between this kind of behavior and modern anorectic self-starvation is manifest in the German word for anorexia nervosa, *die Magersucht*—a longing to be thin. The ascetics who rolled in thorns, flogged themselves and lived on bread and water did not do so to improve their appearance.

Nonetheless, a certain dark, romantic attraction hovers over the emaciated girls whom Lasègue and Gull described in the 19th century, when they became the first physicians to classify anorexia nervosa as an illness. These girls had in common with religious fasters a certain renunciation of common social obligations, as well as enigmatic self-banishment from family comforts that were, in a typical patient's household, generously provided.

It often appeared to therapists that these young women were trying to dodge adulthood, with its menstruation, sex problems and responsibilities, as much as they were fat. A later generation of clinicians, in particular the feminists among them, have adjusted the emphasis, looking instead for evidence that anorectics want above all to exercise control of their bodies and minds—which is to say, of their lives—in a private microcosm from which the threatening world has been excluded. Not to eat is thus their "statement" about society, and serious objections have been raised against tube-feeding anorectics against their will.

Actually, anorexia nervosa of the restrictive or "pure" type, with the patient approaching death by starvation at a weight of 50 pounds or less, has become rare. The eating disorder of the 1980s, bulimia nervosa, did not even acquire its name until 1979. Its growth in recent years has been swift and frightening.

The bulimic does not waste away, so her family usually does not know of the problem until it is well advanced—rounds of overeating followed by purgation to get rid of the dreaded calories. The gorge-purge cycles may rise to a frequency of a half dozen a day. Alcohol, drugs, guilt feelings and depression are familiar companions to the bulimic, contributing to a formidably intricate tangle of behavior that therapists are hard put to treat.

Many anorectic patients, although they diet to the point of emaciation, go through bulimic episodes. As in anorexia, most patients are women, but men in substantial numbers are being treated for bulimia. Many of them are students who need to lose (or have been advised to lose) weight for better athletic performance.

If the restrictive anorectic succeeds too well in establishing control over her little world, the bulimic fails miserably, regaining lost weight, sinking deeper into a private hell of frustration, stimulants and depressants. Since all this indulgence is expensive, debt and forfeited credit often are added to the burden of distress.

What has happened in our century to bring on all this self-destructive—and family-destructive—behavior? Clinicians in the field get used to eating disorders, in the sense of recognizing familiar patterns, but familiarity does not mean that the disorders have been tamed or their healing mastered. One comes to wonder whether the proper subject for treatment is a patient or a whole society.

This book is meant, then, to bring light to certain matters that in some of their aspects are not very well illuminated, and understanding to subjects on which expert researchers have not been able to agree. Under these circumstances it seems to me that the encyclopedic approach is especially useful; for while an encyclopedia cannot give exhaustive information about any subject, it can bring crucial questions about that subject into focus, give the reader a reasonably accurate "bottom line" and list further reading for those who want to know more.

So we believe that this volume is timely and valuable. It aims to be helpful to the young student, the perplexed parent, the confused practitioner and the prospective consumer of a vast variety of goods and services that purport to guide our eating behavior into wholesome paths. We hope that it will provide insights and accurate references to those in need. Last and not least, we recommend that readers consult the list of bibliographic sources appended to the main body of text.

Félix E. F. Larocca, M.D., F.A.P.A.

INTRODUCTION

THE HISTORY OF OBESITY AND EATING DISORDERS

Fashions shift in human beauty as they do in clothes and architecture, a fact pointed out by Anne Scott Beller in her natural history of obesity, *Fat & Thin*. Physical proportions strived for and glorified during one era or generation are avoided, even stigmatized, in another.

HILDE BRUCH, while describing the historical and sociocultural perspectives in *Eating Disorders,* noted that the oldest known representation of the human form, the "Venus of Willendorf" (Paleolithic period [20,000 to 30,000 B.C.], found in Willendorf, Austria), is the figure of "an extremely obese woman with large breasts and an enormous abdomen." Other Paleolithic figures represent similar fat women. The idealization of obesity in women continued into the Neolithic period. Prehistoric Greek, Babylonian and Egyptian sculptures also "indicate preference or artistic admiration for women with large abdomens and heavy hips and thighs," according to Bruch.

It is not known, Bruch adds, whether these archaeological "Venuses" are representations of women's actual appearances or whether they reflect a cultural ideal; they have usually been taken as symbolic representations of abundance and fertility at periods in human history when famine was an ever-present possibility (though some researchers have surmised that these figures were based on actual models). In any case, Bruch explains, in every age and in every land people have starved, and typically, during hard times, obesity has emerged as a kind of cultural goal or desirable state.

In very poor societies, sufficient food is consistently available only to a privileged few. Thus obesity may become a prestigious and admired characteristic. Bruch discovered during her anthropological research that in some Polynesian cultures it was considered a sign of great distinction to be so well nourished as to become fat. "Malayan kings were very large and fat; they were treated with special massages and exercises to keep them in good health."

Anthropologists tell us that in conditions of general scarcity, gluttony was conceived of as a practice to be aspired to, as in expressions from both South Pacific and southern African cultures about anticipated feasts: "We shall be glad, we shall eat until we vomit." "We shall eat until our bellies swell out and we can no longer stand." We are told that the southern African's dream was to be fat himself as well as to have a fat wife and children and fat cattle.

Bruch adds that ancient travelers reported African cultures in which young girls at puberty were sent to fattening houses to make them ready for marriage. The fatter a girl grew, the more beautiful she was considered, although the men were expected to remain athletic and slim. The king's mother and his wives competed with one another as to who should be the fattest. They took no exercise and were carried in litters when going from place to place.

The attitude that "bigger is better" prevailed during hard times earlier in this century among America's immigrants. Having suffered hunger during their own early years, poor mothers saw fat children as symbols of success. These children were not called fat; they were "solid" or "hefty." Author Harry Golden, who grew up in that environment, relates, "I, too, was a husky kid and when I worried about it my mother consoled me with the observation, 'In America, the fat man is the boss and the skinny man is the bookkeeper.' "

Paradoxically, Bruch says, during prosperous times and in affluent societies obesity is commonly associated with poverty and lower-class status. Now the ideal is to be thin, and there is much concern about obesity. The privileged classes of the Western world have been preoccupied through this century with the question of how to stay slim in the face of abundance.

The ancient Greeks of the classical age envied their cultural predecessors, the Cretans, for having known of a drug that permitted them to stay slim while eating as much as they wanted. Leaders in Sparta were stern taskmasters in their attitude toward obesity. Young people were examined in the nude once a month, and those who had gained weight were forced to exercise. The Athenians also frowned upon obesity. Socrates is said to have danced every morning in order to keep slim, and Plato was forgiven his fatness only on account of his brilliance. Hippocrates described obesity in great detail and made observations that are still pertinent today.

The Romans disliked obesity as much as the Greeks; ladies of the upper class literally starved to make themselves look slim as reeds. Yet, as with the Greeks, there were also famous Romans who were fat, and exact descriptions have been preserved of some of their eating habits. It is known that Marius, the defender of Rome, enjoyed enormous quantities of food. Horace, the poet, was famous for the extraordinary variety and elegant preparation of his meals.

During the Middle Ages also, there were conflicting views on obesity. On the one hand, gluttony was counted among the venial sins. But obesity was also considered a sign of the grace of God. In Lochner's painting *The Last Judgment,* the sinners being dragged into Hell are stout, and the blessed being led into Paradise are slender.

Ron Van Deth and Walter Vandereycken, of the University of Leiden, the Netherlands, and the University Psychiatric Center, Kortenberg, Belgium, have noted that despite the enormous number of scientific publications on anorexia nervosa, research into its history is still in its infancy. Believing that historical studies would shed light on the sociocultural genesis of anorexia nervosa, they began research some years ago. In *BASH Magazine* (April 1989) they point out that although the medical concept of anorexia is only about 100 years old, self-starvation has been known in various forms for centuries.

The less severe symptoms of lack of appetite and aversion to food have appeared in a variety of psychiatric illnesses. Also symptomatic have been more serious disorders associated with hysteria, melancholy, lovesickness, chlorosis (greensickness) and atrofia nervosa (nervous consumption).

Of these, Van Deth and Vandereycken consider the only one resembling modern-day anorexia nervosa to be atrofia nervosa, which was described by British physician Richard Morton (1689) as "deliberate starvation due to an ill and morbid state of the spirits." The disorder was accompanied by a lack of appetite and indigestion and was difficult to cure. His two detailed case histories described such symptoms as amenorrhea, constipation, hyperactivity, extreme emaciation and indifference toward both condition and cure, classic symptoms of today's anorectic. But even this description lacks any reference to what is a central feature of modern anorexia: the relentless pursuit of thinness.

According to Joan Brumberg in *Fasting Girls,* Simone Porta of Genoa, Italy wrote the first medical account of anorexia in 1500. A very few similar cases were described in medical literature over the next several hundred years.

But the relative silence in pre-1850 medical literature about a disorder with such remarkable and dramatic manifestations is striking, add Van Deth and Vandereycken. They consider it improbable that anorexia nervosa did exist but went unnoticed because of the low general standard of living, as some authors have suggested.

> The observable features and complications of severe anorexia usually are too obvious, if not horrifying, to go unnoticed, even when a majority of the population is underfed. Furthermore, physicians in previous centuries were rather keen observers; they had to rely almost exclusively on clinical examination. Among social classes where people did not suffer from undernutrition and medical consult[ation] could be afforded, possible cases of anorexia nervosa were scarcely mentioned either.

While anorexia nervosa may be a relatively modern phenomenon, self-starvation has been around throughout history. But our ancestors did not consider it to involve a disease.

Extreme fasting was a practice of many pious Christians throughout history, especially in the late Middle Ages among deeply religious women. Although reports of contemporaries claim these "saints" sometimes ate nothing but the consecrated host for years, these reports are subject to misinterpretation and exaggeration. As Van Deth and Vandereycken explain, "Hagiographers (biographers of saints) showed more zeal in demonstrating the holiness of the candidate-saint than in providing truthful historical facts. . . . [T]hey did not write a historically reliable biography or medical report."

Beginning with the 16th century, "miraculous maids" or "fasting girls" moved self-starvation into a more secular atmosphere. While considered by the pious a sign of God's presence on earth because they could eat virtually nothing yet stay alive, they were regarded by most more as curiosities than as divine manifestations. The popular media of the day publicized them. Thousands of people, including kings and other dignitaries, visited them, even offering them money, in the process turning them into tourist attractions.

Physicians of the day took on the task of investigating these cases for their validity rather than for the purpose of treating them or discovering causes for their starvation. Many of these girls were unmasked as frauds and imprisoned or killed, but not all.

By the 17th and 18th centuries, according to Brumberg, religious reform and changes of attitude led to prolonged fasting's being taken as the work of Satan rather than God. "Women who exhibited anorectic symptoms were said to be possessed by the devil and persecuted as witches." During the 19th century, the alleged extended fasts and the deceit of the maids were both labeled by physicians as signs of hysteria. From this point on, most self-starvation was looked upon as a medical-psychological problem.

It was not until 1873 that anorexia nervosa was established as a clinical diagnosis. In that year, E. C. Lasègue, professor of clinical medicine at the University of Paris, claimed that *"anorexie hysterique"* was caused by emotional disturbances that the patient tended to disguise or conceal. He mentioned the patient's "state of quietude—I might almost say a condition of contentment truly pathological. Not only does she not sigh for recovery, but she is not ill-pleased with her condition, notwithstanding all the unpleasantness it is attended with."

About that same year Sir William W. Gull, one of London's most respected physicians, first used the term "anorexia nervosa" in a paper submitted to the London Clinical Society. He explained, "We might call the state hysterical. . . . I prefer, however, the more general term, 'nervosa,' since the disease occurs in males as well as females, and is probably rather central than peripheral.'' He did note that young girls were especially prone to the disease. Lasègue and Gull were familiar with each other's work and recognized they were dealing with "the same maladie.'' They both insisted that anorexia was a mental rather than an organic disease and achieved a small degree of success by treating it with "rest, nourishment, separation from family and supportive therapy.''

In 1879 a French physician, J. Naudeau, published a lengthy description of a fatal case with significant similarities to modern anorexia. Another French doctor, H. Huchard, differentiated between *"anorexie Gastrique"* and *"anorexie mentale"* in 1883. Six years later J. M. Charcot, the famous French neurologist and teacher of Freud, recommended removal of his anorectic patients from their families. Although still relatively rare, the puzzling malady anorexia nervosa had become a recognized disorder affecting mainly the middle and upper classes.

Recognition, however, did not slow the debates as to the disease's causes; was it a physical disease or a mental disease? During the early 1900s, medical experts for the most part considered all disease to stem from abnormal variation of the body's cells or organs. In the case of anorexia nervosa, this theory found strong support when Morris Simmonds, a pathologist at the University of Hamburg, described pituitary cachexia in 1914. During an autopsy, Simmonds had observed lesions on the pituitary gland of a severely emaciated woman who had shown signs of pituitary failure and died. For the next 15 years, though anorexia might be mentioned in the literature, virtually all cases involving unexplained weight loss were diagnosed and treated as "Simmonds' disease.''

Then in 1930, John Mayo Berkman of the Mayo Clinic in Rochester, Minnesota published the first long-term report on large numbers of anorexia cases. His report outlined treatment of 117 patients at the clinic during a 10-year period. Even though the clinic treated anorexia as a metabolic disorder and rarely administered any kind of psychiatric treatment, researchers have credited Berkman with "rediscovery'' of anorexia as a separate disorder.

In 1942, R. F. Escamilla and H. Lisser searched medical literature worldwide to review cases reported as Simmonds' disease. In their report (*Journal of Clinical Endocrinology 2,* 1942), they determined that 494 of the 595 reported cases were, in all probability, cases of anorexia nervosa and not pituitary disease.

During the 1940s, the theory that anorexia nervosa was a psychological disorder began to gain support, although disagreement as to its exact causes ran rampant for the next 20 years. These psychological theories ranged from fantasies to fears of oral impregnation to emotional disturbance to psychosexual dysfunction.

The start of the modern era in the treatment of anorexia nervosa has been credited to a paper delivered by Hilde Bruch in 1961 and published in *Psychosomatic Medicine* 24:2 (1962): "Perceptual and Conceptual Disturbances in Anorexia Nervosa.'' As Patricia A. Neuman and Patricia A. Halvorson explain *(Anorexia Nervosa and Bulimia)*, "Bruch differentiated between 'primary anorexia nervosa' (the classic form as described by Morton and Gull) and 'atypical anorexia nervosa' (self-starvation due to other psychiatric illnesses).''

The classic or true form, according to Bruch, is characterized by severe disturbances in body image (the way subjects see themselves); misinterpretations of internal and external stimuli, particularly of hunger; and a paralyzing underlying sense of ineffectuality, the subjects' conviction of being helpless to change anything about their lives.

Prior to the 1960s, reports of anorexia nervosa were rare, but since then they have been occurring at a rapidly increasing rate. In addition, anorexia has increased its geographic spread. Cases have been reported in countries as far apart as the former Soviet Union and

Australia, Sweden and Italy, England and the United States. Mara Selvini-Palazzoli, an Italian pioneer in the psychiatric study of anorexia nervosa, reported no cases at all at her clinic during World War II when dire food shortages occurred; yet after the war, as the Italian economy improved and food became plentiful, hospitalizations did occur for anorexia nervosa. Studies in both the United States and Switzerland have indicated that the incidence of anorexia nervosa has doubled since 1960. During the early 1960s, for example, the University of Wisconsin Hospital typically admitted one anorectic a year; in 1982 more than 70 cases were admitted. It is so common today that it represents a substantial problem in high schools and colleges.

Another change Bruch observed over the years was a difference in the way patients approached the illness. Formerly no anorectic had ever heard of the condition; each thought she had invented a form of independence and control. Today most patients have read or heard about anorexia nervosa; some even compare their illness with textbook examples. Moreover, occurrence of anorexia is now often a group phenomenon. It is not unusual for an anorectic to be aware of others in her school classes with the same problem, and to use the others to measure her "success." With the increase in media attention, anorexia nervosa has become a fashionable disease among affluent adolescent and young adult women who are particularly susceptible to peer influence. It has been estimated that as many as 30 percent of all current cases are what Bruch once called "me-too" anorectics.

Just as the incidence of anorexia nervosa has surged since the 1960s, bulimia has also emerged recently as an increasingly common psychophysiological disorder, so much so that there is a widespread misconception that it is of quite recent origin. In fact, bulimia has an extensive history.

Episodic overeating has been a common practice. Primitive peoples dependent on hunting went on one- or two-day binges before spoilage could occur after successful expeditions, in attempts to compensate for long periods of famine.

Two early English references to bulimia were Steven Blankaart's *Physical Dictionary* (1708) and John Quincy's *Dictionary* (1726). Both discuss excessive appetite, but Blankaart refers to an extraordinary appetite usually accompanied by a "defection of the spirits."

In 1743 James, in *A Medicinal Dictionary,* credited the Greek physician Galen (A.D. 130–200) with defining the origins of boulimus, or the "great hunger." Galen considered it a digestive dysfunction, the primary symptom of which was a desire for food "at very short intervals." This, he said, was often coupled with fainting, loss of color, coldness in the extremities, oppressive feeling in the stomach, and weak pulse. According to Galen, boulimus was probably caused by an acidic "humor" lodged in the stomach, causing intense but false hunger signals. In addition, he suspected that the disorder was associated with the too-rapid digestion of food, resulting in inadequate nourishment and chronic hunger.

James added to Galen's and other writers' descriptions in an effort to distinguish boulimous from similar conditions associated with worms, ulcers and normal pregnancy. He noted that shortness of breath and an intense preoccupation with food may be symptoms of true boulimus. He further distinguished between true boulimus and a variant of it complicated by vomiting, "caninus appetitus."

> In the caninus appetitus, there is a desire after much food and great quantities are eaten, which oppressing the stomach, are again discharged by vomit. The patient thus being relieved, his appetite returns, which having gratified, he finds himself obliged to ease his stomach again, like a dog, by vomiting.
>
> In the true boulimis *[sic]*, there is a ravenous hunger and eating, but instead of vomiting, the patient suffers from lipothymy [fainting spells.]

Motherby, in 1785, differentiated three types of bulimia. The first two were bulimia of the pure hunger type and bulimia in which hunger was terminated by vomiting. In the third form, hunger was associated with "swooning."

In 1797, the *Encyclopedia Britannica* included an entry for bulimia under the heading "Bulimy": "a disease in which the patient is affected with an insatiable and perpetual desire of eating; and unless indulged, he often falls into fainting fits."

In the early 1800s, dictionaries described bulimia as featuring violent appetite, vomiting, fainting and canine appetite and occurring most often in hysteria and pregnancy.

During the 19th century, Gull acknowledged that anorexia patients occasionally displayed extremely voracious appetites, quite the opposite of their usual starvation tactics in their pursuit of thinness. Researchers have suggested that Gull's notation of such variations in symptoms, variations also seen by clinicians through the years, probably contributed to the idea of classifying bulimia simply as a subtype of anorexia nervosa.

However, in 1869 in France, P. F. Blanchez identified "boulimie" as a distinct syndrome, while admitting that it might occur as an accessory to another disorder. He described boulimie symptoms as food being an obsession and major preoccupation, yet with hunger sometimes continuing even after enormous quantities of food are eaten. He described the patient as becoming lethargic after a binge until the intense hunger returns a few hours later.

Then in 1894, in Germany, O. Soltmann posited "nutritional neuroses" such as "hyperorexia," of which bulimia was taken to be a symptom. According to Soltmann, hyperorexia, a syndrome, might be partly neurotic and partly biological in origin, affecting "over-excited, hysterical chlorotic young girls".

Purging is also not a recent phenomenon. The ancient Egyptians thought all diseases originated in food and thus purged their bodies every month. Tilmann Habermas writes that "vomiting was one of the most popular nonspecific symptoms in the nineteenth century, so its absence was often noted in cases of anorexia. On the other hand, it was rather unexpected that patients might intentionally induce vomiting."

Many of the physicians reporting on anorectic patients from the 1800s on included among the illness phases purging of some kind to get rid of unwanted food. Some patients learned to vomit immediately after swallowing; at least one was reported to use "a kind of hose to empty her stomach" (Habermas). During the early 1900s, abuse of laxatives or thyroid medication for the purpose of weight control was first mentioned, although vinegar had been drunk as a laxative for centuries.

Bulimia among individuals who did not have histories of weight disorders was first observed in 1976 by Marlene Boskind-White, who coined the term "bulimarexia" to describe this group. Bulimia officially became a distinct diagnostic entity in 1980 with the publication of the third edition of the *Diagnostic and Statistical Manual of Mental Disorders* of the American Medical Association. *DSM-III* suggested that episodic binge eating is not only an isolated symptom but an essential component of a specific syndrome of disordered eating.

REFERENCES

Bell, R. M. *Holy Anorexia*. Chicago: University of Chicago Press, 1985.

Beller, Anne Scott. *Fat & Thin*. New York: McGraw-Hill, 1977.

Bliss, Eugene L., and Branch, C. H. H. *Anorexia Nervosa: Its History, Psychology and Biology*. New York: P. B. Hoeber, 1960.

Bruch, Hilde. *Eating Disorders: Obesity, Anorexia Nervosa, and the Person Within*. New York: Basic Books, 1973.

Brumberg, Joan Jacobs. *Fasting Girls: The Emergence of Anorexia Nervosa as a Modern Disease*. Cambridge: Harvard University Press, 1988.

Bynum, C. W. *Holy Feast and Holy Fast: The Religious Significance of Food to Medieval Women.* Berkeley and Los Angeles: University of California Press, 1987.

Habermas, Tilmann. "The Psychiatric History of Anorexia and Bulimia: Weight Fears and Bulimic Symptoms in Early Cases." *International Journal of Eating Disorders* 8, no. 3 (1989); reprinted in *BASH Magazine,* December 1989.

Neuman, Patricia A., and Halvorson, Patricia A. *Anorexia Nervosa and Bulimia: A Handbook for Counselors and Therapists.* New York: Van Nostrand Reinhold, 1983.

Van Deth, R., and Vandereyecken, W. *From Miraculous Fasts to Morbid Pursuit of Thinness: Anorexia Nervosa in Historical Perspective.* Amsterdam: Boompers, 1988.

A

abdominoplasty A shaping of the abdominal area by surgery, popular since the 1960s. Frequently referred to as a "tummy tuck," this surgery gets rid of stomach fat and tightens flabby muscles and loose abdominal skin. The surgeon cuts seven to 15 inches across the body at the bikini line, lifts the skin, uses sutures to tighten the abdominal muscles and tissue, pulls the skin back down over the tightened area, cuts off excess skin and then closes the incision, making a new "belly button" in the process. The length of the incision depends upon the looseness of the skin. There is some pain and a scar, which usually fades to a thin line within a year. Costs generally range between $1,200 and $8,500. Once an indulgence of the wealthy, such surgery is now advertised to the public. At least one medical consulting firm has even offered an easy monthly-payment plan: the customer can borrow up to $10,000 for a tummy tuck and take as long as five years to pay. This firm claims that nearly 300 doctors nationwide subscribe to such a plan. According to the American Society of Plastic and Reconstructive Surgeons (ASPRS), performance of abdominoplasty procedures increased 215 percent between 1981 and 1988. The ASPRS reported 20,213 such procedures in 1990.

Abdominoplasties are not always without problems. When fat above the incision is not completely removed, bulges can occur above the scar line. These bulges can also appear if circulation is impaired during surgery, resulting in an accumulation of fluid. Because removing fat from the upper part of the abdomen can lead to bleeding and interfere with the skin's blood supply, fat is frequently left in this upper area, giving unsatisfactory results, with the upper abdomen sticking out over the more flattened lower abdomen.

These complications have led to a more frequent use of LIPOSUCTION for abdominal fat removal. However, because successful liposuction depends upon normal elasticity to shrink the skin after surgery, this procedure isn't always satisfactory either where there is excess skin or loose muscle. In many such cases, surgeons first use liposuction to remove the fat and then follow with abdominoplasty to tighten the abdominal muscles and remove excess skin.

acupressure A technique similar to and derived from ACUPUNCTURE, this treatment involves the application of manual pressure to the body rather than the insertion of needles. Acupressure has been recommended by some practitioners to control APPETITE. It is administered by applying pressure with the ball of the thumb and sometimes the fingers to specific points on the body. The main pressure point is on the upper lip; a point midway between the breastbone and navel is said to control HUNGER. Other points on the elbow and the knee are said by practitioners to control the emotions that lead to overeating. Not an instantaneously effective treatment, according to specialists, it is said to take three days for the reflex passages to the brain to become programmed by acupressure. Acupressure is even less well documented and scientifically tested than acupuncture.

acupuncture An ancient practice, used especially by the Chinese, of piercing the skin with extremely fine needles at strategic places on the body to treat disease or relieve pain. Acupuncturists believe that vital energy *(chi)* flows through the body along 12 main pathways (channels or meridians) connected to internal organs and systems like the kidney and respiratory system. They believe that disease occurs when there is an imbalance of energy in one of these systems, and that acupuncture needles inserted at specific points (numbering more than 1,000) on the body correct the flow of energy through the channel and help the body to heal itself.

1

Some medical doctors speculate that acupuncture may produce a state of painlessness partly by stimulating the release of endorphins (natural painkillers). Acupuncture as a treatment has some respectability based on empirical observations, but almost no scientific basis for acceptance. A very few medical doctors use acupuncture to supplement standard treatment.

The origin of acupuncture is unknown, but it is believed to have been practiced in China for more than 3,000 years. When acupuncture is used to help lose weight, the needle is placed in the area of the external ear known as the concha. The vagus nerve, which extends from the brain down the neck and chest to the stomach, branches to the concha. When the sharp point of the needle finds this branch of the vagus nerve, it acts to inhibit the contractions of the stomach.

The acupuncture treatment to the ear does not itself cause a person to lose weight. Rather, it causes the person to feel less HUNGER. Doctors in the United States have used staples and small needles, which are left in the ear to be jiggled when the patient feels the urge to overeat.

Published studies evaluating acupuncture as a treatment for obesity have thus far been inconclusive. In one, the author claimed a good response from 75 percent of 1,030 patients, but few details were given. In another study of 120 volunteers, it was reported that 70 percent treated at the "hunger" point experienced decreased appetite, compared with only 20 percent who had a stud (needle) in another part of the ear. And in a study of 350 obese subjects treated with acupuncture, 66 percent of them lost weight after seven treatment sessions. However, subjects had a variable number of courses of treatment of various duration. There were also no control subjects for comparison, so no final conclusions could be drawn. After reviewing several studies, Vincent and Richardson concluded that even though there are no clear indications for or against the use of acupuncture, an individual patient might derive less tangible psychological benefit from belief in the treatment.

Giller, R. M. "Auricular Acupuncture and Weight Reduction: A Controlled Study." *American Journal of Acupuncture* 3, no. 151 (1975).
Ishida, Yasuo. "Acupuncture Today." *Southern Medical Journal* 81, no. 7 (July 1988).
Lewith, George T. "Acupuncture." *Practitioner* 230 (December 1986).
Sacks, L. L. "Drug Addiction, Alcoholism, Smoking, Obesity, Treated by Auricular Staple Puncture." *American Journal of Acupuncture* 3, no. 147 (1975).
Vincent, C. A., and Richardson, P. H. "Acupuncture for Some Common Disorders: A Review of Evaluative Research." *Journal of the Royal College of General Practitioners* 37 (February 1987).

addiction Physiological or psychological dependence on some substance (e.g., alcohol, drug) or practice, with a tendency to increase its use. Addictions such as smoking and alcoholism share characteristics with binge eating and purging, but the eating-disordered person is addicted to the illness itself rather than to a substance. Food is the agent the addicted eating-disordered person uses to cover up or forget a weight problem (either real or imagined), fear of losing control over eating or other behavior, distorted body image, negative self-image, dissatisfaction in sexual or interpersonal relationships or lack of independence. According to Vandereycken, addiction-like behaviors exhibited by bulimics include "craving, preoccupation with obtaining the substance, loss of control, adverse social and medical consequences, ambivalence towards treatment, and risk of relapse."

The self-starving anorectic's behavior may also include alcoholism, although the binge eater is more likely to be addicted to alcohol or drugs. The way in which bulimics and anorectics (see BULIMIA and ANOREXIA NERVOSA) often tackle exercise and schoolwork also resembles addiction. Alcohol, over-the-counter diet pills, caffeine, barbiturate and amphetamine addictions have been noted by many researchers to be commonly associated with bulimia. In a 1981 study done at the University of Minnesota Adult Outpatient Psychiatric Clinic, bulimic women reported using alcohol to avoid depression associated with binge-purging, to relax and to delay or prevent overeating.

In a 1984–85 survey of 1,100 patients at Hazelden, a Minnesota chemical dependency treatment center, approximately 7 percent of female patients and 3 percent of males reported enough symptoms to be classified as bulimic under DSM-III criteria.

Hazelden reported that its bulimic female patients experienced more adolescent behavior problems and self-destructive behavior than nonbulimic patients. The typical chemically dependent female bulimic at Hazelden is more likely to "be a polydrug user; have had adolescent behavior problems such as school suspension or expulsion, stealing, and fighting; exhibit self-destructive tendencies through self-inflicted injury, suicide attempts, or suicidal thoughts during treatment; have had outpatient or inpatient mental health treatment or medication."

Although these problems could signal difficulty in treatment, Hazelden officials reported similar results for both bulimic and nonbulimic patients in most cases. "Bulimics required the same length of stay in treatment, were discharged with staff approval at similar rates, had about the same number of conflicts with peers during treatment, and saw their counselors with the same frequency as bulimia-asymptomatic patients." Bulimic patients did use mental health services at Hazelden slightly more than nonbulimics.

While Hazelden officials caution that recent changes in the diagnostic criteria for bulimic and Hazelden's pretreatment assessment methods make the data "tentative," conclusions suggest that it is reasonable to work with "manageable" eating disorders in chemical addiction treatment.

See also MULTICOMPULSIVE.

Pyle, Richard L. "The Subtle, Puzzling Affinity of Drugs and Bulimia." *BASH Magazine*, September 1989.

"Study Suggests Some Bulimia Manageable During Chemical Dependency Treatment." *Hazelden Professional Update*, September 1988.

Vandereycken, Walter. "The Addiction Model in Eating Disorders: Some Critical Remarks and a Selected Bibliography." *International Journal of Eating Disorders* 9, no. 1 (1990).

adipose tissue   A layer of fat lying just under the skin and around many internal organs (e.g., the heart and kidneys) to protect them from injury. This tissue acts as a shock absorber, cushioning areas such as the heels and buttocks against the frequent and sudden jolts they receive. Adipose tissue also functions as an insulating thermal blanket, keeping body heat inside. Because adipose tissue accumulates from eating more food than necessary for the body's immediate needs, it stores triglycerides as energy for future needs. When more adipose tissue is accumulated than is needed for cushioning, insulation and energy reserves, OBESITY results.

adolescent obesity   During the early years of adolescence, as their bodies are undergoing dramatic physical growth and biological change, some individuals become plump and may think of themselves as "too fat." But once the growth stops and the biological change is completed, the weight of most will naturally level off until they regain slimmer proportions.

For some, adolescent obesity is a temporary condition. For others, it is the beginning of a lifetime of obesity compounded with severe emotional and personality problems, since experiences during adolescence play such an important role in psychological development.

Just as other segments of America's population are becoming increasingly obese (see OBESITY), there is a growing national health problem of true obesity among young people. Various studies have estimated the number of truly obese adolescents in the United States as high as 10 million, or 11 to 21 percent of the total. The incidence of obesity in the 12- to 17-year age group has increased 39 percent since 1963. Superobese adolescents are an even faster growing group, with a 64 percent increase among children 12 to 17.

Some obese adolescents are simply continuing a history of childhood obesity, becoming even heavier during puberty. Some have not been overweight until adolescence. Others go from extreme thinness to obesity during these years.

This period of rapid growth is usually accompanied by an increase in APPETITE, especially for high-calorie foods, and some adolescent obesity is caused by an apparent inability to restrict food intake. While some adolescents burn off these extra calories in vigorous physical activities, others appear unwilling to exercise. They choose instead to treat their fatness as a "disability," refusing to join in normally active and boisterous adolescent games and activities. Frequently, this refusal to participate derives from feelings of inferiority and shame brought on by taunting and name-calling by their peers. Further exacerbating their difficulty may be parents and teachers who lecture them about their unhealthy weight and social nonparticipation. It soon becomes easy for them to blame all their failures or disappointments on their obesity.

Such feelings, demoralizing at any age but devastating during adolescence, can have serious long-term consequences. Thus, adolescent obesity may often contribute to life-long behavioral and psychological problems.

When obese adolescents do not receive—or accept—help, whether in losing weight or dealing positively and maturely with their weight and emotional problems, they usually withdraw even further from social life. They frequently then turn to food for solace, causing them to put on even more weight.

Obesity in adolescence is also frequently blamed for problems with sexual adjustment.

Although being fat can prevent a person from being considered "attractive" in our weight-conscious society, HILDE BRUCH cautioned that "it is not the weight excess itself but the attitude toward it, or more correctly toward oneself, that interferes with any personal relationships, most of all in the sexual area." Studies of adolescent obesity have described frequent cases of provocativeness and uncontrolled sexual behavior, even to the point of promiscuity.

Adolescents with severe personality problems who are desperately unhappy about being fat are especially easy prey for FAD DIETS and NOVELTIES. The promise and dream of changing a boring, uneventful life to one of exciting activity and romance make the advertised products appear magical.

Members of the American Society of Bariatric Physicians have reported little success in treating younger children for obesity, but they have had increased success with adolescents at about the age of puberty. Emerging interest in the opposite sex and a developing maturity level contribute to the motivation to follow eating restrictions.

Because the adolescent body undergoes so many energy-requiring physical changes, "average" calorie requirement tables are of little use for obese adolescents dieting to lose weight. Following typical calorie requirement tables is likely to result in an unhealthily low calorie intake. Diets are particularly difficult for boys around the age of 15, when their calorie intake may increase five times or more. Adolescent dieting can also be stressful socially because so much of teenage social life revolves around eating. Well-meaning but nagging parents may add to this stress, especially given adolescents' growing independence. Experts suggest that, for this reason, parents may be most helpful in supportive roles.

Bruch, Hilde. "Obesity in Adolescence." In *Eating Disorders: Obesity, Anorexia Nervosa, and the Person Within.* New York: Basic Books, 1973.

Burch, Gwen Weber, and Pearson, Paul H. "Anorexia, Bulimia, and Obesity in Adolescence:

The Sociocultural Perspective.'' In *Eating Disorders: Effective Care and Treatment*, edited by Félix E. F. Larocca. St. Louis: Ishiyaku .EuroAmerica, 1986.

Collipp, Platon J., ed. *Childhood Obesity*. New York: Warner Books, 1986.

adoption and eating disorders   There is some interest in discovering how adoption and the incidence of eating disorders may correlate, since both anorexia and the internal conflicts faced by adoptees manifest themselves in early adolescence and around puberty. However, reports on anorexia nervosa in adopted children are sparse.

A case was reported in 1985 in which three biologically unrelated individuals in one family had severe anorexia: a father, his adopted daughter and an unrelated person living with them. This case suggests the possible importance of environmental factors in the generation of anorexia nervosa and also reveals the special problems underlying the development of the condition in adoptees.

Fry, Richard, and Crisp, Arthur H. ''Adoption and Identity: A Case of Anorexia.'' *British Journal of Medical Psychology* 62 (1989).

adult onset obesity   Obesity that starts at about the age of 25, usually from overeating (especially of high-calorie snack foods) and frequently because of emotional frustration, stress or boredom. It is generally seen in people who did not have weight problems as children. Some of the more common emotion-charged events that can lead to first-time obesity in adults include leaving home for college or career, marriage, pregnancy, divorce, death of a close family member, extended illness or serious injury. In one study, 68 percent of obese adults related the onset of their weight problems to inactivity because of injury or illness; frequently these traumatic events result in unusually excessive eating of high-calorie foods combined with long periods of inactivity. Because these rather common and relatively sudden increases in weight frequently remain even after the stress and and the excessive eating stop, one theory suggests that there may be a resetting of the set-point mechanism during these eating/exercise pattern changes (see SET-POINT THEORY).

aerobic exercise   Exercise that conditions the heart and lungs by increasing the efficiency of oxygen intake by the body, usually through an activity in which oxygen reaches the muscles at the same rate at which it is used up. This type of physical activity is also recommended for weight control and body conditioning. Such exercise involves the large muscles of the upper body, arms and legs, and to be effective it should be continued for periods of at least 20 minutes at least three times a week. Typical aerobic exercise is not too strenuous and can be performed slowly for a long period of time. Such exercise includes walking, jogging, swimming, bicycling, ice-skating, roller-skating, rowing, aerobic dancing, ballroom dancing, rope skipping and cross-country skiing.

Aerobic exercise is effective for weight reduction because it increases the muscles' ability to use oxygen to burn energy from stored fat. Although the exercise itself may seemingly expend few calories, the expenditure is cumulative and continues after exercise ends.

The effectiveness of aerobic exercise in reducing fat deposits depends upon several elements, including body weight and the frequency, intensity and duration of exercise. According to the Exercise Physiology Laboratory at the University of Massachusetts Medical School, the average 150-pound person burns approximately 100 calories walking a mile. Its tests have shown that the average person who takes a brisk 45-minute walk four times a week for a year and does not increase food intake will burn enough calories to lose 18 pounds. Virtually all of this weight loss will be fat, because regular aerobic exercise preserves muscle mass.

Usually, aerobic exercise tends to decrease appetite. Some fitness experts claim that exercising aerobically during the lunch hour reduces appetite sufficiently that a bowl of soup or a cold drink will satisfy hunger, and that some people have lost as much as 20 pounds within five weeks. . . . (See ANAEROBIC EXERCISE.)

Cooper, Kenneth H., *The Aerobics Program for Total Well-being: Exercise, Diet, Emotional Balance.* New York: M. Evans, 1982.

Layman, Donald K., ed. *Nutrition and Aerobic Exercise.* Washington, D.C.: American Chemical Society, 1986.

Rippe, James M., *Fit for Success.* New York: Prentice-Hall, 1989.

affective disorders and eating disorders   Affective disorders are disorders of feelings or emotions, usually involving depression or elation or mood swings between them. They are sometimes related directly to another physical or mental illness. The affective disorders of depression, premenstrual syndrome (PMS) and seasonal affective disorder (SAD) share similar features with eating disorders, including symptoms and development, a genetic or familial tie and neuroendocrinological evidence, and receive similar treatments.

One symptom common to all these disorders is weight fluctuation. Depressed patients and SAD patients usually gain or lose weight as a result of increased or decreased appetite; PMS patients may retain water, causing weight gain, or they may crave foods high in CARBOHYDRATES—and as their snacking increases, so does their weight. Marked weight gain or loss is also often a key symptom to diagnosing eating disorders.

Additional evidence that affective and eating disorders are related is that 20 to 30 percent of all eating-disorder patients are also depressed, and many of them have a family history of depression as well. Patients with anorexia nervosa may also manifest signs of mania such as euphoria and hyperactivity, as well as feelings of sadness, thoughts of suicide and suicidal behavior. In one study, 27 out of 94 anorectic patients were depressed following treatment. Three others had committed suicide. Several other studies have reported incidence of depression among former anorectic patients in the 40 to 45 percent range.

Researchers have also found a biological link between eating and affective disorders. APPETITE is controlled by the same endorphins (hormones secreted in the brain) that control the sense of well-being, pain tolerance levels, irritability, memory, ability to concentrate and other feelings and functions. The hormone melatonin, which affects appetite, aggression and sex drive, may be one culprit in the cases of SAD, PMS and bulimia. Both exposure to light and darkness and premenstrual changes in the body determine the levels of melatonin produced. Disproportionate levels of melatonin seem to be a problem in bulimics and compulsive overeaters, causing them to eat more at certain times of the day. In women with premenstrual syndrome, melatonin may cause heavier eating before the period; in SAD patients it may cause them to eat more at other times. Victims of these disorders often find that after ingesting carbohydrates, they are in a better mood, can concentrate more easily and are less irritable. This theory is being studied more thoroughly, since a craving for carbohydrates, which bring melatonin to more normal levels, is common to all these disorders.

Another problem area may be SEROTONIN, a NEUROTRANSMITTER, which also affects frame of mind, appetite, and sex drive. High levels of serotonin can also cause craving for carbohydrates.

A study conducted by Toner, Garfinkel and Garner investigated the incidence of affective and anxiety disorders in women who had been diagnosed with anorexia nervosa five to 14 years earlier. Results indicated that these disorders developed frequently, regardless of the outcome of the anorexia nervosa. Major depression and anxiety disorders developed before the eating disorder in more than half of these cases.

A genetic or familial tie between eating and affective disorders has also been noted in several studies. In one, a group of 26 anorectic patients had two fathers, 15 mothers and six siblings diagnosed as having affective disorders. In another study, 25 anorexia nervosa patients were compared with 25 nonanorectics. The relatives of those with anorexia had a 22 percent incidence of affective disorder, whereas only 10 percent of the relatives of the control group had such histories. And a University of Minnesota study reported that among patients with bulimia, 34 to 60 percent had first-degree relatives with affective disorders. As with the relatives of the patients with anorexia nervosa, the predominant type of affective disorder among them was major depressive disorder.

Evidence against a connection between eating disorders and affective disorders is that eating disorders and affective disorders have different patterns of recovery; treatments that work for depression do not always work for eating disorders. And according to Dr. Moises Gaviria, professor of psychiatry at the University of Illinois at Chicago, at five-year follow-up, only 3 percent of depressed adolescents are eating-disordered, and their chances of developing an eating disorder in their lifetime is only 2 percent. The chances of their developing another affective disorder are 6 to 10 percent.

Hatsukami, Dorothy K.; Mitchell, James E.; and Eckert, Elke D. "Eating Disorders: A Variant of Mood Disorders?" In *The Psychiatric Clinics of North America*, vol. 7, no. 2: *Symposium on Eating Disorders*, edited by Félix E. F. Larocca. Philadelphia: W. B. Saunders, 1984.
Jewell, Regina. "Affective, Eating Disorders: Their Common Ground." *BASH Magazine*, November 1989.
Munoz, Rodrigo A. "The Basis for the Diagnosis of Anorexia Nervosa." In *The Psychiatric Clinics of North America*, vol. 7, no. 2: *Symposium on Eating Disorders*, edited by Félix E. F. Larocca. Philadelphia: W. B. Saunders, 1984.
Toner, Brenda B.; Garfinkel, Paul E.; and Garner, David M. "Affective and Anxiety Disor-ders in the Long-Term Follow-up of Anorexia Nervosa." *International Journal of Psychiatry in Medicine* 18, no. 4 (1988).

alexithymia   Difficulty in describing or recognizing one's emotions; confusion about one's feelings, or an apparent lack of thought and concern about one's personal experiences. This disturbance is very common in anorexia nervosa. When asked to describe their sensations of SATIETY, anorectics often respond with such statements as "I feel like I have eaten"; "I don't like it"; "I feel guilty." Inquiries about their emotions may result in defensive or hostile responses to what is viewed as an intrusion into an area they do not understand.

A 1988 Canadian study of 95 subjects supported numerous reports of the presence of a high degree of alexithymia in the obese. One theory is that some people have difficulty coping psychologically with stressful, emotionally intense situations and relieve their anxiety through physical action. Eating, already associated with satisfaction and the relief of stress, is by far the most common device.

Legorreta, Gabriela; Bull, Robert H.; and Kiely, Margaret C. "Alexithymia and Symbolic Function in the Obese." *Psychotherapy and Psychosomatics* 50 (1988).

amenorrhea   A suppression or absence of menstruation. It is considered normal after the menopause, during pregnancy and during lactation (secretion of milk after childbirth). Primary amenorrhea is failure of menstruation to occur at puberty; secondary amenorrhea is cessation of menstruation after its establishment. Among the causes of abnormal amenorrhea are metabolic disorders (diabetes or those stemming from OBESITY or malnutrition) and emotional disorders (ANOREXIA NERVOSA or those stemming from excitement, shock, fright or hysteria).

When the amount of fat drops below a critical percentage of body weight (20 percent) for any reason, hormonal release is affected, which in turn results in amenorrhea. Because of this, it is generally considered to be a symptom of anorexia nervosa. At one time the presence of amenorrhea was considered necessary in order for anorexia nervosa to be diagnosed; however, today's emphasis on psychodynamic (psychologically driven) issues has eliminated the requirement, although amenorrhea is usually present. Although drastic weight reduction generally leads to amenorrhea, there have been cases in which amenorrhea has occurred prior to weight loss. In many of these cases, the amenorrhea continues even after the weight has been regained, sometimes for years. For this reason, some suggest that amenorrhea is a response to psychic stress or indicative of an underlying hypothalamic (body temperature) disorder. Others suggest that perhaps poor nutrition or abnormal psychological development can affect hormonal functions and cause these different results.

Irregular menstrual cycles and amenorrhea in bulimic women have been reported by nearly a dozen authors in medical journals, with irregular menstrual cycles reported in as many as 50 percent of cases studied and amenorrhea in 7 to 20 percent of cases studied. (See BULIMIA NERVOSA.)

American Anorexia/Bulimia Association (AABA) An association of support groups and other programs designed to assist anorectics, bulimics and their families. There are several chapter affiliates and task forces; total membership is about 3,000. AABA was founded in 1978 by Estelle Miller, a clinical worker. Its board is comprised of pediatricians, psychiatrists, parents, recovered anorectics and bulimics, teachers, school nurses, social workers and members of the lay community. The organization is tax-exempt and nonprofit. Its newsletter (untitled) is published five times a year and is mailed to all interested persons in the United States and elsewhere. General meetings, held five times a year, are free to members and open to the public by donation. At the meetings, professionals present current theories about eating disorders, and communication workshops are held. The latter are led by mental health professionals and recovered anorectics or bulimics or parents of recovered anorectics or bulimics.

The most active advocacy group for eating disorders, AABA has lobbied the U.S. Food and Drug Administration against over-the-counter sales of IPECAC. The organization works energetically to keep anorexia and bulimia in the public eye.

The association offers anorectics and bulimics, family members and professionals the opportunity to participate together in the effort to cope with and overcome these life-threatening conditions. Membership is open to all interested persons. (See APPENDIX II.)

amitriptyline A tricyclic ANTIDEPRESSANT that has been used to treat bulimic patients for depression and BINGE EATING behavior. In one study, amitriptyline (trade name Elavil) was tested against a PLACEBO in a sample of 32 bulimic subjects. Even though it was discovered that as many as half the subjects receiving amitriptyline may have been inadequately treated, amitriptyline still proved to be significantly superior to the placebo on one rating scale for anxiety and depression, but not significantly superior on another rating scale.

Other studies have reported less favorable results in treating ANOREXIA NERVOSA. Because amitriptyline has been shown to produce carbohydrate cravings in nonanorectics, GARFINKEL AND GARNER cautioned that there may be a significant risk of triggering BULIMIA in anorectics (see CARBOHYDRATES and CRAVINGS). In a 1985 study comparing the effects of amitriptyline and placebo on weight gain, depression, eating attitudes and obsessive-compulsive tendency over a five-week period, no significant differences favoring amitriptyline were found in any of the outcome variables.

Side effects include increased appetite and thirst and constipation.

amphetamines   Amphetamines are central nervous system stimulants whose effects resemble those of the naturally occurring substance adrenalin. They have the temporary effect of increasing energy and apparent mental alertness. Until recent years amphetamines were widely prescribed by physicians for obesity because they lessen the appetite.

Amphetamines were originally formulated in a German laboratory in 1887 but were largely ignored until they were rediscovered in 1932 by Gordon Alles of the University of California, who transferred his patents to the pharmaceutical firm of Smith, Kline & French (SKF) Laboratories. By 1937, amphetamines were being recommended for certain patients whose obesity was accompanied by low-level depression, on the grounds that a patient whose mood improved would no longer need to overeat and thus would lose weight. It wasn't long before amphetamines were being hailed as a painless way to lose weight through appetite suppression. By the time the federal government stepped in to control the manufacture and sale of amphetamines, SKF was selling $30 million worth each year. (See APPETITE SUPPRESSANTS and OBESITY.)

Their use does initially reduce appetite and increase energy levels. Because they induce conditions in the body that mimic a state of alarm or arousal, they may inhibit the digestive functions, causing the body to use fat rather than food for energy. Some practitioners believe this theory shows that weight loss from amphetamines is the result of a lowering of the set point rather than appetite suppression (see SET-POINT THEORY). It has also been suggested that the anorectic effect of these drugs is a consequence of their inhibition of the salivary glands, which causes dry mouth, makes food less palatable and results in a loss of appetite. Amphetamines are frequently misused by anorectics, who experience intense hunger on the one hand yet terror on the other at giving in to the impulse to eat. Amphetamine abusers have experienced difficulty in swallowing, an extreme way to suppress the appetite.

All of these appetite-control mechanisms have only temporary effects. The body soon draws on its immense recuperative powers, learns to adapt to the chemical and restores digestion, salivation and appetite to normal, thus preventing any more loss of tissue. Those who adhere to the lowered-set-point theory also say that the resultant weight loss is temporary: after use of the drug is stopped, the set point returns to its previous level, so weight also rises to its previous level, or higher.

The American Medical Association (AMA) has evaluated amphetamines as hazardous because of their undesirable effects, including a tendency to produce psychic and, occasionally, physical dependence when used indiscriminately and in large doses. The AMA suggests that physicians prescribe them only for temporary use of four to six weeks. The Food and Drug Administration affirms that these common drugs are of limited usefulness and that their use for prolonged periods in the treatment of obesity can lead to drug dependence and abuse and must be avoided.

Amphetamines are marketed under a variety of trade names; Dexamyl, Fastin, Pondmin, Preludin, Sanorex and Tenuate are among the more popular. All of them are closely related chemically.

Lukas, Scott E., *Amphetamines: Danger in the Fast Lane*. New York: Chelsea House, 1985.
O'Brien, Robert, and Cohen, Sidney. *The Encyclopedia of Drug Abuse*. New York: Facts On File, 1984.

amylin   A recently isolated hormone discovered in high levels in the pancreas of Type II (non–insulin-dependent) diabetics. It appears to be responsible for the obesity, the reduced insulin secretion and the reduced effectiveness of insulin observed in Type II diabetes. Until this discovery, obesity had been considered by many to be a major contributor to the disease rather than a result of it.

anaclitic depression   A state of reduced spontaneity and expressiveness in an infant resulting from lack of maternal responsiveness to the infant's demands. Although there is no scientific proof of the theory, some researchers have attributed the sense of emptiness and loss experienced by anorectics to an anaclitic depression that develops because of maternal over- or underinvolvement. During the child's exploratory phase of development, the mother needs to allow and encourage freedom in order to promote the illusion of self-sufficiency, but she should also be available for emotional support. When the mother offers either too much or too little assistance, she can hinder the toddler's development of self-reliance. One theory is that the mother of an anorectic overprotects her daughter rather than encourages her to explore, or is emotionally unavailable for support when her daughter returns for comfort or reassurance. This lack of dependable and consistent maternal responsiveness inhibits the daughter's normal striving for autonomy and slows her separation-individuation process.

This school of thought theorizes that it is specifically because the anorectic's mother had difficulty in allowing or promoting independent behavior in her daughter that the anorectic is later unable to mature and separate. During adolescence, when separation and independence develop, the anorectic's dependency again surfaces, along with the latent psychopathology originating in her infancy.

Anaclitic depression is not a DSM-III diagnosis.

anaerobic exercise   Exercise that demands brief spurts of intense effort, such as calisthenics or weight training. Anaerobic exercise is so intense that the oxygen supplied to the muscles by the blood is insufficient, forcing the muscle cells to work without it. For this reason, it does not burn as many calories as AEROBIC EXERCISE does. Anaerobic exercise is important to include in an overall fitness program because it helps to improve flexibility, toning and firming of the muscles, but it will not contribute a great deal to a weight reduction program.

anorectic behavior   A term used by GARFINKEL AND GARNER to describe the behavior of young women who have weight concerns that interfere with their psychological well-being but do not have full-blown anorexia nervosa. Garfinkel and Garner speculate that these women may be using weight control to deal with issues similar to those of anorectics—the regulation and expression of self, autonomy and self-control; they correspond to Bruch's THIN FAT PEOPLE. Among the features of so-called anorectic behavior are intense preoccupation with food, food fads, mixing unusual food combinations and dawdling over meals.

Garfinkel, Paul E., and Garner, David M. *Anorexia Nervosa: A Multidimensional Perspective.* New York: Brunner/Mazel, 1982.

anorectic bingers   Although most anorectics restrict the amount of food they eat, and never overeat, there are some who alternate between severely restrictive diets and binges. Anorexia accompanied by the BINGE EATING syndrome has been found to affect older age groups more frequently than adolescents.

Bingeing anorectics display less self-discipline and act more impulsively than RESTRICTOR ANORECTICS. They also have greater incidence of MULTICOMPULSIVE behavior such as alcohol and drug abuse and shoplifting, as well as more SUICIDE and SELF-MUTILATION attempts. There is also more VOMITING and LAXATIVE ABUSE among bingers.

In comparing anorectic bingers and nonbingers, Neuman and Halvorson referred to a 1980 study by Casper et al., reported in the scientific journal *Archives of General Psychiatry*, 37, that found that anorectic patients who binge tend to be more depressed, anxious, guilt ridden and preoccupied with food than nonbingers. Anorectic bingers also complain more about aches and pains and have more trouble sleeping, resulting in more complaints of fatigue. Bingers also tend to be more outgoing and sensitive to others. In the Casper study, 86 percent of the anorectic bingers were described as outgoing as children in contrast to only 57 percent of the anorectic nonbingers. Besides being more outgoing, anorectic bingers are often sexually active and concerned with physical attractiveness and attention from the opposite sex, in marked contrast to the restrictor, who denies or avoids sexual feelings. Perhaps not coincidentally, poor father-child relationships have been reported more often in the lives of anorectic bingers than nonbingers.

While restrictor anorectics are able to ignore and even deny hunger, bingers report stronger appetites that are more difficult to control. Possibly because of this feeling of lack of control, the binger is more likely to seek treatment. Yet anorexia accompanied by bingeing is more difficult to treat, since it occurs intermittently and persistently over a longer period of time.

Neuman, Patricia A., and Halvorson, Patricia A. *Anorexia Nervosa and Bulimia: A Handbook for Counselors and Therapists.* New York: Van Nostrand Reinhold, 1983.

anorexia mirabilis The term used by physicians during the High Middle Ages to describe "miraculously inspired" loss of appetite. This was a fairly common occurrence in medieval Europe, especially between 1200 and 1500. It was considered miraculous when women survived prolonged periods of fasting; many insisted they were actually unable to eat normal "earthly fare." Fasting was critical to female sainthood during this time, given medieval culture's association of the female body and food. Catherine of Siena (1347–1380) restricted her diet to a daily handful of herbs; whenever she did partake of other food, she would cause herself to vomit by forcing a stick down her throat.

Other female saints became ill or felt their throats close up around food, fasted for days at a time, ate only orange seeds, and even died of starvation. Anorexia mirabilis, unlike anorexia nervosa, was not restricted to adolescent or young adult women. And today's anorectic strives for the modern ideal of physical perfection or beauty rather than the medieval ideal of spiritual perfection or beauty.

As the Protestant Reformation revolutionized medieval culture, prolonged fasting became a negative practice; it was considered a work of the devil rather than of God. Where fasting females were once venerated as saints, they were now denounced as evil, possessed by the devil or insane.

Brumberg, Joan Jacobs. *Fasting Girls.* Cambridge: Harvard University Press, 1988.

anorexia nervosa A serious psychological disorder characterized by intense fear of gaining weight and the deliberate practice of self-starvation. Anorectics refuse to maintain even a minimal body weight and are pathologically preoccupied with food and dieting. Anorexia literally means "lack of appetite" and thus is actually a misnomer, but it is the generally accepted name for the condition. Anorectics do experience hunger, but they simply refuse to give in to it for fear of becoming fat. Anorexia nervosa affects chiefly young women in their teens and twenties.

Anorexia nervosa has always been overwhelmingly a disorder of upper-class adolescents (the usual age range is from 12 to 25), but studies by GARFINKEL AND GARNER show it to be increasing in older women and in other social classes. Ninety to 95 percent of anorectics are female; those between the ages of 12 and 18 are in the highest risk group.

It is estimated that in the United States, one in every 250 young women as well as one in every 200 adolescent girls is starving herself (source: *Diagnostic and Statistical Manual of Mental Disorders,* 3d ed., Washington, D.C.: American Psychiatric Association, 1980). The Anorexia Nervosa and Related Eating Disorders Organization (ANRED) estimates that approximately one in every 100 white females between the ages of 12 and 18 suffers from anorexia. Incidence in eight- to 11-year-olds is said by ANRED to be increasing. For girls over 16 in private schools or in universities, the figure may be as high as one in 10. Of those patients being treated for anorexia, about 15 of every 100 will actually die. Of the remainder, only half will recover to lead normal lives; the rest are likely to relapse. ARTHUR H. CRISP has reported patients relapsing after being in remission for 50 years. (See ELDERLY, EATING DISORDERS IN THE.) Morbidity and mortality rates in anorexia nervosa are among the highest recorded for psychiatric disorders. The mortality rate of 6 to 18 percent reported frequently in medical journals would make anorexia the most lethal psychiatric illness. However, George Patton reported in the *British Medical Journal* (July 15, 1989) that a comprehensive assessment of 481 patients over 10 years has shown a crude mortality for anorexia nervosa of just over 3 percent, "confirming the recent trend to lower mortality."

Authors, researchers and journals have referred to the "dramatic increase in diagnosed cases of anorexia nervosa in the last 20 years," but actual numbers have been difficult to come by. This is due partly to a lack of a system for collecting and interpreting data and partly to a lack of standardization in diagnostic criteria. However, there is evidence that such an increase has occurred. Two measurements used have been hospital admissions and case reportings around the country. The University of Wisconsin Hospital, for example, showed an average of fewer than one anorectic patient admission per year prior to the 1960s; in 1982, it admitted more than 70. In Monroe County, New York, the number of reported anorexia nervosa cases doubled between 1960 and 1976.

A number of reasons have been given for this apparent surge in diagnosed cases of anorexia nervosa: (1) Both the professional and popular press have published numerous articles and reports on the disorder. This has resulted in both the medical profession and the general population becoming more familiar with the disorder, thereby exposing more cases. (2) There has been a history of inadequate recordkeeping in anorexia cases and lack of agreement regarding criteria for diagnosis. This leaves some question as to the actual incidence of the disorder in years past. (3) Because anorectics do not admit to their illness or even complain about it, there is a belief that many cases prior to the recent increase in press coverage were never brought to the attention of doctors. (4) Some psychologists estimate that as many as 30 percent of today's cases are "copycat" anorectics, responding to a peer group phenomenon rather than suffering true anorexia nervosa.

Although estimates of the incidence of anorexia nervosa in western Europe and the United States have suggested a great increase since 1950 and perhaps even since 1930, a study conducted by the Mayo Clinic showed no significant trend in rates over time. The study was population based and spanned the years from 1935 through 1984; it consisted of a survey of the medical records of residents of Rochester, Minnesota. The incidence rates for females were high during 1935–49, relatively low during 1950–64 and high again during 1965–79. The difference in rates over time, although not statistically significant, was accounted for by changing rates for 10- to 19-year-old girls. For women 20 years of age and older there was no change in the rates over time. Population-based rates are not yet available for 1980–84, but the total of 38 females and three males diagnosed with anorexia nervosa suggests that the incidence rates will be very high. On January 1, 1980, the lifetime prevalence rate for anorexia nervosa among Rochester residents was 204 per 100,000 population for females and 17 per 100,000 population for males. Among 15- to 19-year-old females it occurred in one of every 332 residents.

The person with anorexia nervosa typically begins dieting with a simple goal of losing weight, but over time the achievement of that goal becomes a manifestation of mastery, control and virtue. The anorectic may find dieting easy and rewarding from the start, or at least discover that in a sense she is good at it. Typically she ends up by continuing to diet despite having gone past her target weight. The desire for slenderness becomes secondary to the need for control and mastery over the body and develops into a real fear of fatness and a drive to remain small and childlike.

Because anorexia nervosa patients do not see themselves as abnormal, they do not want any help in reversing their weight loss. When told they cannot live on such a small amount of food, they will insist that they feel better as they become thinner. Because they do not suffer, they must be well. This denial of illness is an important feature early in the disorder. The clinical picture of anorexia nervosa centers on a three-fold denial—denial of hunger, of thinness and of fatigue.

Even if they admit to some weight loss, anorectics will feel that while they may have lost weight generally, some particular part of their body is still too large. When family pressures or social obligations force anorectics to eat, most will use deception to hide their extreme dieting. They'll slip food to the dog, flush it down the toilet or throw it into the garbage. Teenagers will tell parents, "I'm not hungry; I ate at a friend's house." Many will induce vomiting after meals. When undergoing treatment, anorectics will resort to all kinds of deceptions to lead doctors to believe they are gaining weight. Among those that have been documented are drinking enormous amounts of water before being weighed, recalibrating scales and inserting weights in the rectum and vagina.

Anorexia nervosa has been said to develop only in the face of plenty, that it exists only where food is abundant. However, today's researchers are beginning to discover that the stereotype is inaccurate and that it may have come about because such a large proportion of the studies done were of college students and patients who could afford treatment. In a 1989 survey of more than 2,000 adolescent girls and their mothers, University of Michigan psychologist Adam Drewnowski discovered that the frequency of eating disorders is the same in lower-income communities near Detroit as it is in the city's wealthy suburbs—about 2 percent.

Herzog, David B., and Copeland, Paul M. "Eating Disorders." *New England Journal of Medicine* Vol. 313, No. 5 (August 1, 1985).

Knapp, Caroline. "Anorexia: My Story." *New Woman*, March 1990.

Orbach, Susie. *Hunger Strike: The Anorectic's Struggle as a Metaphor for Our Age.* New York: W. W. Norton, 1986.

Causes   There is no known specific cause of anorexia. Several theories do exist, but they are based on individual clinical observations and histories, so none has been accepted as definitive. Researchers do agree that anorexia nervosa is probably a negative response to a number of psychological, environmental and physiological factors rather than a disease that can be traced to a single cause. Although these influencing factors affect virtually all individuals, the anorectic appears to lack the skills necessary to cope with them. Neuman and Halvorson have identified several potential causes of anorexia nervosa:

Stressful Life Situations   These may range from major developments such as family conflict, a change in schools (especially transitions from junior high to high school or from high school to college), a family move, the loss of a boyfriend or girlfriend or a serious illness, to less obvious difficulties such as a casual remark made by an athletic coach or dance instructor about "dropping a few pounds," teasing by classmates or siblings or a rejection, which may be real or perceived. Many stressful situations are caused by or lead to change, and change in general is difficult for an anorectic to handle. One possible explanation for this is the anorectic's obsession with perfection and the fear that she may not be able to achieve her goal in new circumstances. Change may well trigger overwhelming fear that things are out of control.

Adolescence   One hypothesis is that anorexia nervosa is a rejection of female sexuality brought on by the physical development associated with puberty. Neuman and Halvorson explain this as "an attempt to retain 'little girl' status by warding off the adolescent's physical development." HILDE BRUCH described in *Eating Disorders* several of her patients who had had active fantasies as children about being boys—until puberty put a shocking end to them. Other professionals argue that it is the entire *role* of an adult that is being rejected: the responsibilities, decision making, sexual intimacy and so on. To support this, they point out that anorectics avoid intimacy, largely because of their fear of rejection over "mistakes" they might make. Even sexually active anorectics have been described by therapists as withholding feelings and thoughts from partners. It has been suggested that anorectics' sexual activity happens at all only because of their inability to be assertive in that arena—to say no.

Culture   Another reason some feel anorexia is a rejection of the adult female role is that the adolescent of recent years has no clear-cut road to follow into adulthood. Neuman and Halvorson explain that the anorectic adolescent typically has mastered the role of being a "good little girl." But the criteria for being a "good woman" are no longer well defined; in fact, the social messages, these therapists feel, are confusing to the anorectic. No longer do the wedding and first pregnancy define "growing up." Today's adolescent is also encouraged to "be something" or "somebody," at the same

time that biological changes may be reminding her of more traditional roles. And because anorectics are usually good students, they are frequently steered into academic and career paths rather than down a more traditional female road. So, being unassertive and evading decisions, they may retreat into the familiar "child" role where they already mastered the well-defined "rules."

Anorexia nervosa is believed to be primarily a disorder of Western culture. It is rare in China, for example. It has been suggested by Chinese researchers that this could be related to protective sociocultural factors specific to the Chinese. In most Western societies, a strong cultural emphasis is placed on individual success. Neuman and Halvorson explain that until recently Western women's social success was judged by their affiliations—by whose daughter or wife they were. Today's woman has new demands. "Thus many maturing females find themselves caught up in the 'Superwoman' syndrome, trying to be all things to all people." And, they add, girls who are already perfectionists and not good at making decisions can become overwhelmed by feelings of powerlessness. College-age anorectics especially have reported to Neuman and Halvorson these feelings of confusion and being out of control of their own future.

Other cultural factors influencing the recent rise of anorexia nervosa include the growing concern about nutrition and physical fitness and a national obsession with calorie counting and being thin. Television, magazine and newspaper messages bombard women and girls with advice on how to lose weight more quickly, exercise more and eat less in order to be thinner. The messages blatantly state that being thin will make a woman more attractive, improve her popularity, lead to success on the job and snag her an ideal mate because she will then be sexier and more desirable. Fashion models display small waists and busts, narrow hips and thin thighs. This has resulted in a cultural focus on the physical being more than on the inner person. Small wonder, experts say, that some girls in the highly vulnerable adolescent and young adult years take these "thin-or-sorry" messages to heart and carry their responses to them to extremes. (See CULTURAL INFLUENCES ON APPEARANCE and CULTURAL INFLUENCES ON EATING DISORDERS.)

Biological Predisposition While research has shown that women are far more likely than men either to eat more or to lose appetite in response to stress, Neuman and Halvorson suggest that appetite fluctuation in women may also be a learned response. Women have also been found to be more prone to "holding in" negative feelings, which can lead to increased stress. It has been suggested that this stress, in the presence of a biological predisposition to eat more or less because of it, may lead to a greater likelihood of anorexia nervosa.

Many of the physical symptoms associated with anorexia nervosa also occur with a disorder of the hypothalamus, a region of the brain that regulates menstruation, eating, metabolism, body temperature and sleep. Numerous studies have also established that disturbances in hypothalamic function occur in those suffering from anorexia nervosa. What has not been established is whether anorexia causes the hypothalamic disturbance or the hypothalamus directly influences occurrence of anorexia. (See HYPOTHALAMIC DISEASE.)

Family Dynamics It has been noted that there is a greater risk of a person's developing anorexia nervosa when another member of the family has had the disorder or when a parent is either very thin or obese. What has not been established is whether this risk is genetic. Because a few sets of identical twins have been found in which both twins succumbed to anorexia, and because several cases are known of adopted family members matching the patterns of their biological families' histories, this family tendency is believed to be more environmental than inherited. However, research in

this area has been sparse; much more needs to be learned.

Anorectics do tend to come from families placing strong emphasis on food. Neuman and Halvorson explain that "this concern may be the result of the special dietary needs of a family member, an emphasis on nutrition, and/or previous power struggles over eating. The family may also have used food for purposes other than nourishment. Eating may be used when members face problems or unpleasantness, as a sign of love and caring for the providers, to fill time, or to keep the family together and 'happy.' "

Clinicians have found that certain personality types seem to appear frequently among parents of anorectics. Mothers are often found to be domineering, intruding in the anorectic's hour-to-hour life. Mothers of anorectics also frequently suffer from depression, and fathers are described as "aloof or passive." Alcoholism and other addictions, of one or both parents, are not uncommon. However, none of these patterns is always present; some cases even show the exact opposite family dynamics.

But there are medical experts who still insist that family dynamics play an important role in generating the disorder. They cite those family features most likely to encourage anorexia as enmeshment (entanglement in one another's affairs), rigidity, overprotectiveness and inability to resolve conflict within the family. Margo Maine, assistant clinical director of the Eating Disorders Service at Newington Children's Hospital in Connecticut, suggests that a father's emotional or physical absence from the family may be a major influence on both anorexia nervosa and bulimia in adolescent girls. Thirty-six of 39 young female patients questioned by Maine described their fathers as emotionally distant. (See FAMILY THERAPY.)

Peer Relationships The tendency of anorectics not to develop or keep close long-term friendships outside the family group has been theorized to be an important factor in the development of the disorder. Neuman and Halvorson note that when relationships are developed by anorectics, they are usually with only one person at a time, and even then they are short-lived. ARTHUR H. CRISP noted that male anorectics have been found to be inhibited, nonassertive loners—even during their teen years when a group or "gang" affiliation is usual.

Therapists such as Neuman and Halvorson believe that during adolescence peer relationships are essential for the move from a family-centered existence to an adult existence in a social environment. According to Delores Jones, "the anorectic who is overly involved with and dependent upon her family to the exclusion of outside relationships is at a distinct disadvantage. Because she has no peer group to help her make the transition, she is effectively imprisoned within the family." However, her increasingly adult size as she matures elicits social pressure on her for more independent behavior. Jones speculated that the anorectic resolves this conflict by losing weight so that in terms of size and biological functioning, she becomes a child again and can legitimately remain within the family.

Byrne, Katherine. *A Parent's Guide to Anorexia and Bulimia; Understanding and Helping Self-starvers and Binge/Purgers.* New York: Schocken Books, 1987.
Jones, Delores. "Structural Discontinuity and the Development of Anorexia Nervosa." *Sociological Focus* 14(3) (August 1981).
Lee, Sing; Chiu, Helen F. K.; and Chen, Charnie. "Anorexia Nervosa in Hong Kong: Why Not More in China?" *British Journal of Psychiatry* 154 (1989).
Neuman, Patricia A., and Halvorson, Patricia A. *Anorexia Nervosa and Bulimia: A Handbook for Counselors and Therapists.* New York: Van Nostrand Reinhold, 1983.

Clinical Features   The central feature of anorexia nervosa is the overriding pursuit of thinness. This may seem to begin innocently with ordinary adolescent self-consciousness—dieting to lose extra pounds put on during puberty's growth spurts. But after several months, the anorectic will stubbornly refuse to eat normal amounts of food. Typically she limits her intake to about 600–800 calories per day, resulting in a loss of 25 percent or more of body weight. In extreme cases, the loss may be as high as 50 percent.

When questioned about her loss of weight, an anorectic will deny that she is too thin or that there is anything wrong with her. This denial can be an obstacle for doctors during diagnosis and assessment. Because they don't perceive themselves as ill or abnormal, anorectics refuse help. Denial is a typical characteristic of anorexia nervosa and is seen as an early sign of the disorder.

One of the fundamental characteristics of anorexia nervosa is a disturbance in body image, "feeling fat" even when emaciated. During treatment, the anorectic claims that her body is larger than it really is. She seems genuinely unaware of her changed body proportions. Even though her body may appear starved, she may stubbornly insist she is not as thin as another anorectic who is as thin or thinner than she; yet she will recognize the other anorectic as too thin. A few will admit to their emaciated state and even recognize the health dangers, but they will still refuse to eat. Many anorectics argue that their thin bodies are still too fat. Others consider their stick-figure legs and arms to be attractive and "just right."

Overestimation of body size may indicate greater severity of disorder with less hope of recovery. In studies, patients who most grossly overestimated were also those who were the most malnourished, were previous treatment failures, indicated a greater loss of appetite, had a greater tendency to deny their illness, vomited, were more depressed and in general exhibited more symptoms of anorexia nervosa as measured by the EATING ATTITUDES TEST.

In addition to the misperception of body size, the anorectic's body image disturbance can involve her attitude toward her body.

Frequently she manifests self-loathing, particularly of her developing female body parts, such as the normal slight curve of stomach or rounding of hips or buttocks.

HUNGER is usually denied, even in the presence of stomach pains. When she does eat a small bit of food, an anorectic will complain about ensuing acute discomfort.

In contrast to starving nonanorectics, who generally attempt to conserve energy by reducing activity and who usually show symptoms of listlessness and indifference, anorectics are often hyperactive, tending to indulge in heavy or prolonged exercise. Instead of being exhausted while starving, these young women enjoy boundless energy until late in their illness. The anorectic begins exercising in order to burn up calories and lose additional weight. As with dieting, however, exercising over time becomes an issue of self-discipline and control; anorectics cannot allow themselves to miss even one day of the highly structured regimen they have assigned themselves.

If an anorectic was already involved in a sport, she will likely become driven, almost obsessed to excel at it. Anorectics may appear to be in perpetual motion; constantly busy, moving about restlessly until late into the night, almost never sitting down. Studies have shown that anorectics walk an average of 6.8 miles a day compared with the average of 4.0 miles walked by women of normal weight. This hyperactivity is not generally present before the onset of anorectic illness. Just as the anorectic denies hunger, she will deny any difficulty in sitting still and attending to her work.

Often compulsive behavior is exhibited in excessive orderliness, cleaning and studying. As Neuman and Halvorson explain, "Anything less than perfection is upsetting to the anorectic, and everything undertaken seems to be done in excess."

A few years ago anorexia was generally interpreted as reflecting a wish not to grow up, to return to a prepubertal stage; therapists now say that many anorectics appear anxious to exercise authority and to control their lives through regulation of body weight.

Anorectics have been described as suffering from a "weight phobia." Regardless of the original reason for dieting, subsequent weight gain by the anorectic causes severe anxiety and weight loss reduces it. This "phobia" about "normal" body weight appears to intensify as the patient becomes thinner. She weighs herself frequently, becoming anxious if the scales show an increase over the previous reading. In her mind, each drop in weight becomes a new barometer; next time she must weigh less to be normal. Anorectics seem to have a greater fear of becoming obese than of dying from starvation. As the anorectic's weight drops, her fear becomes more entrenched: the thinner she gets, the fatter she thinks she is.

In addition to a phobic attitude toward weight, the anorectic develops another phobia toward food. At first, she fears only high-carbohydrate foods and so deletes them from her diet. Soon she systematically eliminates fats and other foods until only a few vegetables and fruits remain. She also controls food portions rigidly; she must restrict intake to a specific number of pieces or bites a day. If she does exceed her allotted daily portion, the anorectic suffers severe anxiety and sets about to control her eating even more severely.

Anorectic patients often become experts in devious behavior. They will conceal their eating habits by lying about what, when and where they eat. Usually they do not like to eat in front of others and come up with excuses to avoid eating with the family, partly to avoid the food itself and partly to avoid confrontations about their eating habits and their appearance. Because of family pressure to eat, they may take food onto their plate, surreptitiously slipping it to the dog under the table or hiding it in their napkins to flush down the toilet or throw away later. Many pathological behaviors occur in secret: hiding food, self-induced vomiting, laxative and/or diuretic abuse and excessive exercising.

Constipation and abdominal distress typically result from restricted food intake and the starvation state. These in turn lead to further symptoms of bloating and reduced dietary intake. Long-term laxative abuse can produce permanent damage to the colon resulting in malabsorption and loss of ability to evacuate naturally.

Also accompanying anorexia nervosa is delayed psychosexual development. According to Neuman and Halvorson, "Boyfriends may be desired but usually only in a fairy-tale sense—to live 'happily ever after.' " Anorectics exhibit virtually no sexual interest, with low estrogens in female anorectics and low output of testosterone in males. During therapy, anorectics cannot even talk about sex, "not out of embarrassment, but because it is so foreign: anorectics are totally out of touch with the sexual part of their being." (See SEXUALITY AND EATING DISORDERS.)

Anorectics also gradually narrow their interests. Many entirely restrict their activities to exercise, schoolwork and dieting, and all other activities fall by the wayside. Most girls lose interest in their friends early in their dieting; this loss is considered a most important early signal of the problem. By the time the weight loss has progressed to the point of requiring medical attention, an anorectic may be totally isolated from others. This isolation results in loneliness and a sense of social inadequacy.

Other warning signals include dizziness and fainting spells, nervousness around mealtime, excuses during mealtime for not eating, cutting food into small pieces or playing with it, an increased interest in collecting recipes and cooking for others, weighing frequently and wearing multiple layers of clothing (anorectics are frequently cold as a result of the loss of fat and muscle tissue). In some cases obsessive interest in food will result in an anorectic's insisting on

cooking for, and overfeeding, her immediate family. Anorectics have been reported to hoard and conceal food, including food that is rotten or moldy, while refusing fresh food.

Another established feature of anorexia is AMENORRHEA (absence or suppression of menstruation). In a high percentage of cases, this is the first sign of the disorder, appearing before any noticeable loss of weight. Ultimately, it occurs in nearly all cases as weight plummets.

Anorectics have frequent mood swings; when they are most hungry and their blood sugar levels the lowest, they may become quite irritable. They also will sometimes demonstrate an inability to concentrate, and this may be coupled with confused thinking. Initially they will deny all problems, including mood changes; anorectics display a stubborn defiance about most matters, along with a noticeable lack of concern for personal problems. They tend to be highly perfectionistic, particularly about physical appearance, as well as highly self-critical. They tend to be overachievers. They will frequently seem angry, irritable, indecisive, stubborn, tense or overly sensitive. Depression or obsession is common when the disorder becomes chronic.

When asked to describe their anorectic daughters as children, parents refer to most of them as "model children," using terms like introverted, conscientious and well behaved. They are usually nonassertive, reacting passively to others. But although an anorectic may appear outwardly smiling and happy and is usually a highly competent people pleaser, she may actually be miserable. Neuman and Halvorson stress that while a passive personality has been found to be consistently among the most common of anorectics' traits, it is not always present. Anorectics can display irritability, indecisiveness, stubbornness and defiance.

In addition to an emaciated appearance, an anorectic usually has dry, cracking skin and may lose some hair from her scalp. Her nails become brittle. A fine downy growth of fetal-like hair (lanugo) over the cheeks, neck, forearms and thighs is common. Yet she will keep her pubic and underarm hair as well as the shape of her breasts, thus ruling out glandular insufficiency as the root cause of her symptoms. The anorectic's hands and feet usually have a bluish tinge, which may also appear on her nose and ears. Other likely results of anorexia include a slow heartbeat, low blood pressure (hypotension) and a low basal metabolic rate. An anorectic may also have trouble sleeping when the loss of fat tissue padding makes sitting or lying down uncomfortable.

Those anorectics who frequently and over a long period resort to vomiting as a way to control food intake can develop a variety of dental problems, including loss of enamel, decay and enlarged salivary glands. (See DENTAL CARIES.)

Neuman, Patricia A., and Halvorson, Patricia A. *Anorexia Nervosa and Bulimia: A Handbook for Counselors and Therapists.* New York: Van Nostrand Reinhold, 1983.

Complications Most of the medical complications of anorexia are those caused by starvation. The body defends its vital organs, the heart and brain, against a lack of nutrients by slowing down: menstrual periods stop, breathing, pulse and blood pressure rates drop and thyroid function slows.

Particularly critical are the fluid and electrolyte (sodium, potassium, hydrogen, etc.) imbalances that commonly occur, especially among anorectics who induce vomiting or use laxatives extensively. Potassium deficiency can lead to muscle weakness, abdominal bloating, nervous irritability, apathy, fatigue, drowsiness, dizziness, mental confusion and irregular heartbeat. Death from kidney or heart failure may occur. Such electrolyte imbalances are not always outwardly apparent; the person suffering from them may appear to be in relatively good health.

Studies have also raised questions about the possibility of ZINC DEFICIENCY in anorexia nervosa. In 1987, Rebecca Katz et al. reported in the *Journal of Adolescent Health Care* that their evaluation of anorectic adolescents suggested that individuals with anorexia nervosa may be at risk for zinc deficiency, which can impair taste, appetite and physical growth, cause hair loss and delay sexual development. But C. J. M. van Binsbergen et al. reported in the *European Journal of Clinical Nutrition* in 1988 that no significant difference was found in the concentration of zinc in plasma between 20 female anorectics and 20 lean to normal-weight female control subjects.

Mild anemia, swelling joints (from edema), reduced muscle mass, dizziness and light-headedness are also results of anorexia. If the disorder becomes severe, osteoporosis, kidney failure, irregular heart rhythm and heart failure can occur. The anorectic who turns to purging to limit weight is in particular danger; the abuse of drugs to stimulate vomiting (see IPECAC), bowel movements and urination increases the risk of heart failure. In addition, there is a possibility of temporary or even permanent edema (accumulation of fluid in the body's cells, tissues or cavities) once the use of diuretics as an aid to weight reduction is stopped.

Osteoporosis (a loss of bone mass accompanied by mineralization of the remaining bone) is another consequence of anorexia nervosa. A study of anorectics by Anne Klibanski and other Massachusetts General Hospital researchers involving seven adolescent girls and 26 women found that adults with anorexia nervosa had bone density that was 30 percent lower than normal. Those whose menstruation stopped before age 18 had even weaker bones—20 percent weaker than the bones of the older anorexia victims.

A report in the journal *Clinical Endocrinology* states that in 24 anorectic patients who were severely malnourished, the ovaries were small and shapeless, and some hormone levels were very low.

Depression, weakness and obsession with food also accompany starvation. Personality changes can occur. Outbursts of hostility and anger or social withdrawal may surprise those who have become used to the typical "good girl" anorectic. Other complications can include amnesia, generalized fatigue, lowered body temperature (hypothermia), low blood sugar, low white blood cell count and lack of energy.

To determine the range and severity of medical complications encountered in younger patients, a study was made of the medical records of 65 adolescents and preadolescents in the Eating Disorders Clinic of the Children's Hospital at Stanford University. A total of 55 percent of anorectic patients required hospitalization for medical reasons during the study period.

George Patton reported in the *British Medical Journal* (July 15, 1989) that in an assessment of 481 anorexia nervosa patients, half of those who died killed themselves, either accidentally or intentionally through drug overdoses. This challenges the earlier view that death in anorexia nervosa is always a direct consequence of malnutrition.

There have been no clear, consistent predictors of worsening conditions without eventual improvement in anorexia nervosa cases, but factors most often found in these cases include extremely low weight, long periods with the illness, older age at onset, and disturbed family relationship.

Treatment Various treatments have been suggested for anorexia nervosa, including psychoanalysis, PSYCHOTHERAPY, simple supportive therapy, isolation, ACUPUNCTURE, lobotomy, FAMILY THERAPY, BEHAVIOR MODIFICATION, COGNITIVE THERAPY, TUBE FEEDING, FORCED FEEDING, bed rest, HYPERALIMENTATION, PHARMACOTHERAPY, electroshock, psychosurgery and SELF-HELP GROUPS.

Because anorectics and their families tend to deny the presence of the disorder or its severity, the results of treatment of anorexia have been among the most unsatisfactory in clinical medicine. Even patients in treatment tend to resist prescribed medical and psychiatric care; because they don't consider

themselves to be ill or because they don't want their efforts to lose weight thwarted, they make those trying to help them "the enemy."

Virtually every type of therapy known to psychiatry has been proposed and tried at some time in the treatment of anorectics, but no one has been found distinctly effective or definitive. Part of the reason for this is the lack of agreement about the relationship between food and its "host." We know very little of the chemical processing of food by the body and how dieting and purging may affect the appetite center of the brain. To make matters worse, there is body image distortion and an interoceptive (internal sensory receptor) problem. (See INTEROCEPTIVE DISTURBANCE.) In addition, the treatment needs of different patients can vary widely; considerable flexibility is necessary.

Because anorexia nervosa patients differ widely in psychological, social, behavioral and biological functioning, treatment centers most frequently offer integrated and multifaceted programs. Both the physical and psychological aspects of the disorder have to be addressed: the physical aspects take precedence when the weight is low and the starvation strategy is most dominant, and the psychological aspects take precedence later, after weight concerns have been addressed and eating habits have been stabilized. Ideally, internists, nutritionists, individual or group therapists, psychopharmacologists, psychiatrists and family therapists may all be involved in treatment.

Weight gain must occur if psychological treatment is to be meaningful. Garfinkel and Garner explain that there are two reasons for this. First, the effects of starvation must be reduced for the patient truly to benefit from psychotherapy, a learning process that cannot proceed well when a patient's mental functioning is impaired. Second, patients have developed a phobic attitude toward weight and must learn to face it as a precondition for dealing with underlying psychological issues. "As long as a low weight is maintained through rigid dieting, the phobia is being reinforced, as is the avoidance of dealing realistically with significant life problems.'' (The concept of weight phobia is now being questioned by experts such as ARTHUR H. CRISP, who argues that what a patient dreads is facing herself at a normal weight. He believes that what is being reinforced when weight is kept very low is the ''advantage'' of being prepubertally thin so this dread doesn't become an actuality.)

The most difficult and critical factor in treatment is gaining a patient's trust. The problem here is that many anorectics deny their illness; they insist there is nothing wrong with them if only others would leave them alone. They mistrust themselves and especially mistrust medical people they think are interested only in getting them to gain weight, or who represent parental authority. Anorectics feel that treatment represents a betrayal of their trust, fearing a return to being what they consider overweight.

Although controversy has surrounded almost every means of weight restoration, the issue of hospitalization has been far less controversial. Historically, hospital admission has been advocated both to allow the physician to control the situation, and to separate the patient from her parents.

Hospitalization is usually considered if weight is at least 15 percent below a normal standard and is urged if weight is 25 percent or more below normal. When weight loss is 40 percent or more from the norm, emergency action is required. The urgency of hospitalization depends on several factors, including weight loss greater than 30 percent of body weight over three months, severe metabolic disturbance, severe depression or suicide risk, severe purging, psychosis, family crisis or symptoms of severe starvation. Hospitalization is also suggested when outpatient treatment has failed.

Frequently, even when emergency care is not necessary, several days of unstructured hospital rest are ordered to give physicians and psychiatrists a chance to observe the patient. The treatment team can thus learn whether she is a starver or a vomiter, whether she hoards food or secretly throws it away, whether she drinks water or not before weighin. They also observe how much walking and exercising she does, and whether hospitalization has resulted in her becoming agitated and manipulative or passive and withdrawn.

Length of hospitalization usually varies between two and four months. Brief hospitalization of 10 days to two weeks can be helpful for anorectics who are not severely malnourished but who suffer from laxative withdrawal (e.g., dependence on the laxative drug in place of normal bowel action) or uncontrollable binge eating and vomiting.

Application of EXPOSURE AND RESPONSE PREVENTION treatment principles to anorexia nervosa requires a patient to face the twin fears of eating and gaining weight. Reports have shown that psychological improvement does occur with weight gain; to realize it, several approaches to treatment may be effective, including forced feedings and structured diets.

Response prevention can be used to treat anorectic ''rituals'' such as vomiting after meals, food fads, use of laxatives, compulsive exercising and frequent weighing. Response prevention entails forced avoidance of these rituals; for example, the patient might agree to delay vomiting for an increasing amount of time after meals in order eventually to stop vomiting altogether.

In general, it is felt that patients must retain as much control as possible as long as the desired result is achieved. Patients discharged from the hospital while the medical staff is still in control via structured enforced diets or tube feeding usually relapse.

Those patients better motivated to change will sometimes benefit from outpatient treatment. Education about the effects of starvation and application of the principles of exposure and response prevention, coupled with simple support, sometimes will produce weight gain. Individual psychotherapy is the approach most commonly prescribed for outpatient treatment, especially when the patient has stable relationships and adequate self-esteem.

Also beneficial can be the use of behavioral techniques that the patient can apply herself: keeping records of food intake, using structured meal plans and practicing "nonanorectic" eating. In cases in which certain foods are feared, it is recommended that these be left out of the diet initially but introduced later. Eventual exposure to feared foods is important; to avoid it would be to reinforce anorectic behavior. Cognitive behavioral therapy is designed to help the patient gain control of unhealthy eating behaviors and to alter the distorted and rigid thinking that perpetuates the syndrome.

The goals of individual therapy are to help the patient regain physical health, reduce symptoms, increase self-esteem and proceed with personal and social development. Long-term individual therapy may be indicated when the patient has a mild personality disorder, such as irritability, anxiety, depression, mood swings or sleep disturbance.

Group therapy can be helpful to motivated anorectics, allowing them to feel less alone with their symptoms, to get feedback from their peers and to build their social skills. It has been found useful to have patients at varying stages of improvement in a group. The role modeling done by recovering anorectics, as well as the support and appropriate confrontation by an entire group, has proven to be quite powerful.

Family therapy attempts to establish more appropriate eating patterns, facilitate communication and permit family members to feel more connected with one another. It may be helpful even if a patient is able to achieve only a limited degree of autonomy, because of disturbed family relationships.

Anorectics often retreat into denial when experiencing anxiety in therapy and may flee treatment early on.

Many drug therapies have been tried either as the major focus of treatment or as adjuncts to general support and psychological therapies. Among these have been CYPROHEPTADINE, CHLORPROMAZINE, AMITRIPTYLINE and METOCLOPRAMIDE. In one trial, dietary zinc supplementation for anorectic adolescents was followed by a decrease in the levels of depression and anxiety.

The primary aim of such treatment has been to promote food intake and weight restoration. Although drug treatments do have a place in the *management* of eating disorders, they have not yet attained a high enough degree of effectiveness to be considered as useful as they are in the treatment of such disorders as mania or depression.

In a 10-year follow-up of 76 anorectic women in Iowa and Minnesota who had been treated in hospitals and released at normal weight, Cornell University Medical College researchers found that only three women kept their weight within normal range during the 10-year study period. Thirty-one of the 76 women were still below minimum weight for their age and height at the 10-year mark. Five women in the study had died; their average weight at death was 58 pounds.

Anderson, Arnold E. "Inpatient and Outpatient Treatment of Anorexia Nervosa." In *Handbook of Eating Disorders*, edited by Kelly D. Brownell and John Foreyt. New York: Basic Books, 1986.

Garfinkel, Paul E., and Garner, David M. *Anorexia Nervosa: A Multidimensional Perspective*. New York: Brunner/Mazel, 1982.

Levitt, John L. "Treating Adults with Eating Disorders by Using an Inpatient Approach." *Health and Social Work* 11(2) (Spring 1986).

Neuman, Patricia A., and Halvorson, Patricia A. *Anorexia Nervosa and Bulimia: A Handbook for Counselors and Therapists*. New York: Van Nostrand Reinhold, 1983.

Recovery Recovery from anorexia nervosa does occur, but it isn't always the same for every patient—or for every authority of clinic. Generally, recovery involves many factors and may vary from partial to full recovery. The criteria most usually associated with recovery are weight gain, resumption of menstruation and social/emotional maturity. Because different criteria are used by different researchers to indicate recovery, and because different treatment centers select different types of patients, studies reporting recovery rates can be confusing and contradictory.

It is tempting, because it is so noticeable, to consider only weight gain as a measure of recovery, but weight restoration alone is not always a good barometer. Returning a patient to normal weight is certainly important, but it is relatively easy to accomplish simply by hospitalizing the patient and controlling her food intake. The critical and more difficult task is to get the patient to maintain the higher weight in her normal environment. For this reason, the length of time reported in studies between "recovery" and follow-up is important. The longer the time from treatment to follow-up, the higher the reported mortality rates, the more frequent the rehospitalizations, the greater the continuing psychological problems, the more inadequate the marital and social adjustments and the lower the recovery rates. However, researchers hope that newer treatment methods, along with earlier detection (due to educational efforts and publicity), will result in more permanent recoveries.

In terms of nutrition, Neuman and Halvorson correlated various studies to determine that 50 percent of diagnosed and treated anorectics can be expected to recover completely within two to five years. When those anorectics who demonstrate *some* nutritional improvement are included, the rate of recovery increases to 66 percent. Approximately 90 percent of treated anorectics go on to become employed. Between 50 and 87 percent of these anorectics resume menstruation, usually a year or more after body weight has stabilized. Neuman and Halvorson add, "Even for those anorectics who do not experience the return of menstrual periods, the possibility of bearing children remains, since ovaries may still be active."

On the other hand, recovered anorectics may continue to experience problems relating to their disorder. Anorexia can become chronic. In their research, Neuman and Halvorson found that as many as half those affected have a relapse, and up to 38 percent may have to be rehospitalized within two years. But rehospitalization can actually be a step toward recovery; sometimes several setbacks occur before real progress is apparent. Nevertheless, approximately 18 percent of diagnosed anorectics do remain ill and unchanged. Death from complications of the disorder or from suicide has been estimated to occur in anywhere from 3 to 25 percent of cases. Psychologically, approximately 50 percent of anorexia victims, on follow-up, show problems with phobias, depression and social adjustment.

A comparison of several studies indicates that recovery rates may be predicted when body weight is low at the time treatment begins; the older the age at the onset of the disorder the longer the duration of the illness. Other predictors are disturbed family relationships, binge eating and/or purging or a history of previous psychiatric treatment or childhood adjustment problems.

Neuman, Patricia A., and Halvorson, Patricia A. *Anorexia Nervosa and Bulimia: A Handbook for Counselors and Therapists.* New York: Van Nostrand Reinhold, 1983.

Szmukler, George I., and Russell, Gerald F. M. "Outcome and Prognosis of Anorexia Nervosa." In *Handbook of Eating Disorders*, edited by Kelly D. Brownell and John P. Foreyt. New York: Basic Books, 1986.

anorexia nervosa: research   The National Institutes of Health are sponsoring research to determine the causes of anorexia, the best methods of treatment and ways to identify those who might have a high risk of developing the disorder.

University scientists, sponsored by the National Institute of Child Health and Human Development, are examining the various factors in society, personality and family influencing persons who develop anorexia. Other projects are comparing weight gain in patients fed high-protein versus low-protein diets.

Researchers at the National Institute of Mental Health are studying the biological aspects of appetite, particularly brain chemistry. Although psychological or environmental factors may precipitate the disorder, the study indicates that it may be prolonged by starvation-induced changes in body processes. Persons with anorexia are sometimes admitted for study and treatment at the Clinical Center, a research hospital located on the National Institutes of Health campus in Bethesda, Maryland.

The National Institutes of Health, through its Division of Research Resources, supports 10 General Clinical Research Centers throughout the country in which anorexia research is under way. Topics currently under investigation include sexual maturation, endocrine evaluation, hypothalamic and pituitary aspects of anorexia nervosa and potassium levels in persons with anorexia.

The National Institute of Arthritis, Diabetes and Digestive and Kidney Diseases sponsors studies in the endocrine disturbances of the hypothalamic, pituitary and ovarian functions in anorectics.

ANRED (Anorexia Nervosa and Related Eating Disorders, Inc.) A national nonprofit organization that collects information about eating disorders and distributes it to anorectics, bulimics, families, school personnel, students and medical and mental health professionals. The ANRED staff leads workshops and seminars across the United States, helping people identify and understand anorexia nervosa and bulimia. ANRED also participates in professional conferences, helping physicians, psychotherapists and other human services personnel learn effective ways of working with eating-disordered people.

ANRED also works closely with Sacred Heart Hospital in Eugene, Oregon, where its offices are located, to provide an integrated, comprehensive eating-disorders program. The program incorporates inpatient, day-hospital and aftercare modes.

The *ANRED Alert,* a monthly newsletter containing research updates, self-help tips, stories by recovered anorectics and bulimics, encouragement for families and descriptions of therapy techniques, is available for $10 per year. (See APPENDIX II.)

ANRED provides speakers and educational presentations for schools, clubs, civic organizations, churches, counseling agencies and other groups. It also provides training for counselors and psychotherapists who work with anorectic and bulimic clients.

anticonvulsant treatment Anticonvulsants are drugs that suppress convulsions. These include diphenylhydantoin (Dilantin), mephenytoin (Mesantoin) and trimethadione (Tridione). They are used in the treatment of epilepsy and in psychomotor (muscular action resulting from mental activity) and myoclonic (involuntary twitching or spasms of muscles) seizures. A relationship between binge eating and seizure disorders has been suggested because binge eaters typically describe their binges as episodic and uncontrollable. Binge episodes are also frequently preceded by a change in mental state that could be interpreted as an aura (flashes of light, unusual smells, increased tension or fear), a phenomenon that sometimes occurs in nervous disorders. A number of compulsive eaters have had abnormalities of their electroencephalogram (EEG) pattern (an EEG measures electric current generated in the brain). Because of these findings, some doctors have treated bulimic patients with anticonvulsant drugs and have reported success. However, others have found these drugs to

be of no use, and there has not been sufficient compelling evidence to support the
hypothesis that bulimia is a form of seizure
disorder.

Johnson, W., and Brief, D. "Bulimia." *Behav-
ioral Medicine Update* 4, 1982.
Wermuth, B. M.; Davis, K.; Hollister, L.; and
Stunkard, A. J. "Phenytoin Treatment of the
Binge-eating Syndrome." *American Journal of
Psychiatry* 134, 1977.

antidepressants   Drugs used in the treatment of depressive illness. They are among
the most commonly used psychotropic (affecting the mind) agents in the treatment of
anorexia nervosa and bulimia in the United
States. Three types of antidepressants have
been commonly used in this country: tricyclics, monoamine oxidase (MAO) inhibitors and trazodones. They all boost the action
of the neurotransmitters SEROTONIN and norepinephrine, two of the chemicals that transmit impulses through the nervous system.
Tricyclics and MAO inhibitors prolong the
active life of these chemicals; trazodones
have a strong sedative effect.

Each of the three classes of antidepressants has been regarded by some as successful in treatment of bulimic patients of normal
body weight. However, there are a number
of questions raised by others. First, there is
no known way to determine which patients
are likely to respond favorably. Most of the
controlled trials of antidepressant medications have studied bulimia patients who are
chronically and moderately to severely ill.
It is not clear if the same success would be
found in less severely ill patients. Of more
concern to doctors is the fact that little is
known about the long-term outcome of the
drug treatment of bulimia or how best to
combine drug treatment with other forms of
therapy. All of the published controlled studies of antidepressant medication in bulimia
have been of short duration (no longer than
two months), and only limited follow-up
data are available. One study conducted by
Pope, Hudson, Yurgelun-Todd and Jonas in
1985 reported that most of the patients who
participated in their original double-blind
trial of IMIPRAMINE (a tricyclic) were doing
well up to two years later. A majority of the
patients were still on some antidepressant
medication, and most of those who had attempted to discontinue medication had relapsed.

At this point, it is still not known how
many bulimia patients who initially respond
to antidepressant medication will continue
to respond if they remain on medication, and
how many will relapse if medication is dis-
continued after a reasonable course of treatment, for example, of six months.

A new family of antidepressants that can
regulate serotonin, chemically unrelated to
tricyclics, MAO inhibitors and trazodones,
is now becoming available. The first of these
drugs to reach the market in the United
States was fluoxetine, developed by Eli Lilly
& Co. as PROZAC. Others awaiting approval
by the Food and Drug Administration are
sertraline, fluvoxamine and femoxetine. These
drugs have fewer or less severe side effects
than other antidepressants, which can cause
thirst, constipation and a CRAVING for carbohydrates.

Therapists have expressed concern that
tricyclic antidepressants such as imipramine
and AMITRIPTYLINE may actually increase
the already high risk of suicide among eating-disorder patients. Some antidepressants
stimulate APPETITE, which can be particularly difficult for the eating-disordered person, but the new serotonin-regulating drugs
seem to spur weight loss instead. Prozac has
been reported to lead to a weight loss of four
pounds in six weeks for the average overweight depressed patient. A number of researchers say that it shows promise as a
treatment of obesity.

See also DEPRESSION.

Pope, H. G., Hudson, J. I., Jonas, J. M. and
Yusgelun-Todd, M. S. 1983. "Bulimia Treatment With Imipramine: A Placebo-Controlled,

Double-Blind Study.'' American Journal of Psychiatry 140.

antipsychotic medication A group of drugs used to treat psychoses (mental disorders characterized by loss of contact with reality). They were introduced into psychiatry during the early 1960s. Occasionally, anorexia patients, particularly agitated ones, have benefited from low doses of antipsychotic medications. Soon after their introduction, CHLORPROMAZINE began to be used along with insulin to produce weight gain among anorectics.

None of these medications have exhibited much overall success in controlled studies. In addition, the severity of potential side effects of antipsychotic medications, including grand mal seizures, hypertension and the long-term risk of tardive dyskinesia (involuntary movements of the face, mouth, etc., believed to be induced by prolonged use of certain tranquilizers), limits the use of these drugs in treating anorexia. Despite these limitations, they continue to be recommended in the management of particularly physically active or compulsive patients who respond to the sedative properties of antipsychotic drugs.

Although the distortion of body image (see BODY IMAGE DISTURBANCE) characteristic of anorexia nervosa at times approaches delusional proportions, there is no indication that antipsychotic medications reduce this disturbance.

anxiety A feeling of uneasiness, apprehension or dread often characterized by tension, increased pulse and sweating. Most persons find healthy ways to deal with their anxiety, such as social activities, hobbies, music, reading and sports. Anxiety can even be a positive signal, alerting the individual to a situation or event that requires preparation to overcome, such as the anxiety that motivates a student to study for an exam. Some, however, respond in negative or inappropriate ways, having insomnia or recurrent headaches, overindulging in alcohol or drugs, overeating or experiencing a loss of appetite, for example.

Instead of using anxiety as a signal to prepare to cope with some perceived stress, eating-disordered persons see anxiety as a signal of impending doom, a warning that whatever is coming will be emotionally overwhelming. They react to anxiety by trying to get rid of it rather than by heeding it. In them, anxiety is likely to set off a binge or, in anorectics, to further restrict eating.

The central theme of the PSYCHODYNAMIC APPROACH TO OBESITY is that anxiety precedes and triggers the overweight person's overeating response. The anxiety that results in overeating is produced by internal emotional conflicts rather than external stimuli. Eating often serves temporarily to make a person feel better. Because much internal conflict is believed to take place in the subconscious, an individual may often not be aware of the source of the anxiety. Studies have shown that uncontrollable anxiety increases eating in obese individuals, but controllable anxiety does not. Some therapists see the use of food as compensating for life's upsets, replacing what seems to be missing in life and soothing, calming and covering up daily stresses and anxiety. Theories in opposition to this include the EXTERNALITY APPROACH TO OBESITY.

appetite An emotional and physical impulse or desire or urge to eat, regardless of nutritional needs. Appetite is psychological, dependent on memory and associations (social learning), unlike HUNGER, which is physiologically aroused by the body's need for food. Appetite is a complex mechanism involving the METABOLISM, gastric juices, the hypothalamus and the cerebral cortex. It is stimulated by the sight, smell or thought of food and accompanied by the flow of saliva in the mouth and gastric juice in the stomach. Appetite may stimulate a person to eat when no hunger signals are present or to continue eating after physiological SA-

TIETY has been achieved. When appetite is disturbed, an individual consumes more calories than he uses up and thus gains weight.

For many years it was presumed that the stomach held the primary role in appetite control. As surgical techniques developed and gastrectomy (removal of the stomach) became possible, it became apparent that this is not so. Ultimate control of feeding lies in the brain. There are also several mechanisms by which the small intestine is thought to bring about satiety.

appetite-stimulating drugs   Although patients with anorexia nervosa do not have a reduced appetite, a number of researchers have tried appetite-stimulating drugs in the hope that they might induce anorectic patients to eat and gain weight. Only one of these drugs, an antihistamine called CYPRO-HEPTADINE, has actually been studied in detail, and it has been found generally to be useless.

appetite suppressants   Drugs such as AMPHETAMINES, BULKING AGENTS and topical painkillers that lessen or eliminate appetite by slowing gastric emptying, and possibly by increasing a ''full'' feeling following eating. They can also maintain a feeling of fullness long enough to help a patient limit the size of the next meal. Many clinicians strongly advise against the use of any appetite suppressant for bulimics or compulsive overeaters.

One of the most potent gastric decelerators among common appetite suppressants is FENFLURAMINE. L-tryptophan, an amino acid occurring naturally in some high-protein foods, was another dietary supplement used for appetite control, but after it was linked to EMS (an abnormal increase of a blood component, eosinophil, resulting in tissue disease), the U.S. Department of Health and Human Services in 1990 ordered virtually all products containing it recalled.

One theory suggests that appetite suppressants temporarily lower the set point rather than suppress the appetite and that because of this any weight lost while using suppressants is usually rapidly regained once the dieter stops taking them. (See SET-POINT THEORY.)

Appetite suppression by a modest amount of readily assimilable energy, such as a caloric sweetener (''diet candy''), is not likely to last longer than an hour.

Some appetite suppressants use the topical painkiller BENZOCAINE to reduce sensation in the mouth and make eating a less rewarding activity.

art therapy   An outgrowth of work therapy and activation therapies, which serve to foster activity and thus rehabilitation by encouraging some form of occupation. Also referred to as creative therapy, art therapy is an attempt to stimulate patients through the creation of art and design and then to transfer this creativity or expressiveness to the reshaping of the patient's life.

Work created during art therapy is not evaluated for aesthetic merit or artistic skill but for its value in psychotherapeutic exploration. Artistic productions can be interpreted by experienced psychotherapists in the context of a therapy, as with free association, or as is done in psychoanalysis with dreams.

Art therapy has existed in various forms since the 1940s. It has been used alone or to augment other forms of treatment with both individuals and groups. Although the field has been gaining acceptance as a legitimate form of psychotherapy, critics say it has lagged behind other therapies in documenting and evaluating its effectiveness. Art therapy is thought to be especially helpful in the case of young children who may express graphically what they cannot yet communicate verbally.

In the treatment of eating disorders, art therapy can provide anorectics with an opportunity to become more sensitive to their inner selves. They create artwork that originates within themselves and is not under the control of others. Anorectics convey their emotional needs through the use of "body language" (by starving themselves), that is, engaging in a nonverbal form of symbolic communication. Drawing and painting are also forms of nonverbal communication; through these media they can express their emotional conflicts and enhance their self-awareness.

In art therapy, anorectics are encouraged to represent themselves, their families, their feelings, their view of treatment and so on. Interpretation of such work can provide an opportunity to begin more formal PSYCHO-THERAPY.

Green, Bonnie L.; Wehling, Christina; and Talsky, Gerald J. "Group Art Therapy as an Adjunct to Treatment for Chronic Outpatients." *Hospital and Community Psychiatry* Vol. 38, No. 9 (September 1987).

Poldinger, Walter, and Krambeck, K. "The Relevance of Creativity for Psychiatric Therapy and Rehabilitation." *Comprehensive Psychiatry* Vol. 28, No. 5 (September/October 1987).

Wadeson, Harriet. *Art Psychotherapy*. New York: John Wiley & Sons, 1980.

———. *The Dynamics of Art Psychotherapy*. New York: John Wiley & Sons, 1987.

assessment of body fat   As early as 1908, there were reports that the obese had a greater susceptibility than the lean to caisson disease, the decompression sickness now called the bends, suffered by underwater workers and caused by too-rapid decrease in atmospheric pressure. In 1935, it was confirmed that rapid changes in atmospheric pressure did result in more severe attacks of the bends among the obese than the lean. This held practical significance for deep-sea diving and aviation and led to the military's practice of rejecting people whose weight was more than 15 percent above that recommended by the standard body weight/height charts.

But the use of standard body weight/height ratios has limitations for assessment of body fat. Muscular football players have been rejected for military service because they were over the limit even though they were not obese. And there are individuals who have extremely large skeletons.

More recently, SKIN FOLD MEASUREMENTS have emerged as a tool to improve the assessment of body fat for the general population.

athletes   Athletes who compete in certain sports in which body thinness is stressed along with high performance expectations, such as gymnastics, wrestling, swimming and ice-skating, have shown frequent symptoms of eating disorders, as have dancers (see BALLET DANCERS). Likewise, bulimia and other drastic weight-control measures have been described as common among jockeys, who must meet low weight requirements.

Female cheerleaders often experience pressure to attain and maintain weight that is lower than other adolescents of the same height. A study reported in 1986 by Lundholm and Littrell examined cheerleaders' desire for thinness in relationship to disordered eating and weight-control behaviors. A total of 751 high school cheerleaders from the Midwest were tested. Cheerleaders who expressed a strong desire for thinness had significantly higher scores on seven of eight eating-disorder scales. The greater the desire for thinness, the more likely the tendency to report disordered eating and weight-control behaviors associated with bulimia.

A 1989 Associated Press story stated that an "alarming number" of women athletes at the University of Texas had eating disorders, with the problem especially prevalent among members of the swimming team. According to the report, during a period of 18 months, one of every 10 female athletes at the university, a total of 12, had been diagnosed as having a serious eating disorder. Another 20 to 30 percent had shown symptoms of an eating disorder, and 50 to 60 percent expressed above-average concern about their weight. Current and former swimmers blamed the pressure to meet weight guidelines for their routine fasting, induced vomiting, laxative and diuretic abuse and excessive exercising. Tiffany Cohen, a swimmer who won two Olympic gold medals in 1984, was quoted as saying that her fear of being overweight when reporting to workouts led her into bulimic cycles of binges and purges that resulted in a nine-week hospitalization. And many women on the professional tennis circuit are known to suffer from eating disorders, including Zina Garrison and Carling Bassett-Seguso.

Some coaches may be contributing to the development of eating disorders in their athletes by putting too much pressure on them to achieve a preset weight or body form without taking the individual's condition into consideration. Many coaches and athletes estimate optimal body weight to be much lower than what researchers believe to be healthy, and consider a well-formed and graceful body to be much leaner than the medically defined healthy body.

"Eating Disorders Soar among College Team Swimmers." *BASH Magazine,* November 1989.

Hahn, Cindy. "Why Eating Disorders Pervade Women's Tennis." *Tennis,* December 1990.

Lundholm, J. K., and Littrell, J. M. "Desire for Thinness among High School Cheerleaders: Relationship to Disordered Eating and Weight Control Behaviors." *Adolescence* 1986 (Fall; 21(83) 573–9).

Perrone, Vinnie. "Pound for Pound, a Most Dangerous Sport." *Washington Post,* April 28, 1991.

Rucinski, Ann. "Relationship of Body Image and Dietary Intake of Competitive Ice Skaters." *Journal of the American Dietetic Association* 89:1 (January 1989).

ATPase   An enzyme that may in some way control predisposition to weight gain. One theory holds that abnormally low levels of it lowers resting energy expenditure by as much as 25 percent. Obese people typically have 20 to 25 percent less ATPase than do people of normal weight. The more obese a person is, the lower his concentration of ATPase is likely to be. A low level of

ATPase alters caloric efficiency in favor of the obese, who burn fewer calories than normal-weight people when they perform the same amount of activity. The ATPase theory is unproven.

atypical anorexia nervosa   A term used by HILDE BRUCH to describe a condition in which weight loss occurs because of various symbolic misinterpretations of the eating function, rather than because of a preoccupation with weight.

One example Bruch describes is the relationship of eating to the symbolization of pregnancy fantasies. Although this theory of the fear of oral impregnation had been considered, in the early 1940s, the cornerstone in the mental and emotional processes underlying anorexia nervosa, Bruch found this preoccupation only in exceptional cases and thus came to rate patients with this preoccupation as atypical. Others she classified as atypical include those who refuse to eat for fear of abdominal pain or vomiting, those who refuse food because they feel unworthy and those who do not eat in response to events in their lives. This refusal to eat is decidedly different from the true anorectic's loss of appetite.

Patients with atypical anorexia nervosa and those with the genuine disorder look deceptively alike, particularly after the condition has existed for some time. In contrast to genuine anorectics, however, in whom relentless pursuit of thinness and denial of their condition, even of acute emaciation, are key symptoms, atypical anorectics complain about weight loss and do not want to stay thin, or value thinness only secondarily, as a means of manipulating others. Inability to eat is the leading symptom in the atypical group. Often there is an unacknowledged desire to stay sick in order to remain in a dependent role, in contrast to the struggle for an independent identity that occurs in genuine, or primary, anorectics. Bruch described these patients as displaying various degrees of neurotic and hysterical symptoms.

Patients diagnosed as atypical do not display the peculiar features of the primary disorder: pursuit of thinness as a struggle for an independent identity, delusional denial of thinness, preoccupation with food, hyperactivity and striving for perfection.

Of 60 female patients Bruch reported on with the diagnosis of anorexia nervosa, there were 15 (25 percent) diagnosed as atypical. She found few if any differences in the descriptive data between the atypical and genuine group. Weight loss was of the same order of magnitude, age of onset in the atypical group was slightly higher and amenorrhea was not present as frequently with the atypical group. Both groups proved equally resistant to treatment.

Bruch found the one common characteristic among atypical anorexia patients to be a severe sense of inadequacy and discontent with their lives. Eating difficulties developed when the demands of reality became overpowering and their fragile sense of self was further undermined.

See also PSYCHOGENIC MALNUTRITION.

Bruch, Hilde. "Psychogenic Malnutrition and Atypical Anorexia Nervosa." In *Eating Disorders: Obesity, Anorexia Nervosa, and the Person Within*. New York: Basic Books, 1973.

aversion therapy   A type of behavioral therapy based on the experiments of Ivan Pavlov (1849–1936), a Russian scientist who worked extensively in the field of conditioned reflexes. Typically, an aversive experience (a foul odor, an electric shock) is administered to a patient at certain times in order to create a negative reaction toward certain foods or behaviors. This therapy was among the first techniques employed in the treatment of obesity. Repeated pairings of aversive experience with certain foods were assumed to result in decreasing palatability of those foods through a process of "Pavlovian" behavioral conditioning; this shift in preference was assumed to facilitate control over eating and, thus, weight reduction. Taste aversions develop most easily to novel and less-preferred foods and often persist for many years. One limitation of this therapy is the relative difficulty in establishing aversions to familiar, preferred foods, which are the very ones to which dieters may wish to develop aversions. Results with overweight patients have been poor, whether the unpleasant stimuli have been foul smells, electric shocks or unpleasant images.

Although aversion therapy has been used quite frequently in the treatment of patients who are overweight because of compulsive eating, few reports deal specifically with patients identified as bulimic. It is now considered an outdated treatment.

See also BEHAVIOR MODIFICATION.

Avicenna   An 11th-century Persian physician and philosopher, called the "Prince of Physicians," who was the first to write about anorexia nervosa. He described the case of a melancholic young prince who was successfully treated for the disorder. He was the author of more than 100 works, of which his *Canon of Medicine* was the most important and was used for centuries as a medical reference in both the Christian and Islamic worlds.

B

Bahamian Diet   A controversial diet formula promoted by comedian DICK GREGORY, who claims to have kept his weight down over the years via fasting and use of his formula, "a low-calorie, powdered, natural food supplement, taken in juice." Its ingredients are listed as soy protein, soy protein concentrate, tricalcium, phosphate, lecithin, cellulose gel, guar gum, pectin, sesamum indicum seed, cucurbita pepo seed, salvia columbariae seed and sea vegetation.

In 1984 Gregory made an agreement with a Swiss-owned natural foods company and began marketing the product, mainly to the black community. In 1987 he began distributing his product through a Philadelphia-based marketing company called Correction Connection. A company spokesperson has reported that there are 7,000 to 10,000 Bahamian Diet distributors nationwide and that the company moves millions of cans of the product per year.

Packaging on the product gives no recommended caloric intake beyond the 180–270 calories provided by the supplement. The National Association to Advance Fat Acceptance (NAAFA) organization has come out strongly against the Bahamian Diet. (See LIQUID FORMULAS.)

ballet dancers According to various reports in medical literature, between 7 and 38 percent of female dancers in competitive settings have been found to have serious eating problems. Classical ballet demands the same high standards of technical proficiency of its dancers as competitive sports do of first-class athletes. And as in wrestling, gymnastics and swimming, the right body shape and weight are primary concerns. Because ballet is basically nonaerobic and has a low caloric expenditure, weight reduction cannot be achieved and low weight maintained through dancing alone.

In a study of 49 female dancers who performed in national ballet companies in the United States and in the Republic of China (Taiwan), 11 percent of the Americans and 24 percent of the Chinese reported that they had an eating problem. Those dancers chosen from general auditions exhibited significantly more anorectic behaviors and had a higher incidence of eating problems, with 46 percent reporting anorexia nervosa, bulimia or purging behavior, than those taken from a company school such as the School of American Ballet (11 percent), where a strict selection process over a number of years weeds out those who do not

meet the rigid body shape and weight requirements. The study's authors contend that companies choosing by audition, who do not control the early selection process of their dancers, "may be choosing women who have more difficulty maintaining the low body weight demanded by this profession, and so are more at risk for developing eating-related problems than dancers selected from company schools, who may be less susceptible to the development of eating problems because they are more naturally suited to the thin ideal required by this profession." This has been suggested as the reason for the wide disparity of eating disorders reported in different studies of ballet dancers.

See also ATHLETES.

Hamilton, Linda H.; Brooks-Gunn, J.; Warren, Michelle P.; and Hamilton, William G. "The Role of Selectivity in the Pathogenesis of Eating Problems in Ballet Dancers." *Medicine and Science in Sports and Exercise* Vol. 20, No. 6 (December 1988).

Schnitt, Diana. "Psychological Issues in Dancers—An Overview." *Journal of Physical Education, Recreation and Dance*, Vol. 61, No. 9 (November 1990).

Banting, William (1797–1878) The "Father of Dieting"; a 19th-century English mortician whose weight began climbing during his late thirties. When his doctor advised him to exercise to lose weight and suggested rowing, Banting bought a small boat, which he took out onto the Thames each morning. But all this exercise and the fresh air made him hungry; he went home and ate even more.

By age 50 he had become so obese that he couldn't bend to tie his shoes; he could hardly exert any energy without difficulty in breathing. He continued to eat and gain weight. As he wrote later, his body fell into a "low and impoverished state." When his doctor suggested that he sweat off some pounds in Turkish baths, he took 90. They didn't work.

By this time, Banting was 65 years old, stood five feet five inches tall and weighed 230 pounds. Walking down stairs caused such strain on his legs that he had to navigate the stairs backward. Finally, in 1862, he consulted another physician, William Harvey.

Harvey was one of the few scientists and physicians of the day who studied the effects of dieting on general health. Until then, weight-control methods had included bleeding from the arm or jugular vein, applying leeches to the arms, eating vegetables with vinegar, taking hot baths or saltwater baths, staying awake most of the night, taking sea voyages, eating soap, pricking the flesh with needles, walking with naked feet and surgically removing fatty tissue with a scalpel.

Dr. Harvey put Banting on a high-protein, low-carbohydrate diet of 1,200 calories per day. Banting was willing to try anything, and it worked. The first week he lost two pounds, the next week three, and the third week four pounds. After a year he had lost a total of 46 pounds and 14 1/2 inches around his waist. Even his hearing and vision improved.

Banting was so pleased that he decided to tell others about his good fortune. In 1863 he wrote a pamphlet called *Letter on Corpulence, Addressed to the Public,* the first diet book. He gave away the first 2,500 copies, and it became the talk of London. The third edition sold 50,000 copies. By the fourth edition, it had grown from its original 25 pages to 100 pages, with the addition of letters and testimonials praising Banting's success and his diet.

Banting became famous, frequently lecturing while wearing the clothes he had worn when he had weighed 230 pounds. The clothes would fall around him, and he would tell his audiences that this is what a proper diet should do for them.

Several doctors dismissed Banting as a fraud and as the "prototype hypochondriac." Some even started rumors that Banting was dying because of his diet. On two occasions in 1864, Banting found it necessary to write to the *Times* of London to deny that he was dying.

During Banting's lifetime, "Bantingism" and "to bant" became household words. He lived to be 81, dying on March 16, 1878, slim and trim to the end.

bariatrics   A branch of medicine that deals with the causes, prevention and treatment of obesity. There are 9,000 members of the American Society of Bariatric Physicians.

basal metabolic rate (BMR)   The rate at which energy (fuel, the fat and glucose obtained from food) is used by an individual at complete physical and mental rest for basic body functioning (breathing, heart activity, nervous system activity and various other essential organ functions). It is usually measured in the morning when a person is relaxed and has not eaten since the preceding evening. In an average person, this basic functioning accounts for approximately 70 percent of total energy expenditure. The remaining 30 percent is largely a reflection of one's level of physical activity. The BMR varies according to age, sex and weight. It is highest in children and begins to decline in young adults after age 24, dropping approximately 5 to 7 percent each decade after age 20, making it more difficult to lose weight as one gets older. BMR is also lower in hypothyroidism and higher in hyperthyroidism.

The wide variance in basal metabolic rate among individuals is one reason why different people respond differently to identical diet and exercise programs. People with high basal metabolic rates tend to remain slim even while eating large amounts of high-calorie food; those with lower BMRs seem to gain weight merely "looking" at food. The BMR actually decreases when caloric intake is severely restricted by starvation or stringent diet.

See also SET-POINT THEORY.

BASH Acronym for Bulimia/Anorexia Self-Help, Inc., located in St. Louis. Begun in 1981, it runs the largest self-help program of its kind in the United States and the first to combine the techniques of group therapy with the principles of self-help and the various clinical applications of a professional support system.

BASH is a self-help organization providing outpatient information and open-ended group therapy and support for anyone in the community who suffers from an eating disorder, including family members of the victim.

Several hundred people are enrolled, and twice a month up to 400 of them, including patients and their families, gather for the better part of a day. During these meetings, there are educational presentations, usually featuring lectures by experts in some area related to eating disorders. Following these presentations and question-and-answer periods, attendees divide into groups of 12 to 15, each led by two trained leaders, or facilitators.

BASH facilitators are recruited and trained from within the organization and include former victims, family members and professional staff of the Deaconess Hospital BASH Treatment Center. Facilitators are required to attend two additional monthly meetings, one a training session on theories and principles of therapeutic approaches and the other a supervising session, at which facilitators' meeting notes (formulated following each meeting) are critiqued.

In May 1984, additional weekly meetings were instituted for members who felt that they needed augmented support. These also include informational presentations, on proper nutrition, for example, and culminate in meetings of small groups led by facilitators.

Anorectics and bulimics are subject to frequent relapses, and their need for crisis intervention is great. A crisis center for bulimics and anorectics was opened in 1984 in St. Louis under the auspices of BASH. This nonprofit center provides 24-hour service, including a toll-free telephone hotline and overnight sleeping facilities. It is the only such institution of its kind. (See APPENDIX II.)

behavior modification The changing of human behavior through conditioning or other learning techniques. In behavior modification therapy, after determining what behaviors are dysfunctional or self-destructive, therapeutic techniques are used to alter or eliminate them.

These techniques are grounded in the theories of the behavioral school of psychology, which holds that human behavior consists almost entirely of responses to physiological stimuli, and dismisses such concepts as the subconscious or the unconscious and in general, nonphysiological causation of behavior. Therapists of many schools, however, have found techniques developed by behaviorists to be useful in their own practices.

Techniques often used include exposing the patient gradually to the presumed cause of his distress while teaching him to cope with anxiety; flooding the patient with anxiety-producing stimuli and preventing him from responding in the usual manner until feelings of anxiety eventually disappear; and modeling by performing the anxiety-provoking activity for the patient to copy.

Advocates of behavior-modification therapy say that it is a more efficient mode of treatment than psychoanalytic or other psychotherapeutic approaches, which often take years and may never produce clear and unambiguous results. Opponents point out that it treats only the symptoms of a disorder and does not engage the profound causes, so that symptoms frequently reappear.

In Anorexia and Bulimia Use of behavior modification for treatment of anorexia and bulimia was first advocated in 1972. The use of such treatment for anorexia nervosa assumes that food refusal is a learned behavior that needs to be changed. Change is achieved through a reward-and-punishment system. Behavior leading to weight gain is rewarded, or "positively reinforced," by access to desirable activities, and behavior not leading to weight gain is punished by making things unpleasant. Proponents of behavior modification claim it achieves weight gain more rapidly than other methods. Detractors express concern that it often provokes serious psychological damage by increasing the inner turmoil and sense of helplessness in patients who feel tricked into losing control over their bodies. HILDE BRUCH condemned it, pointing out that weight gain in itself is not a cure for anorexia nervosa.

Follow-up observations have shown that weight gain achieved through behavior modification is often short-lived. Some hospitalized patients respond to the therapy in order to gain enough weight to obtain release from the hospital—and then freely resume their noneating behavior pattern. It has been most successful with patients who come to it voluntarily and who make a "contract" to gain weight. (See EATING HABITS MONITORING.)

Behavior therapy has acquired greater respectability in recent years, particularly for the treatment of bulimia nervosa. Behavioral techniques to prevent binge eating include eating slowly by putting the fork down between each bite, and always eating with other people. Although results with behavior therapy have been encouraging during initial treatment, some physicians question its long-term effect. It is most likely to be effective when the patient anticipates an oncoming desire or need to binge eat. "Automatic" binge eating is not as effectively treated with behavior therapy.

In Obesity When behavior modification is used in treatment for obesity, the therapist first analyzes the patient's current eating habits. Usually this involves the patient's maintaining a detailed food diary. Noted in the diary are the types and amounts of food eaten at various times of the day, where the food is eaten (at his desk, dining room table, living room, in his car, etc.), activities involved in at the same time eating takes place

(e.g., reading, watching television, listening to the radio, etc.), the degree of hunger at each time food is eaten and the mood the patient is in when he or she decides to eat. The food diary helps identify particular eating patterns or situations in which the patient is likely to overeat.

After a thorough analysis of eating behavior has been made and recurring patterns identified, other behaviors are substituted for eating when a particular situation arises. For example, if the patient regularly snacks while watching television, he could substitute some other behavior such as chewing gum or sipping on a glass of water. If the patient routinely eats candy when she feels angry or depressed, she can instead do 10 repetitions of a simple exercise or go for a walk or express her thoughts on paper. In this way, a new habit is substituted for the established eating response to certain situations.

If the eating pattern analysis shows that the patient has poor eating habits, such as eating too rapidly, behavior modification is used to alter and control them. New eating patterns might include using smaller dishes, putting the fork down between bites and carefully chewing before swallowing in order to stretch out a meal and allow stimulation of the SATIETY mechanisms, substituting low-calorie foods like fruits and vegetables for high-calorie snacks, eating meals at regular times or avoiding distractions such as television during meals.

A central element of most obesity behavior-modification programs is slowing down the act of eating. It was initially thought that doing so would interrupt the "chaining" of behaviors involved in eating: putting food on the fork, lifting it to the mouth and so on, which occurred largely outside a person's awareness. But it has since been found that slowing down the act of eating has an additional benefit because a larger proportion of the meal remains uneaten at the time when the stomach and intestine have begun to absorb nutrients, thus producing the physiological signals of fullness. These signals add to the effect of the techniques used to eat less.

There are specific techniques to help people slow their rate of eating, enabling them to become aware of all its components and gain control over them. The most frequently suggested one is setting down one's fork or spoon between bites. Another is to count each mouthful, chew or swallow. Those patients who have trouble slowing their eating rate are told to stop eating for one minute late in a meal when a delay is more readily tolerated. They are then instructed to increase the number and duration of delays and begin them earlier.

Patients are also urged to make meals a time of comfort and relaxation and to avoid arguments and the rehashing of problems at the dinner table. They are encouraged to learn to savor food as they eat it, to make a conscious effort to become aware of it as they are chewing and to enjoy the act of swallowing and the feeling of warmth and fullness in their stomach. To the extent that they succeed with this, they may eat less and enjoy it more.

A system of rewards (positive reinforcement) is the key element in a behavioral therapy program. Although the ultimate reward is an improvement in health, personal appearance and self-esteem, interim rewards are important in encouraging faithful adherence to the program. Examples include treating oneself to a movie after a three-pound weight loss or going on a trip after successfully shedding 10 pounds. Charts recording weight loss and changes in body measurements also provide positive reinforcement.

Brownell and Kramer write that

behavior modification is practiced so widely, there is a tendency to believe that it consists of little more than a series of techniques or tricks such as record-keeping and slowing eating. This is mistaken. A modern day, comprehensive program is sophisticated and involves systematic work, not only on eating behavior, but on exercise, attitudes, social relationships, nutrition, and other factors. The better behavioral programs now are producing weight losses in the range of 25 to 30 pounds.

For many people, adherence to a behavior-modification program is easier if it is administered in a group setting. Lay groups devoted to weight loss have been proliferating throughout the world (two of the oldest and most successful are WEIGHT WATCHERS and TOPS (Take Off Pounds Sensibly).

Weight loss with behavioral therapy is slow and undramatic, and the amount of weight lost is usually moderate. Even though the goal of behavior modification is a lifelong change in eating habits, many people gradually return to their old eating behavior and regain the lost weight.

See also AVERSION THERAPY; EXTERNAL CONTROL THERAPY.

Brownell, Kelly D., and Kramer, P. M. "Behavioral Management of Obesity." *Medical Clinics of North America* 73(1) (January 1989).

Brownell, Kelly D., and Wadden, Thomas A. "Behavior Therapy for Obesity: Modern Approaches and Better Results." In *Handbook of Eating Disorders*, edited by Kelly D. Brownell and John P. Foreyt. New York: Basic Books, 1986.

O'Brien, Robert, and Chafetz, Morris. *The Encyclopedia of Alcoholism*. New York: Facts on File, 1982.

benzocaine A crystalline compound used in ointments as a mild local anesthetic. When used in a diet pill, it is supposed to deaden the taste buds and thereby lessen the craving for food. It is often used in "miracle" pills and weight-reducing candies in combination with methyl cellulose, which expands by absorbing water from the stomach to give a false sense of fullness. Researchers are divided over whether benzocaine in such small doses (7.5 mg per tablet) actually has a numbing effect on the salivary glands. But, as Edwin Bayrd wrote in *The Thin Game*, that argument "is quite beside the point, for the salivary glands are a part of the mouth and the pills are already in the stomach.''

Beverly Hills Diet   A diet promoted in a book of the same name (1980) by Judy Mazel. The diet stresses combinations of similar kinds of foods that are digested together. The first week allows only fruit; the second adds a few other items.

In *Journal of School Health* (August 1988), M. Elizabeth Collins states that the Beverly Hills Diet marks the first time an eating disorder—anorexia nervosa—was marketed as a cure for obesity. ''The popularity of the book, which focuses on the reward of being 'skinny' and 'perfect,' is viewed by [Orland] Wooley and [Susan] Wooley (former directors of the Eating Disorders Clinic at the University of Cincinnati College of Medicine) as yet another symptom of 'a weight-obsessed culture in which no price is too high for thinness, including health.' ''

P. Wright also condemned the Beverly Hills Diet, writing in ''The Psychology of Eating and Eating Disorders'' (*Psychology Survey No. 6,* edited by H. Beloff and A. Colmon, 1987): ''[It] actually advocates a form of bulimia in which dieters are advised to counteract an eating binge by consuming large amounts of raw fruit in order to produce diarrhea.''

binge eating   Rapid consumption of large amounts of food during a short period of time. A binge is usually defined as the consumption of 2,000 calories or more during the span of one to two hours. An average binge lasts from 60 to 75 minutes, with 3,400 calories consumed (an entire pecan pie, for instance).

Binge eating (see BULIMIA) gained increased attention during the 1980s. Most research has focused on BULIMIA NERVOSA, the binge-purge syndrome, which typically occurs in normal-weight and underweight individuals.

Although many in the general population admit to binge eating, the eating binges of most nonbulimic people are small relative to those of bulimics. Patients with bulimia have had substantiated binges during which they consumed 5,000 to 20,000 calories in an eight-hour period. Twenty thousand calories is roughly 210 brownies or five and a half layer cakes.

Only a few studies have been conducted that describe the prevalence of binge eating among obese patients. Independent research at Duke and Stanford universities has indicated that approximately 50 percent of obese patients surveyed binged at least once a week.

Binge eating, as defined by the full DSM-III criteria for bulimia, appears to be a frequent problem among the obese and overweight. Researchers have reported binge eating to be most prevalent in young females who have a tendency to be at least slightly overweight. Moreover, binge eating becomes significantly more prevalent as the degree of obesity increases. Studies have suggested the possibility of a never-ending, full-circle relationship between overweight and bingeing. Being overweight leads to excessive dieting, which leads to binge eating and increased caloric intake, which leads to a greater degree of overweight.

A University of Pittsburgh study compared the incidence of psychiatric disorders among 25 obese binge eaters and 25 obese non–binge eaters of similar age and weight. Sixty percent of bingers met the criteria for one or more psychiatric disorders, compared with 28 percent of nonbingers, with differences most apparent in affective (mood) disorder: 32 percent of obese bingers reported a history of affective disorder, compared with only 8 percent of nonbingers. (See AFFECTIVE DISORDERS AND EATING DISORDERS.) Obese binge eaters also reported significantly more psychiatric symptoms, especially symptoms of DEPRESSION, ANXIETY and sexual dysfunction.

Binge eaters have also been reported to do less well with behavioral treatment than nonbingers. This leads to increasing difficulty in treating obesity as weight increases. (See BEHAVIOR MODIFICATION.)

The true binger stops not when she's beginning to feel uncomfortable but only when it becomes impossible to eat more because she has reached the limit of her physical capacity. Binge eating is usually done alone and in secret. Binges tend to be ended by running out of food, loss of energy, physical discomfort, social interruption or sleep. Most bingers feel bad and self-critical after a binge; it is usual for subjects to promise themselves that they will never do it again and to set out on a strict diet or fast. Some bingers find that negative feelings are relieved by vomiting up the food they have eaten, and a few will go to great lengths to make sure that they have purged it all. Thus a binger may eat "marker" foods early in the binge that can be easily recognized when they are vomited. A number of bingers have described their practice of drinking water and then vomiting in an attempt to wash out all the food. The process is repeated until the vomit is "clean."

Bingers typically have an ambivalent attitude toward their behavior, usually predominantly negative. Almost all patients show some attempts to resist binge eating, although the same patients who take specific steps to stop the practice may simultaneously be planning binges. Both types of behavior may be extreme. Thus bingers might prepare elaborate foods and stock up on items especially for a binge; some go so far as to injure their fingers in a desperate attempt to stop themselves from using them to induce vomiting.

Patients with bulimia cite several moods and conditions that may precede individual binges, including tension, CRAVING certain foods, unhappiness, uncontrolled APPETITE, and INSOMNIA. Late afternoon, early evening and late evening are the most common times for binge eating. The foods most commonly ingested are those high in FATS and/or CARBOHYDRATES that can be easily eaten and do not require much preparation, such as ice cream, doughnuts and candy.

Marcus, Marsha D.; Wing, Rena R.; Ewing, Linda; Kern, Edward; Gooding, William; and McDermott, Michael. "Psychiatric Disorders among Obese Binge Eaters." *International Journal of Eating Disorders* 9, 1 (1990).

Hirschmann, Jane R., Munter, Carol H. *Overcoming Overeating*. Reading, Mass.: Addison-Wesley, 1988.

Binge Eating Scale (BES)   A self-test developed in 1982 by Gormally, Black, Daston and Rardin to assess binge eating among the obese. The BES contains 16 items designed to measure the behavioral components of the binge-eating syndrome and the feelings or perceptions that precede or follow a binge.

> Sample items from the BES:
>
> I don't think about food a great deal.
>
> Most of my days seem to be preoccupied with thoughts about food. I feel like I live to eat.
>
> Because I feel so helpless about controlling my eating, I have become very desperate about trying to get in control.

Binge Scale   A self-test developed in 1980 by Hawkins and Clements. It contains nine items designed to measure binge-eating behavior (e.g., frequency, duration, rate of eating) and attitudes associated with BULIMIA. The scale was developed to parallel the diagnostic criteria described in DSM-III.

Sample item from the Binge Scale:

> How often do you binge?
>   A. Seldom
>   B. Once or twice a month
>   C. Once a week
>   D. Almost every day

biofeedback   A technique that seeks to control certain emotional states, such as ANXIETY or DEPRESSION, by modifying, with the aid of electronic devices, involuntary body functions such as blood pressure or heartbeat.

This technique has been experimented with in the treatment of ANOREXIA NERVOSA, but it is not yet widely used. Its basic benefit is the teaching of relaxation techniques to counteract the typically high activity level of anorectics, who tend to deny fatigue and typically are unable to relax. They pursue their activities compulsively, producing excessive levels of autonomic arousal (heart, blood pressure and so on), which can lead to psychophysiological stress reactions.

Through connection to the biofeedback machines by muscle or temperature sensors, the patients learn to become active participants in the process of relaxation training. Patients find it difficult to deny their condition when the evidence can be seen on a sound or light monitor. Biofeedback may make it easier for the therapist to break through the denial process of anorectic patients.

Gross, Meir. "Anorexia Nervosa—Treatment Perspectives." In *Eating Disorders: Effective Care and Treatment,* edited by Félix E. F. Larocca. St. Louis: Ishiyaku EuroAmerica, 1986.

body fat   Body fat is a reservoir of available fuel for energy needs. When we eat CALORIES in excess of immediate needs, the body converts this fuel into a storable form (FAT). When we eat an insufficient number of calories, the body takes some of the stored fat and metabolizes it into available fuel. (See METABOLISM.)

Some body fat is desirable. For example, fat cushions the balls of our feet and protects the bony structure. Fat insulates our organs from cold during winter months and protects them against damage from outside the body. Too-low body fat reduces resistance to viral infection.

Excess body fat, however, is harmful. Excess fat requires the heart to pump harder and at higher pressures simply because the arterial circuit is longer. Fat also chokes down the available passageways, forcing the heart to pump still harder. This extra strain significantly increases the risk of heart attacks, strokes, hypertension and other cardiovascular diseases. In addition, excess fat puts undue strain on other body organs and has proven to increase significantly the risk of diabetes and even certain types of cancers.

Compare a five-foot seven-inch football player weighing 200 pounds and a sedentary executive of the same height and weight. The athlete may have 6 to 7 percent body fat (at the low end of the recommended range), while the executive may have 25 percent (over the recommended maximum). What *is* recommended? According to the University of California *Wellness Letter* (January 1991), the ideal amount of body fat varies from person to person, depending on age, sex, fitness level and genetic makeup. It can also vary according to who sets the standards. Many researchers suggest a desirable range for men of between 11 and 18 percent; for women, between 16 and 23 percent. Others say that up to 23 percent is acceptable for men and up to 30 percent for women.

Recent data indicate that simple DIETING reduces lean body material (muscle) and predisposes the individual to regain lost weight with even higher percentages of body fat (see YO-YO DIETING). However, simultaneous dieting and exercise retains and even increases muscle, initially at the expense of water, then fatty tissue. Studies are under way exploring techniques that could increase thermogenesis and permit obese people to burn off their excess fat.

During World War II, the U.S. Navy sought submariners with low body fat for their greater ability to withstand nitrogen uptake and discharge, which protected them against the "bends"). Thus began the search for a reliable means to measure body fat.

Until recently, the methods most often used were hydrostatic testing (water pressure), SKIN FOLD MEASUREMENT, blood analysis and impedance measurements (sound waves).

The direct method for measuring body fat is through biopsies. However, other measurements have been developed and are now used more frequently. Densitometric analysis (hydrostatic weighing) compares regular weight with underwater weight in calculating the amount of lean body mass and body fat. (Because fat weighs less than water, a fatter person weighs proportionately less underwater than a lean one.) This method has become the "control" against which other fat-measuring methods are compared and standardized. However, equipment to perform these tests can usually be found only at certain hospitals or university labs.

Anthropometric measurements such as body circumference and thickness of skin fold provide more practical assessments for measuring body fat. In particular, caliper measurements of skin folds have been advocated for use in behavioral research. In this procedure, calipers are used to measure the thickness of skin and underlying fat at several locations on the body, with results calculated in an equation. However, some researchers have found measurement of height and weight to have a smaller standard deviation than skin folds, so they are frequently the anthropometric measurements of choice in assessing fatness. In addition, some clinicians have found height and weight measurements more convenient, practical and reliable in treatment than the caliper assessments.

Recently developed instruments offer the ability to determine an accurate measurement of body fat and lean body mass with no discomfort, with results in seconds. These fitness and body fat analyzers are based on a technology developed by the U.S. Department of Agriculture. By touching the biceps, a fiberoptic wand emitting infrared light senses a spectrum change (because fat absorbs more light than muscle or bone) and displays an accurate body-fat percentage on a digital readout.

Still another recent development is the bioelectrical impedance analysis (BIA). This sends a mild electrical current through electrodes attached to the foot and hand; the greater the resistance to electricity, the more body fat. Researchers do not agree about the reliability of the BIA and infrared tests.

Garrow, J. S., et al. "Comparison of Estimates of Fat-free Mass in Normal and Obese Women from Measurements of Body Potassium, Body Water and Body Density." *European Journal of Clinical Nutrition* 44(3) (March 1990).

Gray, D. S., "Skinfold Thickness Measurements in Obese Subjects." *American Journal of Clinical Nutrition* 51(4) (April 1990).

Westrate, J. A., et al. "Body Composition in Children: Proposal for a Method for Calculating Body Fat Percentage from Total Body Density or Skinfold-thickness Measurements." *American Journal of Clinical Nutrition* 49(11) (November 1989).

body image disturbance An inability to judge one's appearance realistically, particularly common in anorectics, ballet dancers, jockeys and pregnant women. For the AN-OREXIA NERVOSA patient, misperception reaches quasi-delusional proportions and is evident in the anorectic's lack of concern about, stubborn defense of or inability to recognize an emaciated condition. Some patients display a variation of this disturbance in which their misperception is restricted to a particular part or parts of the body. Stomach or thighs are magnified in a patient's mind and seem disproportionate to the rest of the body. These patients will acknowledge that in general they appear emaciated but believe that further dieting is necessary to eliminate a protruding belly or some other perceived unattractive feature. HILDE BRUCH first recognized body image disturbance to be an essential characteristic of anorexia nervosa, and she considered its correction necessary for recovery.

In a study of both eating-disordered and normal women at Douglas Hospital in Montreal in 1989, anorectics, but not bulimics, exhibited body image distortion.

Another investigation, of the relationship between body image distortion and self-esteem among normal-weight college students, revealed that females had significantly higher body image distortion scores than males and significantly lower self-esteem scores. These were women who were within 10 percent of "ideal" (recommended) weight and had no history of eating-disorder behavior.

Many obese individuals perceive themselves as larger than they are and have very negative attitudes toward their body. Patients who have been obese as children or adolescents and who subsequently lose weight often retain a distorted perception of themselves as very obese. (See OBESITY; CHILDHOOD OBESITY; ADOLESCENT OBESITY.)

There has been a large accumulation of data on body image perception, distorted and undistorted, by eating-disordered patients, but as Peter J. V. Beumont, head of psychiatry at the University of Sydney in Australia, told a BASH audience in 1989,

> All assessments of body image to date have been too subjective. They all depend on what the patient chooses to tell us about her perception, and there is no way of being sure she is reporting this accurately. . . . [A]s yet no one has confronted the issue of directly correcting body size overestimation in therapy, or showing that this affects prognosis. It is as if research workers are repeatedly rediscovering the wheel, without finding a practical use for it.

Ben-Tovim, David I.; Walker, M. K.; Murray, H.; and Chin, G. "Body Size Estimates: Body Image or Body Attitude Measures." *International Journal of Eating Disorders* 9:1 (1990).

Beumont, Peter J. V. "Trying to Make Sense of Body Image Data." *BASH Magazine*, 8: 6 June 1989.

Rucinski, Ann. "Relationship of Body Image and Dietary Intake of Competitive Ice Skaters." *Journal of the American Dietetic Association* 89: 1 (January 1989).

Steiger, H.; Fraenkel, L.; Leichner, P. P. "Relationship of Body-Image Distortion to Sex-Role Identifications, Irrational Cognitions, and Body Weight in Eating-disordered Females." *Journal of Clinical Psychology* 45: 1 (January 1989).

body types   Typologizing the human body, or classifying bodies by shape and size, has been proposed since Hippocrates, who described the basic Greek physiques as phthisic (linear and vertical) and apoplectic (broad and horizontal). Ernst Kretschmer, a 19th-century psychiatrist, divided the population into pyknics (short and round) and asthenics (lean and long legged), with athletes falling somewhere in between. After analyzing thousands of specially posed photographs, William Sheldon devised a three-part classification of body types in 1940. He named them ENDOMORPHS (soft, round, fleshy, light boned, well padded), MESOMORPHS (muscular, square, broad shouldered, sturdy) and ECTOMORPHS (long legged, fragile, thin, skeletal, linear). Sheldon also claimed that body type is an unalterable inheritance, demonstrating by his elaborate measurement system that people retained the same basic body type after weight changes of as much as 100 pounds. He demonstrated that even after subjects underwent semistarvation for six months and changed outward signs of body type, they all returned to their original shapes within two years. Forced-weight-gain tests produced similar results. Kretschmer's and Sheldon's studies are not considered scientifically sound today.

body wrapping   A technique claimed by hucksters on late-night television and in magazine ads to cause layers of fat to disappear without dieting. Common body-wrapping devices include sauna suits or heated belts that are strapped to the waist or stomach or whatever area needs reduction. The heat produced by these gadgets, either alone or when used in conjunction with exercise, supposedly melts away fat much as a hot stove burner melts lard or butter in a saucepan. The advertisements do not explain how the body can withstand temperatures high enough to melt deposited fat, or how the melted fat will be eliminated from the body. In fact, of course, such temperatures are not generated, and any loss of bulk or weight from using these devices is due strictly to a temporary reduction in water content of the wrapped area, which will be reversed as the tissue becomes rehydrated.

See also FRAUDULENT PRODUCTS.

McCurdy, John A., Jr. *Sculpturing Your Body: Diet, Exercise and Lipo (Fat) Suction.* Hollywood, Fla. Frederick Fell Publishers, 1987.

brown fat   A type of tissue named for its brownish color, caused by the numerous blood vessels that course through it. In humans, thermogenesis takes place in brown fat tissue. Thermogenesis is a process, induced by food intake or by cold temperatures, whereby calories are converted to heat. An impairment in thermogenesis can result in greater efficiency in energy storage, which could lead to excess fat.

Abundant in newborn infants, brown fat can be found under the arms, across the back, near the kidneys and around large blood vessels in the chest. Research suggests that defective brown fat cells might be the cause of obesity in some people. Heavy people appear to have less brown fat than average-weight people, and what they do have seems to work inefficiently. All this is conjecture, with nothing proven scientifically.

Bruch, Hilde (1904–1984)   A practicing psychiatrist and professor of psychiatry at Baylor College of Medicine in Houston. In the years following World War II, she was the most influential person in the United States in shaping the conception of eating disorders as psychiatric illnesses and in formulating psychotherapeutic approaches to their treatment. Throughout her work Bruch stresses the formation of individual personality and factors within the family that precondition victims of these disorders to respond

to certain kinds of problems by self-starvation or overeating.

Bruch did not regard obesity as a single condition but distinguished three main forms: in some individuals obesity is due to physical factors, and their weight has no association with emotional problems. Others have "reactive obesity," brought about by overeating in situations of psychological stress. The third type, "developmental obesity," has its onset in childhood and is associated with a disturbance in the maturation of the individual's personality.

Bruch was one of the first to stress that many cognitive defects in anorectics are directly related to starvation. Therefore, a meaningful psychiatric evaluation is possible only after the worst effects of malnutrition have been corrected.

Bruch's principal works include *Eating Disorders: Obesity, Anorexia Nervosa, and the Person Within* (New York: Basic Books, 1973); *The Golden Cage: The Enigma of Anorexia Nervosa* (Cambridge: Harvard University Press, 1978; New York: Vintage Books, 1979); *Conversations with Anorexics/Hilde Bruch,* edited by Danita Czyzewski and Melanie A. Sur (New York: Basic Books, 1988).

bruxism   The habitual grinding of the teeth, either during sleep or as an unconscious habit while awake. The most common causes of bruxism are said to be psychological factors such as fear, rage, rejection by others and emotional tension. The condition is sometimes seen in patients with eating disorders and results in loosening or drifting of the teeth. Bruxism causes even worse damage in bulimic patients, whose protective tooth enamel has been dissolved by bathings in gastric acid from VOMITING.

See also DENTAL CARIES.

bulimarexia   A term coined in 1976 by Marlene Boskind-White to cover the compulsive practice of bingeing and purging; at the time BULIMIA was officially described as bingeing without purging (DSM-II). Bulimarexia was called a "nomenclature atrocity" by HILDE BRUCH. Though still used by some researchers and clinicians as interchangeable with "bulimia" or "BULIMIA NERVOSA," the term is not listed in any standard manual of diagnosis.

Boskind-White, Marlene, and White, William C., Jr. "Bulimarexia: A Historical-Sociocultural Perspective." In *Handbook of Eating Disorders*, edited by Kelly D. Brownell and John P. Foreyt. New York: Basic Books, 1986.

bulimia The word *bulimia* literally means "oxen appetite" or gorging. It refers to the compulsive practice of binge eating. The term has been used in various ways by different medical authors, for example, to describe a subgroup of patients with anorexia nervosa who also binge eat. It is now frequently used to indicate the compulsive practice of bingeing and PURGING, interchangeably with the term BULIMIA NERVOSA as defined in DSM-III.

bulimia nervosa An eating disorder characterized by an intense fear of becoming obese. It involves a recurrent pattern of BINGE EATING followed by purging. It is not known to be caused by any physical illness. It usually begins in adolescence or early adult life and is mainly found in females.

A number of terms have been used to describe this disorder, but the term "bulimia nervosa," introduced by GERALD F. M. RUSSELL, is the most widely accepted and frequently used because it implies a link to ANOREXIA NERVOSA and differentiates the syndrome from simple binge eating (bulimia). In moments of stress, bulimics turn toward food, not away from it as anorectics do. Bulimic patients are usually more distressed and humiliated by their behavior than anorectics, swinging between intense feelings of self-control while dieting and total self-loathing when bulimic.

Sometimes eating behavior becomes bizarre. A young woman from a financially secure background may search through garbage for food. Another may shoplift food or steal money from friends and family to buy it. The behavior that supports the "habit" of recurring bulimia can resemble that of alcoholism, and its cost may also be similar.

Bulimics usually control their eating while busy with other things, but during solitary leisure time they may eat to the point of exhaustion. Enormous amounts of food may be eaten at one time, as many as 20,000 calories a day. Studies have shown the average binge to last slightly less than 1 1/4 hours and to include slightly more than 3,400 calories. This gorging will be followed by purging via vomiting (induced by gagging, emetics or simply willing it), diuretics or laxatives (from 50 to 100 or more tablets at one time).

Although it is common in other countries, bulimia is said to be epidemic in the United States. It is harder to detect than anorexia because there is no obvious physical evidence such as emaciation, and thus the extent of bulimia is less clear than that of anorexia, but medical experts estimate that as many as 16 to 30 percent of all women may have practiced bulimic behaviors to some degree. As many as 18 percent of young women between the ages of 17 and 23 are thought to suffer from bulimia in one form or another. When Drewnowski, Yee and Krahn of the University of Michigan conducted a survey of college freshman in 1988, they found the incidence of bulimia nervosa to be 4.2 cases per 100 women per year. The rate remained stable (2.9–3.3 percent) as new cases were offset by partial remissions. Some women continued bulimic behaviors without meeting full DSM-III-R criteria. In a survey conducted of 1,728 10th-grade students, 13 percent reported purging behavior. Female purgers outnumbered male two to one. Until recently, anorexia was more common, but bulimia became the eating disorder of the 1980s, achieving almost celebrity status.

Yet David E. Schotte and Albert J. Stunkard reported in 1987 in the *Journal of the American Medical Association* a different view of the "sweeping epidemic" of bulimia. They interviewed a sample of 1,965 students at the University of Pennsylvania, using a 15-item self-report questionnaire. Only 1.3 percent of the female and 0.1 percent of the male respondents met DSM-III-R diagnostic criteria for bulimia. From this study they determined that whether there is an epidemic of bulimia on the college campus or not depends on the definition of bulimia. "If bulimia is defined as self-reported overeating, or even as self-reported overeating in combination with occasional purging, then the answer is an emphatic 'yes.' If, however, the term 'bulimia' is restricted to the diagnosis of a clinically significant disorder, the answer is 'no.' "

Bulimia has been called the disease of success because the typical bulimic is a professional woman in her mid- to late-twenties, college educated, single and working and living in a big city—an overachiever. Increasing numbers of men are being reported with bulimia nervosa, estimated at between 5 and 10 percent of adult males, although it is theorized that there are many more who do not reveal their bulimic activities because of its status as a "woman's disease."

Many of these men form a bona fide subgroup of overeaters and compulsive exercisers. Rather than following the typical binge-purge cycle, they are preoccupied with physical activity. After exercising for hours, they will become ravenously hungry and eat uncontrollably. Sometimes the food will be a reward for the frantic workout, but afterward the thought of the calories ingested will cause them to begin the cycle again with even more exercising.

The disorder can go undetected for years, even by close family members. Both the gorging and purging are carried out in secret,

with all evidence destroyed. Because the bulimic appears outwardly to be quite successful in school or career, no one suspects that she doesn't feel as good as she may appear to be. It is not unusual for a diagnosis not to be made until a patient is well into her thirties or forties.

Bulimia typically begins during the late teens or early twenties, after the patient has unsuccessfully tried to lose weight via several reducing diets, especially when restrictive dieting results in hunger. The hunger is satisfied by bingeing. Either through reading about it or hearing a fellow student or co-worker talk about it, the patient learns that self-induced VOMITING or laxative use will get rid of the extra calories, thereby relieving feelings of guilt brought on by the binge eating. However, self-induced vomiting leads to further hunger. Ultimately, a vicious cycle is established, perpetuated by emotional disturbances and the continuing desire to lose weight. Some bulimics begin with vomiting after regular meals to lose weight and only binge eat later when their hunger and cravings increase because of the lowered energy intake. During a binge, bulimics typically eat foods high in CARBOHYDRATES, foods they would normally not be allowed to eat on healthy or weight-reduction diets, setting aside time each day for solitary, secret binge eating. However, therapists have reported patients eating salads, vegetables, cheese, meat and yogurt during a binge.

University of Alabama researchers report that more women who were college freshmen in the mid-1960s are engaging in extreme weight-control measures such as bulimia-like behavior today than they did in their high school and college years. Bulimia-like behaviors reported in the study included the use of DIET PILLS, laxatives and diuretics, self-induced vomiting, FASTING and bingeing. This study was conducted to determine if the increase in bulimia-like behaviors reported by psychologists was real or just a reflection of greater awareness of such problems. Results showed that there is indeed a real increase and that those at risk are not just college women overly concerned with dating and appearance but older women as well.

The researchers surveyed 159 women, ranging in age from 35 to 45, who were college freshmen in 1964. Subjects were asked about their weight-control practices during high school, college and today. Most reported an increase in the use of extreme weight-control measures (diet pills, fasting, laxatives, etc.) during the years since high school. For example, 84.7 percent said that they had never used diet pills when they were in college, but that figure has dropped to 77.4 percent today.

Comparing these results with those of a similar study in 1983, researchers found that a large proportion of both age groups saw themselves as heavier than they were, a problem that is linked to bulimia, anorexia and other eating disorders. (See BODY IMAGE DISTURBANCE.) The study indicates that older women, as well as adolescents, are feeling more pressure about their weight. Researchers related this to the fact that we live in a very youth-oriented society and that cultural pressures to be thin are great. Many women are trying to conform to an ideal body image that is almost impossible to obtain without these extreme unhealthy measures.

The role of the family is also being looked at closely by researchers attempting to determine the causes or origins of bulimia and other eating disorders. A 1989 study comparing 50 bulimic women with 40 non–eating-disordered women, all from the same geographic area, revealed no significant differences between the two groups in social class, family size, birth position or sibling sex ratio, but the parents of bulimic women were found to have been significantly older than those of the control group at the time of birth of their daughters. An earlier study (1983) had found no significant difference in this area. Researchers determined that further study is needed in order to determine

what signficance these later findings may have.

Drewnowski, A., Yee, D. K., Krahn, D. D. "Bulimia in College Women: Incidence of Recovery Rates." *American Journal of Psychiatry* (June 1988) 145:6.

Schotte, D. E., Stunkard, A. J. "Bulimia: A Sweeping Epidemic?" *Journal of the American Medical Association* 1987: 258.

Clinical Features Typical physical signs of bulimia include dark circles under the eyes, tooth decay, puffiness around the face (eyes and below cheeks), facial pallor, red knuckles, dull and lifeless hair and loss of hair. In many bulimics, the menstrual cycle becomes irregular. Bulimics may be—but rarely are—emaciated; they are most usually of normal weight but sometimes are overweight.

Bulimic behavior is to be suspected where there is evidence of consumption of unusually large amounts of high-calorie foods, especially if consumed alone or secretly. A diagnosis of bulimia nervosa requires binge eating at least twice a week for three months. Other signs include excessive exercise or fasting, a preoccupation with food, weight and bodily concerns, frequent weight fluctuations due to alternative binges and fasts or purges, increased time spent alone and less with family and friends, theft of money for binges and frequent trips to the bathroom, especially after meals. Sexual interest may also diminish, but not always.

Emotionally, bulimic patients have feelings of depression and self-loathing after eating binges, feel unable to control eating behavior and may appear embarrassed, angry, tense and oversensitive. COGNITIVE DISTORTIONS may also exist:

• *Denial* Bulimics seek acceptable reasons for unacceptable behavior. Whereas others say obesity results from a simple lack of willpower, the bulimic will have excuses or even lie about his overeating ("I eat because . . .") ("I don't know why I'm fat . . . I never eat."). Bulimics hide their purging by using breath sprays, mints and chewing gum. They will often seek "magic" cures for their problems (depression or obesity) through such gimmicks as mail-order BODY WRAPPING.

- *Distorted Body Image* Although more anorectics than bulimics appear to have body image disturbances, the bulimic also may not have an accurate grasp of her weight. Bulimics sometimes believe themselves fatter than they actually are. (See BODY IMAGE DISTURBANCE.)
- *Fictional Finalism* Bulimics often believe that there is a "magic" weight, and that once they attain it, they will have happiness and success ("If I were 120 pounds, everything would be perfect"). They usually find that everything is the same except that they do not have food as a bar against reality.
- *Demandingness* Bulimics often make infantile demands ("I want what I want, when I want it"). The demands are often not met, and they develop an oversensitivity to rejection and a childlike insecurity. Bulimics' demandingness usually provokes the most anger in others involved in their lives.
- *Rigidity and Inflexibility* Bulimics develop an attitude of intransigence, characterized by an air of "I'm right and you're not." This is most obvious in their refusal to try suggested cures or in their rigid persistence with diets that do not work.

Psychologists Barbara Bauer and Wayne Anderson have identified nine irrational beliefs commonly held by bulimics that are related to these emotional distortions: (1) Becoming overweight is the worst thing that can happen to me. (2) There are good foods, such as vegetables and fish, and bad foods, such as sweets and carbohydrates. (3) I must have control over all of my actions to feel safe. (4) I must do everything perfectly or what I do is worthless. (5) Everyone is aware of, and interested in, what I am doing. (6)

Everyone must love me and approve of what I do. (7) External validation is crucial to me. (8) As soon as a particular event such as graduation or marriage occurs, my bulimic behavior will disappear. (9) I must be dependent and subservient yet competitive and aggressive.

The most universal belief, and the one most difficult to modify, appears to be the fear of becoming fat and the failure it represents. Bulimics obsess about and belittle themselves over the slightest weight gain. Although not everyone with bulimia holds all these beliefs, therapists say all are likely to believe in some of them.

A bulimic's weight may fluctuate but not necessarily to the dangerously low levels seen in anorectics. Also unlike anorectics, bulimics are commonly upset by their actions and willing to accept help; they frequently join self-help groups or even seek medical help. Furthermore, they are usually outgoing and have developed attachments, whereas anorectics are isolated and asexual. (See SEXUALITY AND EATING DISORDERS.)

According to Herzog and Copeland, bulimics often have a history of other compulsive behaviors, such as alcohol or drug abuse, and some have features in common with drug or alcohol addicts. They may spend $50 or more a day on food to support their habitual bingeing and often resort to stealing money or shoplifting food. (See MULTICOMPULSIVE.)

A California School of Professional Psychology study in 1987 compared two groups of bulimic women: bulimics who compensate for binges by purging through laxatives, diuretics, vomiting and spitting out food, and bulimics who compensate by fasting. These two groups were compared with each other and with a third group of nonbulimic women for self-esteem and self-role concept. All were of normal weight and were selected from a nonclinical population of undergraduate college students.

Prior to the study, researchers hypothesized that the three groups would differ on self-esteem, with the purging group having the lowest; that the groups would differ on components of gender-related behavior patterns, with the purging group having the lowest score on real-self "femininity" and the highest on ideal-self and imagined male-ideal "femininity"; and that low self-esteem would relate to discrepancies between components of gender-related behavior patterns.

Contrary to expectations, although the bulimic groups combined had lower self-esteem than the nonbulimic group, when the two bulimic groups were examined separately, only the fasting group had lower self-esteem than the nonbulimic group. Moreover, while results indicated that low self-esteem correlates with certain discrepancies for nonbulimics, and that in both fasting bulimics and nonbulimics high self-esteem correlates with a real-self sex-role concept incorporating masculine and feminine gender characteristics, no correlation was found among these variables for purging bulimics.

Bauer, Barbara, and Anderson, Wayne. "Bulimic Beliefs: Food for Thought." *Journal of Counseling and Development* (March 1989).

Herzog, David, and Copeland, Paul. "Eating Disorders." *New England Journal of Medicine* (August 1, 1985).

Complications Menstrual irregularities occur in more than 40 percent of bulimics; for those whose weight falls below 92 percent of ideal body weight, there is an increased likelihood of AMENORRHEA. Repeated VOMITING dissolves tooth enamel and makes the gums recede, can tear the esophagus and stomach and may cause the salivary glands to swell. BINGE EATING can overload the stomach, causing it to expand and even rupture. Low potassium in the blood can lead to heart problems and death and can upset the body's balance of electrolytes (sodium, magnesium, potassium and calcium), causing fatigue, seizures, muscle cramps, irregular heartbeat and decreased bone density (see OSTEOPENIA). Other complications include digestive problems, bursting blood

vessels in the eyes and cheeks, headaches, rashes, swelling around the eyes, ankles and feet, weakness, kidney failure and heart failure. Bulimia can also cause scarring on the backs of hands when fingers are pushed down the throat to induce vomiting. For diabetics, bingeing on high-carbohydrate foods and sweets is particularly hazardous, because their pancreas may not be able to metabolize properly the starches and sugars.

Bulimics speak of being "hooked" on certain foods (particularly CARBOHYDRATES) and needing to feed their "habit." This so-called addictive tendency seems to carry over into other areas, including abuse of drugs and alcohol and KLEPTOMANIA (compulsive stealing). (See MULTICOMPULSIVE.) Many bulimics suffer from serious DEPRESSION, which, combined with their impulsive tendencies, places them at increased risk for SUICIDE. Depression is a problem especially among bulimic students, whose self-esteem plummets when they engage in these extreme behaviors. When they get depressed, their grades fail and they lose their self-confidence.

To determine the range and severity of medical complications encountered in younger patients, researchers reviewed the medical records of 65 adolescents and preadolescents in the Eating Disorders Clinic of the Children's Hospital at Stanford University. Twenty-two percent of bulimic patients required hospitalization for medical reasons during the study period.

Treatment Although bulimic patients are for the most part more likely than anorectics to accept, even seek, treatment, they usually expect quick solutions and become frustrated if treatment does not produce immediate relief of their symptoms. They may deal with their frustration and anxiety in therapy through increased binge eating and may also leave treatment prematurely. GROUP THERAPY is particularly useful for bulimics who feel isolated by their symptoms.

Among the treatments used by psychologists to counter the PERFECTIONISM exhibited by many bulimics is assigning them "unfinished" tasks such as balancing half a checkbook, leaving one corner of a bed unmade or starting a letter and stopping in the middle of a sentence. Other approaches help bulimics deal with irrational belief patterns and include teaching about nutrition, encouraging them to bring food to eat during therapy and helping them to choose activities to fail at in order to overcome their fear of failure.

ANTIDEPRESSANT medication has been used in treatment for bulimia. The two classes of antidepressant drugs most commonly used in the treatment of bulimia have been the monoamine oxidase inhibitors and the tricyclics. The newer fluoxetine (see PROZAC) is now being used frequently. Some controlled studies of antidepressants in bulimia have been promising; IMIPRAMINE and phenelzine have been shown to be significantly successful in reducing bulimic and depressive symptoms.

During controlled testing, the tricyclic antidepressant imipramine produced, on average, a 70 percent reduction in binge frequency. A similar drug, desipramine, resulted in a mean reduction of 91 percent in binge frequency. A third tricyclic antidepressant, AMITRIPTYLINE, was associated with a 72 percent reduction in binge frequency. A controlled trial of phenelzine, a monoamine oxidase inhibitor, found a 66 percent reduction in binge frequency. However, the long-term outcome of drug treatment for bulimia remains unknown. The longest of the published controlled trials used only 10 weeks of treatment, and only limited follow-up data are available.

Medication has proved useful when a bulimic patient also has an associated mood disorder and has failed to respond to PSYCHOTHERAPY. Treatment for bulimia nervosa is most successful when medical therapy and psychotherapy are combined.

Recently, Canadian scientists have reported on preliminary studies showing that bulimic patients also suffering from seasonal mood swings and treated with light therapy (exposure to bright light) have improved both in their depression and in their bulimia. However, these studies have thus far been too limited to yield any serious data. (See AFFECTIVE DISORDERS AND EATING DISORDERS.)

Levitt, John L. "Treating Adults with Eating Disorders by Using an Inpatient Approach." *Health and Social Work* (Spring 1986) 11 (2).
Neuman, Patricia A., and Halvorson, Patricia A. *Anorexia Nervosa and Bulimia: A Handbook for Counselors and Therapists.* New York: Van Nostrand Reinhold, 1983.
Root, Maria P. P.; Fallon, Patricia; and Friedrich, William N. *Bulimia: A Systems Approach to Treatment.* New York: W. W. Norton, 1986.

Bulimia Test (BULIT)   A Self-test developed in 1984 by M. S. Smith and M. H. Thelen. Based on the DSM-III criteria for bulimia, the BULIT is a 32-item multiple-choice scale designed to identify individuals with symptoms of bulimia.

Sample items from the BULIT:

I prefer to eat:
   A. At home alone
   B. At home with others
   C. In a public restaurant
   D. At a friend's home
   E. Doesn't matter

What is the most weight you've lost in one month?
   A. Over 20 pounds
   B. 12–20 pounds
   C. 8–11 pounds
   D. 4–7 pounds
   E. Less than 4 pounds

bulking agents   APPETITE SUPPRESSANTS made from food fiber, taken before meals because they swell up in the stomach, creating a sense of fullness that is supposed to inhibit excess eating. Some doctors dispute the effectiveness and discourage the use of these.

Bulk producers or fillers come in a number of forms: powders, capsules or pills. At most, the Food and Drug Administration says, bulk producers absorb liquid and swell the stomach, thereby reducing HUNGER. There is no proof that they are any more effective than ordinary bulking foods such as whole grains, apples, carrots and sprouts, all of which can provide the same feeling of fullness.

bypass surgery   In use since 1957 to reduce and control weight, bypass surgery offers a rapid weight loss without giving up food by reducing absorptive capacity, thus reducing the amount of food digested or absorbed.

There are two types of bypass surgery used for weight control: intestinal (JEJUNO-ILEAL BYPASS) and gastric. Intestinal bypass shortens the small intestine. As a result, food is not fully absorbed, so the body begins to burn stored energy (fat). Gastric bypass divides the stomach, closing off a large segment by stapling it shut. Because the stomach is smaller, it cannot hold as much, and weight loss results because the patient becomes "full" rapidly. If he continues eating, vomiting occurs, frequently reason enough for the patient to eat less.

Bypass surgery is intended to reduce calorie intake without necessarily reducing food consumption. It is reserved for extremely obese persons and produces substantial and lasting losses of as much as 100 pounds. Side effects such as frequent diarrhea are common, and there is a mortality rate of about 3 percent. In addition, acid-related gastroduodenal disease may occur in the bypassed gastrointestinal tract. Some bypass patients develop BULIMIA, and others become obese again.

Bypass surgery was widely used in treating morbid obesity in the 1970s but is now uncommon because of the frequency and variety of side effects, including cirrhosis of the liver and perforated duodenal ulcers.

C

---

caffeine   An alkaloid, found naturally in coffee and tea, that is a central nervous system stimulant and a diuretic. About 100 to 150 milligrams (mg) are found in a strong cup of tea or coffee.

When researchers at King's College, University of London administered caffeine orally to human volunteers in single doses of 100 mg, it increased the resting metabolic rate of both lean and postobese subjects by 3 to 4 percent over a period of 150 minutes. (See METABOLISM.) It also improved the diet-induced defective thermogenesis observed in the postobese subjects. Measurements of energy expenditure indicated that repeated caffeine administration at two-hour intervals over a 12-hour day increased the energy expenditure of both subject groups by 8 to 11 percent during that period but had no influence on the subsequent 12-hour night energy expenditure. The net effect was a significant increase in daily energy expenditure of 150 calories in the lean subjects and 79 calories in the postobese. The researchers feel that caffeine at commonly consumed doses can have a significant influence on energy balance and may promote thermogenesis in the treatment of obesity.

Robert O'Brien and Sidney Cohen, writing in *The Encyclopedia of Drug Abuse* (New York: Facts On File, 1984), cautioned that regular use of 350 mg or more of caffeine a day results in a form of physical dependence. Regular use of more than 600 mg a day may cause chronic insomnia, breathlessness, persistent anxiety and depression, mild delirium and stomach upset. Heavy caffeine use is also suspected of association with heart disease and some forms of cancer.

Dulloo, A. G.; Geissler, C. A.; Horton, T.; Collins, A.; and Miller, D.S. "Normal Caffeine Consumption: Influence on Thermogenesis and Daily Energy Expenditure in Lean and Postobese Human Volunteers." *American Journal of Clinical Nutrition* (January 1989) 49:1.

Hamilton, Kim. "The Weight-Loss Perk." *Health,* July 1989.

calorie   A unit of measurement of heat. One large, or great, calorie (kilogram calorie) is the amount of heat required to raise the temperature of one kilogram (2.2046 pounds) of water by one degree Celsius (1.8 degrees Fahrenheit); this is the calorie commonly used in metabolic studies. One small calorie (gram calorie) is the amount of heat required to raise the temperature of one gram of water one degree Celsius. In writings on human nutrition the large or kilogram calorie is used. In medical literature, it is occasionally capitalized in order to distinguish it from a small calorie; sometimes it is abbreviated as kcal.

It is possible to calculate the amount of energy contained in a certain food by measuring the amount of heat units, or calories, in that food. (See CALORIMETRY.) Every bodily process—the building up of cells, motion of the muscles, the maintenance of body temperature—requires energy, and the body derives this energy from the food it consumes. Digestive processes reduce food to usable "fuel," which the body "burns" in the complex chemical reactions that sustain life.

From its daily intake of energy converted from food, the body uses only the amount it needs for current activity. The remainder is stored as FAT. If a person consumes more calories than necessary for daily bodily processes, he or she will gain weight. If he or she consumes less than necessary, the body will supplement it by drawing on energy stored as fat, and he or she will lose weight.

Bonnie Liebman, director of nutrition at the Center for Science in the Public Interest,

Washington, D.C., told *Boardroom Reports* (May 15, 1989) that all calories are not alike.

Nutritionists used to say that a calorie was a calorie no matter what kind of food it was—protein, fat or carbohydrate. It didn't matter whether one ate 3,000 calories of fat or 3,000 calories of carbohydrates, the calories the body didn't use were turned into fat. Thus, calorie-counting was the key to dieting. But a growing body of scientific evidence shows that, once inside the body, calories are not treated alike. Fat is handled very differently from protein and carbohydrates, with the fat calories being the most problematic.

Studies conducted by biochemist Jean-Pierre Flatt at the University of Massachusetts Medical School showed that fewer calories are required for the body to turn food fat into body fat than to turn PROTEINS and CARBOHYDRATES into body fat. In the case of food fat, only 3 percent of the calories taken in are burned off in the process of storing it as body fat. In the case of complex carbohydrates, 23 percent of the calories are used up in converting it to body fat.

It is also more difficult for the body to turn proteins and carbohydrates into fat, doing so only when massive amounts have been ingested and using a great amount of energy to do so. The body can store about 1,500 calories' worth of carbohydrates and protein (the rest are burned), but it can store 100,000 to 200,000 calories' worth of fat, according to Flatt. Whereas the normal body attempts to use food fat as energy before storing it in fat cells, the bodies of formerly obese people appear to put fat calories directly into storage, thereby contributing to their weight problem.

Researchers at Harvard Medical School studied 141 women aged 34 to 59 and found no correlation between caloric intake and body weight. The fattest women did not necessarily eat the most. The researchers did find, however, that the women whose diets were highest in fat, particularly saturated fats from red meat and dairy products, were the most overweight regardless of the number of calories they consumed.

Americans today are heavier than ever but consume fewer calories than at the turn of the century. One of the reasons given for this is that we have become a more sedentary society. But it has also been noted that while we may eat less than our ancestors did, the percentage of fats in our diet is 31 percent greater today than it used to be.

See also FAT CELLS; FATS; OBESITY.

calorimetry   A method of measuring the amount of energy (CALORIE) value in food via a burning process. First a small amount of food is weighed and placed in a sealed container, called a bomb calorimeter. Then the food is set on fire with an electric fuse. The calorimeter is then submerged in a premeasured amount of water. The rise in the temperature of the water when the food item is completely burned measures the calorie value of that amount and kind of food. This calorie value is then used to calculate the number of calories in a typical serving.

carbohydrates   A group of chemical substances that make up one of the three sources of nutrients (the others are proteins and fats) and contain only carbon, oxygen and hydrogen. Usually the ratio of hydrogen to oxygen is 2:1. The most common carbohydrates are sugar and starches; others include glycogen, dextrins and celluloses.

Carbohydrates are formed by green plants, which utilize sunlight energy to combine carbon dioxide and water in forming them. Carbohydrates are a basic source of energy. (See CALORIE). One gram yields approximately four calories. Carbohydrate is stored in the body as glycogen (a polysaccharide consisting of sugar molecules) in virtually all tissues, but principally in the liver and muscles, where it becomes a source of reserve energy. Whole grains, vegetables, legumes (peas and beans), tubers (potatoes), fruits, honey and refined sugar are all excellent sources of carbohydrates. Calories

derived from sugar and candy, however, have been termed "empty'" calories because these foods lack essential amino acids, vitamins and minerals.

Carpenter, Karen (1950–1983)   A popular singer and recording star (with her brother Richard) during the 1970s, who died in 1983 at the age of 32 as a consequence of cardiomyopathy, secondary to the effects of the toxic substance emetine. She suffered from ANOREXIA NERVOSA, possibly with bulimic episodes, and abused syrup of IPECAC. Building up over time, the alkaloid emetine in the ipecac irreversibly damaged her heart muscle, eventually leading to her death by cardiac arrest. Because of her popularity, her death brought more attention to eating disorders than anything before or since. A TV movie, *The Karen Carpenter Story*, was first shown January 1, 1989.

cellulite   A term first used in the 1950s to refer to the tenacious FAT that forms bumps and ridges on thighs and buttocks, giving them a dimpled or "cottage cheese" look. It is especially common in women. According to Michael O'Shea, founder and chairman of the Sports Training Institute in New York City, the lumpiness is caused by fat deposits located directly beneath the skin pushing up between the tiny ligaments running from the skin's surface through the fat layer to the muscles underneath. When the fat cells increase in size, as they do during weight gain, they cause the fat deposits to bulge, giving the skin a dimpled look.

Edwin Bayrd, author of *The Thin Game*, writes, however, that "this dimpling is a result of aging rather than overindulgence. It manifests itself when the subdermal connective tissue that forms a sort of honeycomb around the body's adipose cells begins to lose its elasticity and shrinks with age. When this happens, the overlying skin also contracts—and if the encased fat cells cannot shrink, they cannot help but pucker.''

Early promoters of cellulite "therapy" claimed that cellulite is caused by a thickening of this connective tissue, which then traps fluids and "toxic materials" in that fat itself, causing the lumpy look. They promoted a variety of treatments and gimmicks to "melt" these fatty pockets, including balms, creams, lotions, injections, plastic wraps, massage, mineral baths, air hoses and wrappings of cheesecloth soaked in paraffin.

None of these "cures" proved consistently successful for a number of reasons. Primary among these is the very protective nature of the skin, which prevents penetration of most salves, ointments and other substances applied to its surface. Even if one of these "miracle extracts" were able to break through the skin and break down fat stores, this would not necessarily lead to the elimination of fat from the body. Fat cells constantly dispense fat into the bloodstream and simultaneously resynthesize triglyceride (storage fat) from circulating fatty acids. Circulating fat will be burned only if muscle or other tissue extracts it from the bloodstream. If the tissues do not need fuel, circulating fat is redeposited in fat cells.

There is no scientific evidence to support cellulite therapies or the theories on which they are based. Studies have found no detectable difference between so-called cellulite and fat in other areas.

See also FRAUDULENT PRODUCTS.

Bayrd, Edwin. *The Thin Game.* New York: Newsweek Books, 1978.

McCurdy, John A., Jr. *Sculpturing Your Body: Diet, Exercise and Lipo (Fat) Suction.* Hollywood, Fla.: Frederick Fell Publishers, 1987.

chemical dependency and eating disorders In a survey of 1,100 patients at Hazelden, a Minnesota chemical dependency treatment center, approximately 7 percent of female patients and 3 percent of males reported enough symptoms to be classified as bulimic under DSM-III criteria.

An audit of treatment files of bulimic female patients revealed that they had experienced more adolescent behavior problems and self-destructive behavior than their nonbulimic peers. The typical female chemical-dependent bulimic patient at Hazelden differed markedly from her asymptomatic peers. She was more likely to be a polydrug user; to have had adolescent behavior problems such as school suspension or expulsion, stealing and fighting; to have exhibited self-destructive tendencies through self-inflicted injury, suicide attempts or suicidal thoughts during treatment; and to have had outpatient or inpatient mental health treatment or medication.

Although a group of patients with these problems could be expected to have difficulty in treatment, the course of treatment for both groups was similar in most areas of comparison. Bulimics required the same length of stay in treatment, were discharged with staff approval at similar rates, had about the same number of conflicts with peers during treatment and saw their counselors with the same frequency as asymptomatic patients. Bulimic patients did use mental health services at Hazelden slightly more than nonbulimics.

While cautioning that recent changes in the diagnostic criteria for bulimia and in Hazelden's pretreatment assessment methods make the data "tentative," researchers concluded that research and clinical experience demonstrate that it is possible to work with manageable eating disorders in chemical dependency treatment.

childhood anorexia Anorexia nervosa has been reported in children as early as age four; it is estimated that 3 percent of reported anorexia cases occur before the age of puberty. Because prepubertal children, especially girls, have less body fat than adolescents, they become emaciated more quickly than older anorectics. GERALD F. M. RUSSELL examined a series of 20 girls whose anorexia nervosa began before their first menstrual period (menarche), concluding that anorexia nervosa can be devastating to physical development. There is prolonged delay of puberty (late menarche) and interference with growth in stature and breast development. Young children with anorexia have exhibited clinging behavior upon entering school, difficulty in maintaining peer relations, physical and psychological immaturity, depression and an inability to translate feelings into words.

Blinder, Barton J, and Goodman, Stanley L. "Atypical Eating Disorders." In *Eating Disorders*, edited by Félix E. F. Larocca. San Francisco: Jossey-Bass, 1986.

childhood obesity   Childhood obesity is a growing concern among physicians and researchers. According to a study reported by Tufts University Medical Center, the incidence of obesity in children aged six to 11 has increased as much as 54 percent since 1963. The numbers of superobese children in that age group has doubled, the research showed. The overall rate of obesity for children in preschool through adolescence is estimated to be as high as 15 percent (See SUPEROBESITY.)

In one study conducted in New York City, more than 13 percent of 700 children aged three to five were found to be obese. Because parents frequently think their small children will "outgrow their baby fat" or that a chubby child is a healthy child, most of them do not believe their children have a medical problem. But one study in England showed a definite correlation between weight at six months of age and adult weight.

There are relatively complex methods of determining obesity in childhood; pediatricians generally obtain this information from charts giving accepted or "normal" weight ranges based on sex, height and age.

The relationship between obesity in childhood and disease has not been fully examined. However, childhood obesity appears to be related to decreased release of the growth hormone, increased insulin secretion, and intolerance of carbohydrates and hypertension. Most serum lipid (fatty substance) disorders that cause fatty cysts on the walls of arteries appear to have their origin in childhood.

In a 1989 report on the effect of weight control on lipid changes in obese children, researchers stated that childhood obesity is related to increased total cholesterol and triglyceride levels and decreased high-density lipoprotein (HDL) levels. Given the relationship between obesity and serum lipid levels, obese children are at risk of becoming obese adults, with raised serum cholesterol and triglyceride levels and decreased HDL levels, who will be at risk for coronary disease.

Psychological Effects   Because of the psychological trauma of feeling different, inferior, laughed-at, unattractive and ashamed, obese children tend to withdraw from peer group situations and social activities. Tests have shown that personality characteristics of obese girls are similar to those of people who have been subjected to intense discrimination because of their race or ethnic origin: passivity, obsessive concern with self-image and expectation of rejection. These lead to awkwardness in social situations, social isolation and actual rejection, and thus less activity outside the home, increased eating and, consequently greater obesity. Obese girls also consider obesity—and hence their own bodies—undesirable and in extreme cases repulsive. They consider obesity to be a handicap and the reason for all their disappointments.

When an adolescent feels inferior in group situations, he or she tends to withdraw to solitary and usually sedentary activities, such as TV viewing and eating. Food has been described as a "feel-good drug" for the apathetic and unsure adolescent, whose appetite is also increasing to accompany normal physical growth. Coupled with less-than-normal exercise, this usually leads to even more excess fat and often to severe obesity in adulthood. In extreme cases, the obese child may also suffer from depression, leading to total isolation and an incapacity to become emotionally attached to other persons.

Routine and necessary activities like shopping for clothes can upset obese adolescents. Clothes made for "typical" children don't begin to cover their frames. In order to locate pants that fit around his waist, the fat boy must shop in the men's department. But the rest of these pants are far out of proportion, creating a humiliating situation for already self-conscious children. The owners of a Norwood, Massachusetts mail-order company, Kids At Large, offering oversize clothes for youngsters, reported on in the *Wall Street Journal,* say their catalog approach is successful because it is a means for children to escape the embarrassment of going to a special shop for the overweight or facing slimmer youngsters over the clothing racks at the local shopping mall.

Treatment Childhood obesity is usually found to be accompanied by one or more other physical or psychological disorders. Thus it is often treated most successfully by a combination of therapies, including low-calorie diet, behavior modification, nutrition education and increased physical activity.

Children as young as three months have been placed on diets intended to control weight gain. Doctors at the Clinical Research Center of Mt. Sinai Hospital in New York have hospitalized obese children aged two through 11 and successfully treated them with a diet of 400 calories a day, together with iron and vitamin supplements. The diet consists of 46 grams of carbohydrates, 28 grams of protein and 12 grams of fat.

The premise underlying behavioral approaches to obesity—that effective weight control requires major changes in eating behavior—is considered by some to be even more important for children than for adults because it is usually easier to change the habits of children than those of adults, who are more set in their ways. (See BEHAVIOR MODIFICATION.) These behavioral techniques

involve the manipulation of the physical and social environment to decrease the probability of overeating. This is achieved in the case of diet by keeping track of what is eaten, noting various internal and external cues that lead to eating, immediate positive reinforcements of desirable behaviors, dissociation of eating from other experiences and, in some cases, emphasis on eating styles. Behavior therapy in combination with diet restrictions, has been shown in studies to be superior to diet alone, and maintenance of weight loss has been more successful. It is most helpful for those with one or more "obese eating style" problems: rapid eating, few but large bites, short-duration meals, exaggerated sensitivity to external stimuli.

A child's level of involvement in a weight loss program depends, in large part, on his or her level of mental development. Leonard H. Epstein has outlined four age ranges as a guideline for placing increasing responsibility for weight control on a child. At ages one to five, any weight program must rely on parental control. A child is generally not able to read or write and thus is unable to keep track of calories consumed, burned through exercise and so on. Motivation to lose weight is absent. During this time, parents are the major influences on a child's eating and activity habits. At ages five to eight, a child's ability to monitor calorie consumption/expenditure and eating patterns is still limited, although simple diet control can begin. Children at this age can start learning nutritionally sound eating habits and can be trained to handle social situations in which food is offered. In addition, these children can also begin learning to solicit praise and encouragement for healthy eating from adults close to them. Parents will still be involved significantly. At ages eight to 12, a child can set goals and self-monitor. Peer pressure may provide motivation to lose weight; however, children at this age still benefit substantially from parental involvement. From age 13 on, children can use programs similar to those of adults, though they may be helped through social groups. At this stage of development, children are becoming independent of their parents, and too much parental guidance or interference may be counterproductive.

In the attempt to monitor and control types and amounts of food intake, color coding of foods to show calorie amounts can be understood by children as young as age five. The nutritionally balanced TRAFFIC LIGHT DIET developed by Epstein in 1978 separates premeasured food portions into red, yellow and green categories corresponding to traffic signals (stop eating reds, be careful of the amounts of yellows, and go ahead and eat lots of greens). With young children, colored stars corresponding to foods eaten may then be exchanged for reinforcers. This method of encouraging healthy low-calorie eating by obese children has been shown to be useful in school as well as home settings. The New American Eating Guide, a color-coded poster similar in concept to the Traffic Light Diet, and the Nutrition Scoreboard (Center for Science in the Public Interest, 1977) have also been useful in programs of weight control and eating-habit change for children. The Food Exchange Diet prepared by the American Dietetic Association is also applicable to children, with help from adults in learning the procedures. Pediatricians have used colored tokens to represent the food exchanges in this diet; tokens are transferred from one plastic box to another following consumption of food in their color groups. These color-coded systems provide effective visual representation of diet for children too young to read and write. Premeasured portions also eliminate the need for calorie counting.

Numerous food-related factors influence a child's eating pattern and treatment for obesity: the parents' food-buying habits, another family member's eating disorder, contradictory messages to the child regarding eating, the child's attitude toward diet and exercise change and his knowledge of nutrition.

Although exercise is an important component in assessing and treating childhood obesity, some evidence suggests that it may be less important than diet in maintaining weight loss. Some authors recommend "lifestyle" exercise (walking, cycling, etc.) with little structure or intensity over structured aerobic exercise in weight loss programs for children, for two reasons. First, if caloric expenditure and not aerobic fitness is the goal of the program, life-style exercise will accomplish that goal. More important, studies have found that life-style exercise is more likely to be adhered to, and lack of adherence is recognized as a major obstacle to effective treatment.

Parents' involvement in children's weight loss programs has been found to be a barometer of their success. Some programs have achieved their best initial weight losses when parents were active participants, especially when the parents were obese and also involved in losing weight. Interestingly, the effectiveness of these parent-child treatments may be greater when the parent and children are worked with separately rather than together.

For older children, there is some evidence suggesting that maintenance of weight loss is most readily achieved when they engage in self-regulation of food intake and exercise, self-reinforcement and self-imposed restrictions in tempting situations. For younger children, treatment may be enhanced by teaching self-control skills and in changing attitudes toward diet and exercise that may undermine self-control, since parents cannot control what children eat all of the time. As children mature, more responsibility for weight loss can be shifted to them.

Collipp, Platon J., ed. *Childhood Obesity*. New York: Warner Books, 1986.

Epstein, Leonard H. "Treatment of Childhood Obesity." In *Handbook of Eating Disorders*, edited by Kelly D. Brownell and John P. Foreyt. New York: Basic Books, 1986.

Epstein, Leonard H., and Squires, Sally. *The Stop-Light Diet for Children.* Boston: Little, Brown, 1988.

Marin, Roselyn. *Helping Obese Children.* Montreal and Holmes Beach, Fla.: Learning Publications, 1990.

Meisels, Samuel J., and Shonkoff, Jack P., ed. *Handbook of Early Childhood Intervention.* Cambridge and New York: Cambridge University Press, 1990.

Rotatori, Anthony F., and Fox, Robert A., comps. *Obesity in Children and Youth: Measurement, Characteristics, Causes, and Treatment.* Springfield, Ill.: C. C. Thomas, 1989.

Chipley, William Stout (1810–1880) Chief medical officer of the Eastern Lunatic Asylum of Kentucky, who published the first American description of SITOMANIA in 1859 in the *American Journal of Insanity.* His observations were based on his clinical experience at the asylum, where a number of young girls who would not eat were finally brought by their desperate families, always after treatment by their family doctors had failed. Chipley's commentary was significant because of his identification of a specific type of food refuser and because it called attention to the behavior of adolescent girls. He strongly believed that their refusal to eat was an intentional attempt to draw attention, elicit sympathy and exert power within a small circle of friends and family.

chlorpromazine A tranquilizing drug used during the 1960s in conjunction with insulin to treat anorexia nervosa. Garfinkel and Garner wrote that it reduced a patient's initial anxiety and resistance to eating and weight gain. It also sometimes sedated the patient enough to help her tolerate bed rest or other enforced reduction of activity. Although this resulted in rapid weight gain, there were a number of serious problems, including lowered blood pressure and reduced body temperature.

In a comparison of two similar groups of hospitalized anorectic patients, one group treated with chlorpromazine and insulin and the other group treated without chlorpromazine, the patients treated with chlorpromazine gained weight substantially faster and left the hospital significantly sooner. After two years, 33 percent of each group required readmission. However, 45 percent of the patients treated with chlorpromazine had developed bulimia, compared with 12 percent of the patients treated without it. Furthermore, the chlorpromazine treatment was associated with significant side effects, including grand mal seizures.

Chlorpromazine was sometimes recommended only for patients who showed marked anxiety about food and an inability to eat after general supportive measures had been attempted. Insulin therapy with chlorpromazine is not used today.

Garfinkel, Paul E., and Garner, David M. *Anorexia Nervosa: A Multidimensional Perspective.* New York: Brunner/Mazel, 1982.

cholecystokinin (CCK) A hormone released from the intestine within five minutes after eating, which stimulates gallbladder contraction and pancreatic secretion. First isolated more than 60 years ago, it is now said also to send a signal from the stomach to the brain when the stomach is full. All mammals have CCK in varying amounts. In a U.S. Agriculture Department study, scientists discovered that they can block the hormone in pigs by injecting them with a vaccine that makes their appetite insatiable, in effect producing bigger pigs. In less than three months, the injected animals consumed an average of 22 more pounds of corn and soybean meal than untreated pigs, while putting on 11 pounds, of mostly meat rather than fat.

Medical researchers and psychiatrists are monitoring the animal experiments to see if the principle could help anorectics. Studies are also under way to develop drugs to block the CCK hormone in the hope of curbing food cravings.

In 1988, Thomas D. Geracioto, Jr., a clinical neuroendocrinologist at the National

Institute of Mental Health, and Rodger A. Liddle of the University of California at San Francisco released results of a study on bulimia in which they compared several measurements of cholecystokinin in both bulimics and control subjects. They found that, on average, the bulimics secreted half as much cholecystokinin as the controls did, indicating that bulimics may not reach a reasonable satiety level. Some scientists speculate that lowered CCK may be an effect of disturbed eating behavior rather than its cause, others that CCK is but one of a group of hormones acting together in complex fashion. CCK can also cause nausea. Studies are now under way on infusing CCK in bulimics and normal volunteers and then exposing them to unlimited food. But results so far are inconclusive.

Since CCK is produced in the intestine and in the brain, scientists are searching to discover which parts of SATIETY are physiological and which are psychological, and how they interconnect. Doctors have discovered that certain ANTIDEPRESSANT drugs, which help bulimics to stop binge eating, also raise their CCK levels.

Chase, Marilyn, "Pigs May Provide Hints for Humans on Not Being Hogs." *Wall Street Journal*, December 8, 1988.

Geracioti, Thomas D., Jr., and Liddle, Rodger A. "Impaired Cholecystokinin Secretion in Bulimia Nervosa." *New England Journal of Medicine* (September 15, 1988) 319: 11.

Moore, Beth O., and Deutsch, J. A. "An Antiemetic Is Antidotal to the Satiety Effects of Cholecystokinin." *Nature*, May 23, 1985.

cholesterol A pearly white crystalline substance that is found in all foods derived from animals. It is an essential building block of our cells, but when present in high levels in the blood, it can lead to atherosclerosis (impeded blood flow due to thickening of the arteries). Cholesterol helps carry fats in the bloodstream to tissues throughout the body. Most cholesterol in the blood is made by the liver from saturated fats (see FATS

SATURATED); some is absorbed directly from cholesterol-rich foods such as egg yolks.

cognitive distortions Illogical, faulty thinking and irrational beliefs. Neuman and Halvorson determined from their studies of medical literature that one of the most critical tasks facing therapists and anorectics is the correction of cognitive distortions, which are numerous in anorectics. These distortions include an inability to perceive their body shapes and sizes accurately and may even affect their understanding of the body's biological functions. ("For instance, anorectics often have strange ideas about what happens to the food they eat, imagining that it goes 'directly' to their thighs, hips, or abdomens.")

A perfectionistic way of thinking is commonly found in anorectics. Burns gives the following patterns for illogical or distorted thought in perfectionists:

• *Dichotomous Thinking* All-or-nothing thinking in which perfectionists evaluate their experiences in a dichotomous manner, seeing things in black-or-white terms. ("If I don't choose a major before school starts, I'll probably end up just being a bum," or "If I gain any weight, I'll be fat.")

• *Overgeneralization* Perfectionists tend to jump dogmatically to the conclusion that a negative event will be repeated endlessly. An anorectic may have a small lapse in her eating and conclude, "I'll never get better, my eating will never improve."

• *"Should" Statements* When perfectionists fall short of a goal, they berate themselves ("I shouldn't have goofed up! I ought to do better! I mustn't do that again!").

Two other reasoning errors were identified by Garner and Bemis as common to victims of anorexia: superstitious thinking and personalization. Superstitious thinking assumes a cause-effect relationship of unrelated events.

This kind of thinking may play a part in the emergence of anorectic behavior, with the anorectic believing that weight loss will solve other problems in her life. Superstitious thinking can also lead to other bizarre behavior rituals. Personalization involves seeing oneself as the focus of other people's attention and taking events and comments personally whether or not they are so intended. ("Two people laughed and whispered something to each other when I walked by. They were probably saying that I looked unattractive. I *have* gained three pounds.")

Burns, D. "The Perfectionist's Script for Self-denial." *Psychology Today*, November 1980.

Neuman, Patricia A., and Halvorson, Patricia A. *Anorexia Nervosa and Bulimia: A Handbook for Counselors and Therapists.* New York: Van Nostrand Reinhold, 1983.

Polivy, Janet; Herman, C. Peter; and Garner, David M. "Cognitive Assessment." In *Assessment of Addictive Behaviors,* edited by Dennis M. Donovan and G. Alan Marlatt. New York: Guilford Press, 1988.

Garner, D. M. and Bemis, K. M. "A Cognitive Behavioral Approach to Anorexia Nervosa," *Cognitive Therapy and Research* (1982) 6: 1.

Cognitive Factors Scale (CFS)

A self-test developed in 1982 by Gormally, Black, Daston and Rardin containing 14 items designed to assess specific dieting problems. The scale measures two factors: Strict Dieting Standards, and Self-Efficacy Expectations to Sustain a Diet. In general, cognitive factors play a crucial role in leading from an isolated slip (just one piece of pie) to a full-blown relapse (an all-out binge).

Sample items from the CFS:

When I start a diet, I say to myself that I will have absolutely no "forbidden foods."

I don't persist very long on diets I set for myself.

Gormally, J.; Black, S.; Daston, S.; and Rardin, D. "The Assessment of Binge Eating Severity among Obese Persons." *Addictive Behaviors* 7 (1982).

cognitive therapy A treatment method for mental disorders founded on the premise that the way we think about the world and ourselves affects our emotions and behavior. Therapists work with patients' thoughts, senses, memories and perceptions, as expressed in their internal monologues about their behavior.

For example, internal monologues about weight reduction can play a critical role in the maintenance and control of obesity. An internal monologue may say, "It's taking me so long to lose the weight." A therapist will counsel the patient to replace that negative thought with the more positive, "But I am losing it. And this time I'm learning how to keep it off." Simple repetition of counterstatements over a period of time helps to change people's views of themselves, even if they do not completely believe them at the outset.

In a British study, a cognitive-behavioral approach was applied to the individual treatment of 11 bulimic women. First the binge-purge cycle was interrupted, and then cognitive strategies were taught for self-control. Next the patients were helped to modify abnormal attitudes toward food, eating and body weight and shape. Normally restricted foods, such as carbohydrates, were gradually introduced into the diet to lessen the desire to binge on these foods. Patients were also helped to identify situations in which loss of control occurred. Finally, patients were prepared for future relapse events. Duration of treatment was seven months. Nine of the 11 patients reduced their binge eating and vomiting from three times daily to less than once a month. Anxiety and depression decreased, as did dysfunctional attitudes concerning shape and weight. At one-year follow-up of six of the patients, one had stopped bingeing and vomiting completely, four reported that these behaviors occurred two to three times a month, and one showed no improvement. Follow-up data were not available for the other five patients. The research team later reported that subsequent experience with more than

50 patients has confirmed that the majority do indeed benefit from the cognitive therapy approach, with most remaining well and requiring no further treatment.

David Garner (see GARFINKEL AND GARNER) has written that because attitude change is an important element in recovery of ANOREXIA NERVOSA, cognitive therapy has promise as a valuable treatment strategy for it.

Fairburn, Christopher. "Binge Eating and Its Management." *British Journal of Psychiatry* 141 (1982).

Garner, David M., "Cognitive Therapy for Anorexia Nervosa." In *Handbook of Eating Disorders,* edited by Kelly D. Brownell and John P. Foreyt. New York: Basic Books, 1986.

Wilson, G. Terence. "Cognitive-Behavioral and Pharmacological Therapies for Bulimia." In *Handbook of Eating Disorders,* edited by Kelly D. Brownell and John P. Foreyt. New York: Basic Books, 1986.

complement factors Immune system proteins believed to play a role in obesity; they are so called because they are necessary to complete certain hemolytic reactions (the removal of hemoglobin from red blood corpuscles). The term derives from the Latin *compere,* "to fill up."

Findings in a 1989 study of mice conducted by a team of researchers from the Harvard Medical School and the University of Alabama confirmed what scientists had suspected for some time: the system that helps an animal defend itself against infarction (death of tissue from lack of blood supply) may influence how it stores and burns energy. These results are helping researchers investigate the causes of obesity in animals and humans.

The researchers reported that families of obese mice had unusually low levels of complement factors. Human and mouse complement factors appear to be very similar, so researchers believe obese people may show similar deficiencies. This was the first time anybody had established the possibility of a connection between complements and energy metabolism.

Most complement factors—humans have 30—are proteins produced and secreted by the liver. Many of these proteins circulate in the blood like roaming security guards and provide an immediate defense against invading bacteria or viruses. Other complements cannot mobilize until the body produces antibodies, the molecules that recognize and bind to foreign bodies.

The first evidence for a link between complements and the metabolic system appeared several years ago when doctors discovered that human fat cells secrete a protein named Complement Factor D.

In humans, Factor D is among those complements that do not need to unite with antibodies before activating. As the bottleneck in the series of reactions that trigger inflammation, Factor D helps regulate the first response to an attack on the immune system.

The research team compared a mouse complement factor, adipsin, with human Factor D. Like the human protein, adipsin is secreted primarily by the mouse fat cells. Earlier research had shown that 60 percent of adipsin's structure is identical to that of Factor D. When they compared the levels of adipsin in normal and obese mice, they found that obese mice had dramatically less circulating adipsin.

Because human Factor D so closely resembles the mouse protein, scientists suspect that people with certain kinds of obesity will also show Factor D deficiency.

Rosen, Barry S; Cook, Kathleen S.; Yaglom, Julia; Groves, Douglas L.; Volanakis, John E.; et al. "Adipsin and Complement Factor D Activity: An Immune-related Defect in Obesity." *Science,* June 23, 1989.

compulsive eating An eating disorder characterized by symptoms similar to those of bulimia nervosa, but without the purging. Much of the compulsive eater's life is centered on food, what she (most are women) can or cannot eat, what she will or will not eat, what she has or has not eaten and when she will or will not eat next. Typically, she eats continuously from morning until night, much of the time in secret. Her obsession with food is coupled with self-disgust, loathing and shame because of her total lack of self-control around food. Frequently a compulsive eater thinks that if she does not have access to food, she will be all right, and she will therefore keep her home almost bare of food, except for the "health food" variety. But her compulsion will drive her out even in the night to look for food to satisfy her uncontrollable urges. Typically, she will continue to eat long after she is full. She eats not because she's hungry or even because she enjoys it but to satisfy an unacknowledged psychological need.

Not all compulsive eaters are obese; some control their weight by constant EXERCISE, FASTING for a few days at a time or even dieting. There are compulsive eaters at all levels of society, from shop floor to executive suite.

Because many compulsive eaters do have weight problems, they run a high risk of hypertension, heart disease and diabetes. And they usually ingest high levels of fat, cholesterol and sugar, which increase their risk of heart disease, cancer and iron-deficiency anemia.

So-called cures, ranging from hypnosis to hospitalization, do not help many compulsive eaters. Most helpful thus far have been clinics, both inpatient and outpatient, that address both physical and psychological aspects of the problem. Such treatment centers work on the premise that compulsive eating is an addiction similar to drug or alcohol addictions.

Unlike anorexia or bulimia, compulsive overeating generally has a more gradual beginning, according to Siegel, Brisman and Weinshel. They explain that it often starts in early childhood when eating patterns are being formed. Sometimes a family focuses on food as a retreat from feelings, as a way to feel good or as an activity to fill otherwise empty time. Eating patterns that do not cause problems for growing children can cause them in adulthood. When compulsive overeating starts in young adulthood, it is often at times of stress when young people are ill prepared to handle certain kinds of frustration and emotion. Soon they begin to use food inappropriately (often against their better judgment) and eventually become addicted to it, losing control over the amounts of food they eat. HILDE BRUCH says that compulsive eaters often eat more when they feel worried or tense, and they feel less effective and competent when they try to control their food intake; she referred to their compulsion as a "neurotic need for food."

Bruch, Hilde. *Eating Disorders.* New York: Basic Books, 1973.

Hirschmann, Jane R., and Munter, Carol H. *Overcoming Overeating.* Reading, Mass.: Addison-Wesley, 1988.

Koontz, Katy. "Women Who Love Food Too Much." *Health,* February 1988.

Siegel, Michele; Brisman, Judith; and Weinshell, Margot. *Surviving an Eating Disorder.* New York: Harper & Row, 1988.

compulsive eating scale (CES)   A self-test designed by Dunn and Ondercin to assess emotional states related to eating and specific aspects of binge behavior. The CES includes 32 items and provides data related to degree of compulsive eating. In addition, it assesses general information about the frequency of binges, alternations of BINGE EATING with FASTING and DIETING, and emotional reactions following a binge episode.

Sample items from the CES:

I eat when I'm not hungry.

My weight varies and I am usually gaining or losing weight.

Dunn, P. K., and Ondercin, P. "Personality Variables Related to Compulsive Eating in College Women." *Journal of Clinical Psychology* 37 (1981).

control group A group used as a basis of comparison with an experimental group. In a study of the effectiveness of a drug, the experimental group would take the drug, and the control group would take either nothing or a PLACEBO.

See also DOUBLE-BLIND STUDY.

cortisol An adrenal cortical hormone released in response to stress. It is usually referred to pharmaceutically as hydrocortisone.

A good deal of study has been devoted to cortisol levels, particularly as they relate to depression. Recently, scientists have been able to show that the excess of cortisol in both depressed and anorectic people is due to a problem that occurs in a region of the brain near or in the hypothalamus. The hypothalamus regulates many bodily functions—hormonal secretions, temperature, water balance and sugar and fat metabolism; thus, it is certain that there is a link between abnormality in the hypothalamus and the problems associated with eating disorders. Questions remain about cause and effect. Some scientists believe that prolonged stress causes the neurotransmitter/hormone imbalances, which then "drive" the eating disorder.

cosmetic surgery A surgical procedure, usually plastic surgery, performed for the sake of a patient's appearance is called cosmetic surgery. It may be intended to enhance a patient's looks or disguise the effects of aging or to repair damage resulting from accident or injury, such as disfiguring scars or burns.

Dr. Ivo Pitangy described a procedure for removing fat from the outer thighs in 1970. Surgical reconstruction of the inner thigh was developed in 1973, and the "tummy tuck" operation (see ABDOMINOPLASTY) for removing excess skin and fat from the abdomen has been a popular procedure since the 1960s.

Negative aspects of these procedures that involve removal of fat and overlying skin are large scars, prolonged healing periods, hospitalization and occasional necessity for blood transfusion. However, fat does not appear to reaccumulate in the treated areas; rather, those patients who gain weight following surgery (because of failure to follow nutrition and exercise programs) tend to deposit fat more evenly throughout their bodies than before. These observations, made during the early days of cosmetic surgery, provided evidence that "permanent" surgical removal of localized fat deposits was possible and encouraged research.

In the mid-1970s, several European surgeons devised methods for removing localized fat deposits via small incisions. Unfortunately, these techniques were complicated by problems similar to those associated with other available body sculpturing techniques—bleeding, prolonged wound drainage and unsatisfactory healing. Such complications led to experimentation with other forms of cosmetic surgery. Giorgio Fischer, a surgeon in Italy, devised an instrument to remove fat by suction and became the first surgeon to perform LIPOSUCTION surgery.

Most of the more than three million Americans who undergo cosmetic surgery each year are satisfied with the results, but many are mutilated. Most of the blame for this unsuccessful surgery is placed on unscrupulous and unskilled practitioners who often operate in offices with inadequate emergency equipment or with inexperienced anesthetists. Doctors' credentials can be checked with the American Society of Plastic and Reconstructive Surgeons or the American Board of Medical Specialties.

Cosmetic surgeons argue that "vanity" surgery can be as important to psychological health as other surgery is to physical health, and they see little difference between removing fat in an hour on an operating table and doing it over three months in a gym. However, cosmetic surgery is a $3.5 billion-a-year industry, and ethical questions have been raised about the amount of money and medical resources devoted to cosmetic surgery not necessary for health or reconstruction following injury.

Anyone who does decide to have this type of procedure should deal only with certified doctors who are candid about the numbers of procedures they've performed, who will give out names of patients you can talk to, who detail risks and complications, who are on the staffs of major hospitals and have privileges to perform the prospective surgery at those hospitals, who do not advertise that the procedure is always safe or easy and who take thorough medical histories and do thorough preoperative physical exams.

"Cosmetic Surgery: The Price of Beauty." *Economist*, January 11, 1992.

Karlsberg, Elizabeth. "Cosmetic Surgery Update." *Teen*, January 1991.

McCurdy, John A., Jr. *Sculpturing Your Body: Diet, Exercise and Lipo (Fat) Suction.* Hollywood, Fla.: Frederick Fell Publishers, 1987.

Robinson, Donald. "The Truth about Cosmetic Surgery." *Reader's Digest*, February 1991.

"Unmasked: The Very Honest Plastic-Surgery Report." *Mademoiselle*, June 1991.

Council on Size and Weight Discrimination, Inc.

An organization formed in 1991 to influence public policy and opinion in order to fight discrimination based on body weight, size or shape. It is a nonprofit project-oriented advocacy group with a board of directors rather than a membership organization. It depends on contributions and grants to support its efforts. Future projects are said to include negotiations with architects' groups over the standard size of theater seats, testimony before regulatory agencies dealing with diet fraud and discussions with writers and editors of medical textbooks on what the next generation of doctors will be taught concerning weight and dieting.

couples therapy

Psychological therapy involving both a patient and another person with whom the patient has a uniquely close relationship; those involved may be a patient's parent or his or her spouse or life partner. Couples therapy is used in a variety of settings and is recommended for treating eating disorders when there is significant conflict in a couple's relationship. The conflict may be caused by the personalities involved, the eating disorder itself or a combination. The purpose of couples therapy is to strengthen the relationship and to assist couples in problem solving and successfully resolving conflict.

Root, Maria; Fallon, Patricia; and Friedrich, William. *Bulimia: A Systems Approach to Treatment.* New York: W. W. Norton, 1986.

craving

A frequent compulsive and uncontrollable desire to consume a particular food, such as chocolate, or foods from a specific group, such as starches. Consumption of this food gives both a physical and psychological sense of well-being and satisfaction. Research on both animals and humans has demonstrated that cravings can be caused by biochemical needs. A food craving may be the body's signal that something is out of balance. Although eating foods one craves makes one feel better for the moment, the resulting "high" eventually is followed by fatigue, depression, headaches, moodiness, unclear or confused thinking and the weight problems that frequently accompany the abuse of any food. Cravings have sometimes been found to be caused by nutritional deficiencies, food allergies or diseases.

Recent studies have shown that overweight people tend to crave fatty foods; the fatter people are, the more they prefer the taste of fat. In studies, when given a choice of milk shakes made with varying amounts of cream and sugar, overweight people have chosen fattier shakes than their lean counterparts. Overweight people report eating no more calories than others, but more of those calories come from fat.

The effect of fatty foods on the brain—and the way people think about fats—undermine Americans' attempts to stay trim, according to one school of thought. When the brain gets used to the sudden rush of fat/sugar mixtures, a physical craving develops similar to opiate drug addiction, according to research conducted at the University of Michigan. New research indicates that a drug for opiate overdoses can also block craving for such foods as cookies and candy, but it is not a practical or proven treatment.

Writing for *Scientific American* (January 1989), two researchers from the Massachusetts Institute of Technology, R. J. Wurtman and J. J. Wurtman, classified carbohydrate craving obesity as a distinct behavioral disorder. They named as symptoms depression, lethargy and an inability to concentrate, combined with episodic bouts of overeating and excessive weight gain. They also found these cravings to be cyclic, occurring usually in the late afternoons or evenings. They say it appears that this disorder is affected by biochemical disturbances in the neurotransmitter serotonin, which regulates appetite for carbohydrate-rich foods.

Hunt, Douglas. *No More Cravings*. New York: Warner Books, 1987.

creeping obesity   A term used by some researchers to describe the gradual but frequent weight gain affecting people in middle age. According to proponents of the theory that creeping obesity is a specific form of obesity, the average American gains one-half to one pound per year between the ages of 20 and 60. One of the major causes of this creeping obesity, they say, is the lack of physical activity. They support their argument by noting that it affects many residents of industrialized nations.

On the other side of the debate, HILDE BRUCH writes,

In my own experience with this age group there has not been one instance in which obesity had developed in this gradual way. When-

ever a detailed history was taken, weight increases were found to be related to certain events or changes in life patterns. This weight then became stable until some new event precipitated a new increase, such as incapacitating illness, surgery, or states of emotional disatisfaction. The increase at any one time may not have been large, usually in the five to ten pound range. But these episodic increases added up to "overweight."

Crisp, Arthur H.   The leading British researcher and specialist in the field of eating disorders. Chairman of the Department of Mental Health Sciences at St. George's Hospital Medical School, University of London, Crisp is the author of an influential work on anorexia nervosa, *Anorexia Nervosa: Let Me Be* (London: Academic Press, 1982; New York: Grune & Stratton, 1980).

crystal methamphetamine   An illegal appetite-suppressing amphetamine. (See ICE.)

cultural influences on appearance Attitudes toward physical appearance and standards of beauty and desirability have varied over time and from culture to culture. In prerevolutionary China, for example, tiny feet represented the ideal for women of the upper classes, leading to widespread deformities caused by the practice of foot binding. In Greek and Roman representations of the ideal in the form of sculpted gods and goddesses, women often have ample thighs, hips and waists. During the Renaissance, full-bodied women were also the ideal. Plumpness was admired; in some cultures it was an appealing sexual characteristic. But in the 19th century, corsets were invented to enable women to achieve the then-ideal hourglass appearance. It became rude, among the genteel, to eat heartily. It was even glamorous, in some quarters, to look sickly. Because tuberculosis was thought especially to afflict artists and other creative people, a tubercular appearance came to signify a romantic personality. Men preferred delicate, pale women, and women used whitening powders rather than rouge.

In Western society during the 20th century's early years, a buxom appearance was preferred. Then the "flat-chested" flappers became the ideal in the 1920s. Bustiness and the hourglass figure returned in the 1950s. This was followed once again by the still-current ideal of thinness. Researchers have documented recent shifts in our cultural image of women by using data from *Playboy* magazine centerfolds and statistics from Miss America Pageant contestants. The average weight of centerfold models in 1960 was approximately 90 percent of expected average weight, based on the Society of Actuaries 1959 norm; in 1978, it was approximately 83 percent. This decline occurred even while the expected averages of weight and height for young women were increasing. Today a thin look denotes self-control and success; the desire to conform to this slim physical model is one of the social variables that may lead to anorexia.

The culturally generated compulsion to be thin is also reflected in the proliferation of articles about dieting in magazines published principally for women. Fear of being fat, fear of losing control over eating and fear of not being as slim as possible are important social concerns. As far back as 1966, studies found that 70 percent of high school girls were unhappy with their bodies and wanted to lose weight. Particularly for women, thinness has become synonymous with attractiveness.

Studies examining changing standards of attractiveness for men and women portrayed in 20th-century media have indicated that female television characters are more likely to be slim and less likely to be fat than male characters; that women receive more messages through magazine articles and advertisements to be slim and stay in shape than do men; that the prominence of curvaceous females portrayed in popular women's magazines has decreased dramatically since 1901; and that the standard of bodily attractiveness

of movie actresses has become significantly thinner during the past 50 years.

Not all researchers believe that "ideal" appearances have changed in Western culture. Hillel Schwartz, author of *Never Satisfied: A Cultural History of Diets, Fantasies, and Fat,* says that the image of beauty in the United States has *not* changed much over the years. He claims that for men and women alike the ideal woman has long been thin, with a long, thin neck, long arms, thin wrists, a very thin waist and thin ankles. These proportions have also been desirable for young men. (It was only around 1850 that a plump, full-faced look became the ideal for children. Before then, the image of a healthy young child was thin as well.)

Not only slim proportions were considered beautiful for women; as the popular 1890s image of the Gibson girls shows, it was also considered desirable for them to be assertive and athletic, too. This led to the belief that even as people age, they must retain their youthfulness and remain thin, although the body does not naturally keep these proportions. This belief, Schwartz asserts, rather than health or fashion, is at the root of our dieting problems.

Pervasive cultural images linking slenderness with beauty and health have convinced many normal-weight young children into believing that they are overweight. Some start dieting before they are out of elementary school. A Canadian study found that between the ages of five and seven, children begin to apply adult standards of attractiveness to themselves and to one another—and to view fat negatively. By that age they start relating to fat people differently, and the difference is markedly more significant with girls than with boys. They see images equating slenderness with health and beauty, thin adult models in magazines and on television, and they perceive themselves to be fat because they have plump little faces and hands.

Collins reported that most people who worry about their weight are women, and the current standard of beauty is so thin that, almost without exception, they consider themselves "overweight." Clinicians have remarked that the weight problems of most women "would be defined out of existence if a health criterion were used to define obesity" rather than cultural beliefs.

It has also been observed that wherever and whenever food is scarce or not sufficient for all, obesity becomes a symbol of success and is viewed with admiration; where and when food is plentiful, thinness becomes the goal and dieting commonplace. (See CULTURAL INFLUENCES ON EATING DISORDERS.)

Brumberg, Joan Jacobs. *Fasting Girls.* Cambridge: Harvard University Press, 1988.

Collins, M. Elizabeth. "Education for Healthy Body Weight: Helping Adolescents Balance the Cultural Pressure for Thinness." *Journal of School Health* (August 1988) 58:6.

Mazur, A. "U.S. Trends in Feminine Beauty and Overadaptation." *Journal of Sexual Research* 22 (1986).

Schwartz, Hillel. *Never Satisfied: A Cultural History of Diets, Fantasies, and Fat.* New York: Free Press, 1986.

cultural influences on eating disorders

People with eating disorders have come mostly from white middle- or upper-class families, leading researchers to determine that higher socioeconomic status is an important risk factor. International studies offer further evidence to support this notion: eating disorders have increased dramatically in industrialized nations during the last 20 years, while remaining practically unheard of in the Third World countries. "Thinness" is not an ideal among people whose hunger is not a matter of choice. Concern over the shape of one's body is an indulgence of the affluent.

The shift toward a thinner ideal body shape in Western societies has been marked by the increasingly pervasive practice of dieting, especially among women. An estimated 90 percent of the customers of the "diet" industry are women. Though the benefits of slenderness have been extolled by health professionals, the potentially

harmful side effects of dieting have received considerably less attention. Several researchers have connected the cultural pursuit of thinness with eating disorders:

- Data presented by Polivy and Herman indicate that dieting usually precedes binge eating; thus they speculate that dieting is the disorder in need of cure.
- Similarly, Garner (see GARFINKEL AND GARNER) states that bulimia may become a problem in psychologically normal individuals after a period of intensive caloric restriction.
- Katz identifies weight loss by itself as a precipitate for the appearance of anorexia nervosa in vulnerable individuals.
- Mazur identifies anorexia nervosa and bulimia, as well as extreme diet and exercise regimens among "normal" women, as examples of often dangerous attempts to match the ever-changing ideal of feminine beauty.

In addition, Japanese researchers have reported that during the past 20 years, a slim body has become increasingly desirable for young women as a sign of beauty and success in Japan; dieting is now common among them. Research suggests that this dieting is a factor contributing to bulimia among young women in Japan.

While Garner and his team reiterated that cultural influences do not cause eating disorders and that culture is mediated by the psychology of the individual as well as the social context of the family, M. Elizabeth Collins cautioned in *Journal of School Health* that the potential impact of the media in establishing identifiable role models should not be underestimated.

Collins, M. Elizabeth. "Education for Healthy Body Weight: Helping Adolescents Balance the Cultural Pressure for Thinness." *Journal of School Health* (August 1988) 58:6.

Feldman, W.; Feldman, E.; and Goodman, J. Y. "Culture versus Biology: Children's Attitudes toward Thinness and Fatness." *Pediatrics* (February 1988) 81.

Garner, D. M.; Rockert, W.; Olmsted, M. P.; et al. "Psychoeducational Principles in the Treatment of Bulimia and Anorexia." In *Handbook of Psychotherapy for Anorexia Nervosa and Bulimia*. New York: Guilford Press, 1985.

Katz, J. L. "Some Reflections on the Nature of the Eating Disorders: On the Need for Humility." *International Journal of Eating Disorders* 4 (1985).

Mazur, A. "U.S. Trends in Feminine Beauty and Overadaptation." *Journal of Sexual Research* 22 (1986).

Polivy, J., and Herman, C. P. "Dieting and Binging: A Causal Analysis." *American Psychology* 40 (1985).

Cushing's disease

A disease caused by overactivity of the pituitary gland, which influences growth, metabolism and other glands. The disease is characterized by a form of obesity and muscular weakness. It is much more common in women than in men. Obesity is confined almost exclusively to the trunk; any obesity involving the upper arms and the upper thighs is disproportionately small. Patients with Cushing's disease frequently have hypertension and are more susceptible to infection. There may be minor hirsutism in women, particularly on the upper lip and chin, and some in the periareolar region of the breast. Increased hair growth also often occurs over the lower abdomen, extending up from the pubic region.

cyproheptadine

An appetite-stimulating antihistamine used primarily for the treatment of allergic conditions.

An early study in Peru found that cyproheptadine caused anorectics to gain significant weight, but two subsequent studies in the United States failed to replicate this result. In one, there was a differential drug effect related to the presence of bulimia, so that cyproheptadine significantly increased treatment efficiency in the nonbulimic patients and impaired treatment efficiency in the bulimic patients.

There are indications that cyproheptadine in relatively large doses may have some mild effect in promoting weight gain and relieving depression in anorexia nervosa. One major advantage of cyproheptadine is that it appears to have few side effects even in relatively large doses.

D

dental caries (or cavities)

Tooth decay; the progressive destruction of the hard tissues of the teeth through a process initiated by bacterially produced acids at the tooth surface. Dental caries are seen extensively in patients with eating disorders. This is due to an excessive CARBOHYDRATE intake, poor oral hygiene and changes that occur in the saliva.

During binge periods (see BINGE EATING), huge amounts of sugar can be consumed, followed by sugar drinks, often used to relieve thirst after vomiting. Thus, bulimics tend to have higher sugar intake than anorectics, whose diet is limited. But anorectics under the care of physicians also are susceptible to dental caries, because some medications given to them, such as dextrose tablets, dietary supplements, and vitamin C drinks, contain sugar.

Neglect of oral hygiene can be seen in both anorectic and bulimic patients, due mainly to the upset in daily routine. Their eating habits get most of their attention. Meticulous oral hygiene is a necessity in these patients, because of excess acid present in the oral cavity, excess sugar intake and disturbances in the saliva.

Anorectics have been found to have decreased salivary pH and decreased buffering action, with the low pH contributing to the occurrence of dental caries. Patients with anorexia typically have decreased salivary flow as well. Fear and DEPRESSION decrease salivary flow and affect its composition, thus potentially contributing to the formation of caries. Often this decreased flow of saliva is multiplied by the misuse of laxatives and diuretics (see DIURETIC ABUSE, LAXATIVE ABUSE) or by ANTIDEPRESSANT drugs. These drugs decrease total fluid volumes and affect electrolyte balance, causing an even further diminished salivary flow. Anorectic patients, with virtually no natural defense against caries, have monumental decay problems.

Bulimics and anorectics who vomit repeatedly (see VOMITING) to purge themselves of consumed food risk erosion of the enamel of their teeth, particularly on the inner surfaces, from hydrochloric acid in the vomit. This erosion may result in severe gum disease, cavities and tooth loss. The dentist may be the first to encounter actual indications of bulimia. The dental manifestations—although not life threatening and not evident until the later stages of illness—are effects of eating disorders that cannot be reversed.

Dalin, Jeffrey B. D.D.S. "Oral Manifestations of Eating Disorders." In *Eating Disorders: Effective Care and Treatment*. St. Louis: Ishiyaku EuroAmerica, 1986.

depression A mental state characterized by dejection, lack of hope and a general loss of interest in life. It is distinguished from grief, which is a response to a real loss and generally proportionate to its importance. Symptoms vary with the severity of the illness. With mild depression, the main symptoms are anxiety, mood changes and sometimes inexplicable crying spells. Serious depression is usually accompanied by appetite and sleep disturbances, social withdrawal, increasingly poor performance in school, at home or at work, lack of energy and loss of concentration. Severely depressed persons may wish for death or even consider SUICIDE, exhibit phobias and dwell on thoughts of guilt or worthlessness.

In bulimics, depression may be obvious, evidenced by apathy, lethargy, joylessness, suicidal thoughts, sleep disturbances and general lack of pleasure in life. The severity

of depressive symptoms in bulimics is similar to that of patients with MAJOR AFFECTIVE DISORDER.

The relationship between depression and eating disorders has been under considerable study. Many people with eating disorders also appear to suffer from depression, and scientists have wondered whether depression could trigger an eating disorder. There are similarities in neurochemical abnormalities in both disorders. Low levels of SEROTONIN and norepinephrine are associated with depressive disorders as well as eating disorders, and ANTIDEPRESSANT medications may help some people with eating disorders, particularly bulimics. In addition, both the depressed and anorectic tend to have higher than normal levels of the hormone CORTISOL, which is released in response to stress. Depression is commonly seen in patients with bulimia; it is unclear, however, whether the depression leads to bulimia or vice versa.

Researchers have concluded that there is not enough support to prove a relationship between bulimia and depression. To date, they feel, properly designed tests and family history investigations have failed to find differences between bulimic and control samples. But it is generally agreed that it is possible that bulimic patients with family histories of depression are at greater risk of developing depression than bulimics without such a history.

HILDE BRUCH stated that people who use food to combat anxiety and loneliness are likely to become depressed when dieting is enforced. "Even without marked obesity, the secure knowledge that one's appetite and needs will be fulfilled is necessary for a sense of well-being. Mildly depressed patients are often concerned with the loss of satisfaction from ordinary activities. They often complain of having lost all interest, or of finding activities no longer worthwhile. The immediate enjoyment of food serves as reassurance that life still holds some satisfactions. People with this depressive mood are apt to eat between meals, often quite impulsively, as soon as the idea strikes them that something might be tasty or enjoyable.''

One study of 5,600 high school students found that 500 of them suffered from depression, with girls more likely to be depressed than boys. Researchers have concluded that an important factor in adolescent depression is poor body image. In another study of 850 young women, aged 12 to 23, more than two-thirds were unhappy with their weight and more than half with their shape.

"Great Bodies Come in Many Shapes." *University of California, Berkeley Wellness Letter* 7:5, February 1991.

diabetes and eating disorders   People who combine disordered eating with diabetes face significantly more health risks than non-diabetics with similar eating patterns in the general population.

Some studies have identified a higher incidence of eating disorders among diabetics. For example, a British study reported in 1987 that of 208 young women with insulin-dependent diabetes, 15 (7 percent) had a clinically apparent eating disorder, a rate much higher than that reported in nondiabetic women. However, in a survey conducted at the International Diabetes Center, of the 70 percent (385) of 550 females aged 13 to 45 who returned their surveys, the number of individuals who met criteria for a clinical eating disorder was found to be similar to the number obtained in the general population.

But the diabetic's necessary focus on food, his deprivation of certain foods, his guilt over nonadherence to his diet, his unhealthy relationship with food and his rebelliousness toward dietary restrictions can all provoke a disordered eating pattern. The starvation of anorexia nervosa and the purging of bulimia can both lead to serious hypoglycemia (deficiency of sugar in the blood). And binge eating can lead to seriously elevated blood glucose levels and diabetic ketoacidosis.

Birk, Randi. "Eating Disorders and Diabetes." *Diabetes Self-Management*, September/October 1988.

dichotomous reasoning   A faulty thinking pattern that occurs in anorexia nervosa. Dichotomous reasoning involves thinking in extreme, absolute, all-or-none terms and is typically applied to food, eating and weight. The patient divides food into good (low calorie) and bad (fattening) categories. A one-pound weight gain may be equated with incipient obesity. Breaking a rigid eating routine produces panic because it means a complete loss of control. Rigid attitudes and behaviors are not restricted to food and weight but extend to the pursuit of sports, studies and careers.

diet centers and programs   The frustration of continuously striving to achieve the elusive "ideal" weight is a prime motivator for the overweight to turn to other "sufferers," seeking help, understanding, empathy. And when those other sufferers number about 65 million people, according to the National Center for Health Statistics, it is small wonder that an entire industry of diet centers, clubs and programs bringing these obsessive dieters together has flourished. Some, like TOPS (Take Off Pounds Sensibly) and Overeaters Anonymous, are nonprofit organizations; others, like Weight Watchers, Diet Workshop, Diet Center and Slimming Magazine Clubs, are commercial enterprises. Diet centers provide dietary advice and social support and are especially helpful for those people who find that the only way to lose weight is to have others pushing and pulling them along toward their goals. Diet centers provide psychological motivation and "good examples" of others who have succeeded, as well as supervised diet programs with step-by-step daily routines, exercises, menus, weigh-ins and so on. One analysis of such diet centers found that short-term outcomes are at least equivalent to medically prescribed therapies. The average length of membership is about 26 weeks and the mean weight loss about 20 pounds. Little is known about long-term results. The reducing diet, group pressures, BEHAVIOR MODIFICATION techniques, a supportive group, and financial commitments all play a part in accounting for their success.

Scientific interest in dieting for obesity began in the mid-1800s with the Harvey-Banting diet (see BANTING, WILLIAM). The novel aspect of Harvey's diet was the emphasis on meat, the "strong food," which had just been recognized as being less fattening than the "innocent" foodstuffs, such as breads and sweets. Proteins were considered necessary for restoration of body substances, carbohydrates for the acute combustion process.

With Harvey's diet program achieving popular success, other metabolism experts quickly developed their own diets. In additon to the Harvey-Banting "high-protein" diet, Ebstein's method (high fat content) and the Dancel-Oertel cure (fluid restriction and systematic exercise) also proved popular during the 1880s.

But there were difficulties with all three programs, with unsuccessful cases being attributed to their "mechanical" application; presumably more flexibility would have led to success. Despite better understanding of metabolic processes, most of the same problems remain unsolved by today's programs.

HILDE BRUCH wrote that

> every "new" diet program uses the hook of offering nutrient essentials in an unexpected, interesting, and convenient combination so that weight conscious people become curious, follow it for a week or two, and proudly proclaim its effectiveness. An important factor in the diet game is publicity and packaging; scientifically designed diets are taken over by commercial enterprises and advertising, and then become highly successful.

She used as examples a fluid low-protein diet designed for in-hospital metabolic stud-

ies, which became the "Metrecal" diet; and a high-protein diet prescribed for years by the New York City Health Department in its obesity clinic, a diet that became the basis of a multimillion-dollar business called WEIGHT WATCHERS.

In very recent years, the use of celebrities to endorse diet products has helped revolutionize the promotion of weight reduction programs. Elliott Gould, Ed Koch, Susan St. James, Lynn Redgrave and Tommy Lasorda are a few celebrities who have earned as much as $100,000 to $300,000 a year touting diet products and programs. Their endorsements have boosted diet company sales by up to 100 percent; the powdered-diet portion of the industry alone has reached the billion-dollar mark in annual sales.

A January 1990 *New York Times* article quoted a survey conducted for the Calorie Control Council in Atlanta, a trade group in the diet-food industry, as having found a 26 percent drop over the previous three years in the number of people who said that they were dieting. However, the article also said that despite "numerous studies" showing that "the vast majority of people regain weight after dieting, the market for diet products and programs is still booming." Many diet groups are now marketing themselves using new terms such as "nutritional programs."

In the May/June 1989 issue of the *Walking Magazine*, author Madeline Chinnici described common-sense criteria for acceptable commercial diets: 1,000 or more calories per day; at least 50 percent carbohydrate, less than 30 percent fat, and 15 to 20 percent protein; a variety of foods from the four basic food groups; promotion of a weight loss of not more than one to two pounds per week; promotion of permanent loss of fat, especially combined with regular exercise; no vitamin supplementation and no specialized medical supervision, for otherwise healthy people; no side effects in healthy people.

See also FAD DIETS.

diet pills Commonly available over-the-counter diet pills contain the active appetite suppressor phenylpropanolamine (PPA) and are usually packaged and sold with a recommended daily dosage of 75 mg. Brand names include Acutrim, Control, Dexatrim, Dietac, Prolamine and Odrinex.

Although diet pills are commonly used by patients with ANOREXIA NERVOSA and BULIMIA, many bulimics experiment with diet pills but do not take them on an ongoing basis because of their side effects or because they find their use relatively ineffective as a weight-control technique.

These drugs have been shown to facilitate weight loss on a short-term basis in individuals with OBESITY. Studies suggest that diet pills are relatively safe, but habit-forming. There have also been reports of side effects and toxicities for these drugs, including elevated blood pressure, renal failure, seizures, anxiety and agitation, memory loss, transient neurological deficits and intracranial hemorrhage. For some allergic or hypersensitive individuals, the pills are dangerous even when taken according to directions.

In 1990 the Food and Drug Administration ruled that a diet pill known as Cal-Ban 3000 was potentially lethal and recommended that anyone using it stop immediately. The FDA recalled the product and blocked its sale after a man died when Cal-Ban tablets swelled in his throat. At least 50 other users experienced obstructions in the stomach, intestines and other parts of the digestive tract after taking the product. Cal-Ban 3000 diet tablets were advertised as creating a sense of fullness when they swell in the stomach. Their primary ingredient was guar gum, a dietary fiber that absorbs five to 10 times its weight in water. However, in some instances, the tablets began to swell in the digestive tract before reaching the stomach, causing injury. Under normal use, in small doses, as a laxative or food thickener, guar gum is harmless; but the suggested dosage with the Cal-Ban 3000 program was 15 grams a day, or about 30 tablets with each meal.

Manufacturers claim that pills made from the amino acids arginine and ornithine stimulate human growth hormone, causing the user to "burn fat" overnight. No data has been submitted to the Food and Drug Administration to support this claim. Some very preliminary studies show that these amino acids may be able to stimulate human growth hormone, but whether this causes a person to lose weight is not known. If these pills did what the manufacturers claim, they would be dangerous, because in the process they would also stimulate other hormones, altering insulin levels and carbohydrate metabolism, among other things.

In early 1990, researchers at Louisiana State University announced a pill that they say can cause weight loss without exercise and dieting. Its active ingredient is bromocryptine, which works by preventing the secretion of prolactin. This hormone is associated with the body's use of insulin and production of fat. Researchers studied 33 patients who, after receiving doses of bromocryptine, lost approximately 25 percent of their fat within six weeks without exercising or dieting. They said the timing of the dose is crucial, however, and it may be difficult to determine the correct time in humans.

Albert Meier, professor of zoology at LSU, initiated the study after 25 years of research on animals' body rhythm biology during migration and hibernation. What he attempted to translate to humans was the finding that many animals reduce or increase their body fat without altering food intake or activity levels. The procedure is now undergoing clinical trials before application to the Food and Drug Administration for approval.

A 1990 congressional inquiry focused attention on the role diet pills play in eating disorders. It was brought out that many otherwise healthy teenagers think of pills as the standard way to diet. In a survey conducted by *Sassy* magazine, 49 percent of teenage girls responding reported using diet pills. A 1988 study by the National Institute of Drug

Abuse revealed that 22 percent of high school seniors, boys and girls, currently use diet pills. Young people have no trouble buying diet pills, which are available throughout the country with no age restrictions.

See also FAD DIETS.

"Better Dieting through Chemistry?" *U.S. News & World Report*, Feb. 3, 1992.
"Diet Drug Ingredients Facing Ban by FDA." *Chemical Marketing Reporter*, Nov. 5, 1990.
"FDA Bans 111 Diet Drug Ingredients." *Los Angeles Times*, August 8, 1991.
"FDA Wants Diet Pill Taken off Market." *Los Angeles Times*, July 28, 1990.
Gillam, Jerry. "Bill to Limit Diet Pill Sales Moves Ahead." *Los Angeles Times*, May 3, 1991.

dietary chaos syndrome A term used by British researcher R. L. Palmer to describe bulimia.

dietary fiber The edible but indigestible fibrous components of plants. Fiber adds bulk to the diet and can aid normal bowel function by enabling the large intestine to work effectively and by helping regulate the absorption of nutrients in the small intestine. Dietary fiber is not a single substance, and there are significant differences in the physiological effects of the various fibers. A Recommended Dietary Allowance has not been established; however, an adequate amount can be obtained by eating several servings daily of whole-grain breads and cereals, fruits, root vegetables, legumes and nuts.

A report of the Council on Scientific Affairs of the American Medical Association stated that some scientists believe that excessive energy (caloric) intake may be inevitable when diets are low in fiber, with high-fiber diets possibly reducing energy intake, even when more food is eaten. Studies suggest that when people are allowed to eat unlimited amounts of high-fiber food, but not foods containing sugar and other refined carbohydrates, the amount eaten decreases

significantly, and appetites are satisfied. Although fiber has no magical effects in promoting weight loss, it can be an important part of a balanced but low-calorie diet. High-fiber diets are also beneficial because they help prevent constipation, a common result of reduced food intake. Limited data from clinical trials that suggest that fiber supplements or high-fiber diets are useful for weight reduction are contradictory. Dietary fiber may have a limited role as an adjunct in the treatment of obesity, but controlled, long-term trials are needed before this can be established.

dieting A word used to denote the restriction of food intake. Counting CALORIES and restricting food intake has become an obsession with Americans. DIET CENTERS AND PROGRAMS, "slimnastics" classes, weight reduction support groups and "figure salons" can be found in most neighborhoods. In fact, dieting has been called the fastest-growing industry in the United States. It is estimated that more than 20 million Americans are seriously dieting at any given moment, spending $25 billion to $33 billion a year in the process.

And dieting is no longer practiced only by adults. A study of fourth grade girls in California found that 80 percent said they were dieting. The practice of young girls' dieting to get from a size 8 to a size 7 can establish patterns of deprivation, BINGE EATING and weight gain that will haunt them all their lives. The director of one hospital eating-disorders unit estimates that more than 50 percent of the patients there—mostly women in their late teens and early twenties—began dieting before they were teenagers. A survey in London revealed that girls as young as 12 felt too fat, attempted to restrict food intake and expressed guilt about eating. Even nonobese girls of five and six express concern about their body image and fear gaining weight. In extreme cases, children's attempts at dieting can actually stunt their growth: if they occur just before the main growth spurt of early adolescence, they can jeopardize the increase in height that would automatically rectify an obesity problem. Zinc deficiencies and anemia also can result from improper dieting.

One unconfirmed, and possibly unconfirmable, hypothesis is that dieting may begin accidentally during infancy, when dieting mothers unintentionally put their infants on and off diets by attempting to limit the children's food intake when they themselves are not dieting and by becoming more lenient when they are dieting. This theory derives from a single study in which mothers who reported the strongest inclination to diet were most likely to interpret tape-recorded episodes of a baby's crying as a reflection of hunger. The same study showed that fat mothers preferred thinner babies and planned to make more efforts to prevent obesity by limiting intake than thin mothers.

Remedies for obesity have always been a part of American culture. But while there are fad diets, in the United States dieting itself is not a fad; rather, it is a culturally embedded practice, a permanent social feature. Hillel Schwartz explains that

> fashion will not bring a diet to popularity, but rather dieting and fashion evolve from society's and the individual's desires. The history of dieting is a combination of the way we see our bodies and the way society sees our body, and of our fantasies and fears about ourselves, and desires for our society.

The growing weight-consciousness of American society became evident with the appearance of the first public penny scales during the 1890s. These had bells that rang and music that played when people stepped on them; the faces were large so that anyone could see the weight. Then charts began to appear with the scales. These initially showed the average weight for a given height, and later the suggested weight. As scales and weight-consciousness became more widespread, the faces shrunk. Soon, public scales were out of vogue and bathroom scales became popular—one could weigh in private, and without clothes that added extra pounds.

The Vicious Circle Dieting among the obese has a history of failure. When obese people are given dietary advice as the main source of help, combined with programs of regular weighing and counseling, they generally lose weight—while attending. One study reported a mean loss of 25 pounds over an average 24 weeks of treatment. Long-term results are rarely reported. VERY LOW CALORIE DIETS, whether composed of ordinary or specially prepared food, achieve losses similar in size to those produced by starvation, but being safer, they can be employed with outpatients. However, studies of the long-term effects of very low calorie diets have found fairly rapid replacement of lost weight. Within two to five years, 40 percent of people who lose weight actually end up heavier than when they started. Jane R. Hirshmann, coauthor with Carol H. Munter of *Overcoming Overeating,* has been quoted as saying, "Every single diet results in a binge. It doesn't matter what you're on. Everyone who is involved with them knows they don't work."

The increasing evidence is that weight loss achieved exclusively through diet restriction can "prime" for future weight gain. This is because a decrease in the resting metabolic rate occurs when energy intake is reduced, possibly as a result of the loss of lean body mass. A repeated cycle of weight loss and gain may lower the resting metabolic rate, and persons with a history of weight cycling may require significantly fewer calories than persons without such a history. (See SET-POINT THEORY; YO-YO DIETING.)

But a later study reported by the University of Pennsylvania Medical School disputes this "starvation response" theory. Researchers tracked 18 dieting obese women for 48 weeks, all of whom also increased their levels of physical activity. Half the women ate 1,200 calories daily; the other half took 420-calories-a-day OPTIFAST for 16 weeks, gradually returning to solid food.

The Optifast patients had a mean loss of 47 pounds, the others 22. The resting metabolism dropped dramatically for the very low calorie dieters early in the program, but it was only slightly lower by the end because of a reduction in lean body mass. The study determined that when dieters lose weight, they lose both fat and lean body mass; thus, for every 25 pounds lost, the dieter needs to decrease calorie intake by 100 calories a day.

There is some evidence that by dieting, the obese may actually shorten their life span. Japanese men in Hawaii who were heavy at age 25 but succeeded in losing weight by middle age had a higher mortality than those who maintained a high and steady weight. On the other hand, men who had been lean at age 25 and became even thinner fared no worse than those who maintained a low steady weight. Weight reduction was associated with a near doubling of mortality for fat men but was not nearly as hazardous for thin men. Nearly identical results have been obtained in studies of French government workers and Harvard alumni. In an American Cancer Society Study, persons who reported having lost weight by intent prior to entering the study were more likely to die of stroke and coronary artery disease over the ensuing five years of follow-up. In another study, victims of myocardial infarction who successfully lost 10 pounds or more were twice as likely to die as those who maintained stable weights. And in a Dutch survey, obese women who were dieting to lose weight reported an average of 12 health complaints, whereas nondieters reported an average of only eight. These findings have raised questions about the widespread assumption that dieting for weight loss improves health.

Janet Polivy, professor of psychology at the University of Toronto, has been studying dieting for nearly 20 years. She is convinced that dieting to lose weight can be as much of a problem as the one it is supposed to alleviate. Her research suggests that attempts to lose weight may result in both weight gain and poorer health, mental as well as physical. She and her research team have, via their 10-item RESTRAINT SCALE, developed a picture of the chronic dieter as someone who is easily upset and easily distracted, who is obsessed with weight and eating, who is eager to please and generally has lower-than-normal self-esteem.

Polivy has also cautioned that fatigue, weakness, dizziness, irritability, changes in texture of hair and skin and occasionally more severe problems resulting from malnutrition occur as a result of inadequate caloric intake during dieting.

In addition to these physical effects, psychological aspects of dieting also are being studied by health professionals. A University of Vermont study attempted to correlate the daily and major life stress, psychological symptoms and dieting behavior in 143 adolescent girls aged 14 to 18 over a four-month period. The results of this study indicate that there is a correlation between stress and dieting behavior in adolescents, which was also found to be the case in previous studies of adults. The Vermont study also supported the idea that dieting behavior is related to certain psychological symptoms in adolescents.

Hillel Schwartz has noted that the reason most dieters fail to lose weight or keep it off is that they are dieting in order to change their personalities, and when their personalities do not change, they lose confidence and return to their earlier habits. He stresses that being happy with one's body and having a beautiful body has little to do with weight or fat and more with physical grace.

Weight-Loss Strategies: Questions   Considerable attention has been devoted to the identification of behavioral changes that facilitate short-term and long-term weight loss. This research has largely concentrated on the interventions of clinical practitioners in nutrition, medicine and psychology. Most efforts to lose weight, however, are made by individuals independently of professional supervision and counseling and without physical aids such as drugs or surgery.

Dieting has become an informal institution deeply embedded in Western culture and economy. The media, official bodies and product marketers ply the public with information, sometimes inaccurate, about ways to reduce weight. On the basis of such information, as well as from personal experience, many people construct personal programs of eating practices and physical activity with the intention of losing weight. They also continue some of these practices, perhaps conceived as generally healthful eating and exercise, when they are no longer trying to lose weight.

Recent research has attempted to relate people's knowledge of diet and nutrition to issues of health and weight control. One study, for example, found that good knowledge of nutrition seldom correlated with good weight control in the overweight. Others have found differences between men and women in their use of dieting strategies. Women have been found to be more likely than men to use both physical activity and food-restriction strategies. However, another study, while noting that women more often used reduced-calorie diets than men, found that men engaged in physical activity for weight control more frequently than women.

A British research team led by Alan Blair reported in *Psychology and Health* on a study of the relationship between professed beliefs about dieting and reported body weight before and after dieting. Among respondents to their questionnaire, strategies of increasing exercise, avoiding alcohol and cutting down on fat were positively correlated with success in reducing weight. General avoidance of calories between meals was positively correlated with success in maintaining weight loss. Among practices whose use was not correlated with weight loss were conventional slimming strategies such as fast-

ing, skipping meals, using liquid meal replacements and attending diet centers. In addition, effective weight control was directly related to high expectations of success, no matter the weight loss strategy. The researchers suggested that adjustments may be called for in the content of educational messages and clinical therapy for the overweight.

Some recent studies have reexamined the relationships between nutrient intake and overweight. In one, researchers found that high body mass index was most strongly associated with low bread consumption and use of low-fat milk. (Body mass index, or BMI, is the standard scale of obesity measurement. The formula for deriving a measurement is weight-to-height squared.) Another found that average daily alcohol consumption was unrelated to adiposity, and still another reported evidence that fat intake may contribute to overweight independently of total energy intake.

One researcher has hypothesized, on the basis of satiety physiology and surveys of sugar use, that calories in and with drinks consumed after and between meals make a major contribution to difficulties in weight control.

In *Sculpturing Your Body: Diet, Exercise and Lipo (Fat) Suction*, John A. McCurdy says, "The most effective method to assist in sculpturing your body by diet is to formulate a plan that is balanced but utilizes smaller portions of all basic food groups. If a diet is to be skewed in the direction of any one nutrient, it should be constructed to be high in complex carbohydrates because of the many benefits provided by these substances." He cited a study on a college campus that showed that overweight students effectively reduced on a diet *requiring* 12 slices of low-calorie, high-fiber bread per day in addition to virtually anything else they wished (except alcoholic beverages), including between-meals snacks. The high-fiber bulk of the bread appeared to reduce the intake of other high-calorie foods, presumably by increasing satiety or the feeling of fullness.

Many questions, therefore, remain about which energy-related strategies facilitate weight loss in the short-term and, more important, for the rest of one's life. In a representative sample of 100 adult dieters in the English Midlands, only reduction of fatty foods was associated with a decrease in weight after intensive dieting. Exercise was also associated with weight loss. There is also some clinical evidence that exercise, particularly vigorous exercise, can aid weight loss.

Weight Loss: A Sensible Approach The U.S. Department of Health and Human Services suggests the following "sensible approach" to dieting:

Before embarking on any weight loss program, would-be dieters should consult their physicians to be sure there are no underlying medical problems and that the diet and exercise program they are contemplating is right for them. Talking to a registered dietitian or qualified nutritionist can also be helpful.

Women should be aware that they face more of a challenge in losing weight than men do. Because they generally need fewer calories than men simply to maintain their weight, women have to reduce calories to a lower level in order to lose. For example, most men can lose one to two pounds a week consuming 1,500 to 1,600 calories a day, whereas many women may have to cut down to 1,000 to 1,200 calories a day to achieve the same result.

Because she is consuming fewer calories, a female dieter needs to pay especially close attention to the nutrient value of the foods she eats. Anyone, male or female, considering a diet of 1,000 calories or less should discuss with a physician whether a vitamin-mineral supplement at the level of U.S. Recommended Daily Allowances is advisable.

Although women may have more of a battle than men when it comes to weight loss, the same basic principles apply to both:

- Consult a physician and, if possible, a dietitian before embarking on a very restricted diet.
- Aim for a moderate weight loss of one or two pounds a week. Research has shown that losses in excess of this tend to be losses not of body fat but of water and lean muscle.
- Reduce portion sizes, but maintain a balanced diet from the four basic food groups: grains and cereals; eggs and dairy products; fruits and vegetables; meat, poultry and fish.
- Limit intake of fats, sweets and high-calorie foods.
- Exercise regularly—increase exercise if possible.

Some dieters also find it helpful to count calories in order to keep track of how much they're taking in. It also can be helpful to eat several smaller meals, rather than three large meals a day.

Garrow, J. S. "The Safety of Dieting." *Proceedings of the Nutrition Society* (August 1991) Vol. 50. No. 2.

Polivy, Janet. "Is Dieting Itself an Eating Disorder?"*BASH Magazine,* July 1989.

Safer, D. J. "Diet, Behavior Modification, and Exercise: A Review of Obesity Treatments from a Long-Term Perspective." *Southern Medical Journal* (December 1991) Vol. 84 No. 12.

Schwartz, Hillel. *Never Satisfied: A Cultural History of Diets, Fantasies, and Fat.* New York: Free Press, 1986.

Willis, Judith Levine. "How to Take Weight Off (and Keep It Off) without Getting Ripped Off." *FDA Consumer,* U.S. Department of Health and Human Services (Write to Public Health Service, Food and Drug Administration, Office of Public Affairs, 5600 Fishers Lane, Rockville, MD 20857).

dissociation A mental condition in which, under severe emotional stress or trauma, ideas or mental activities are split off from consciousness and relegated to the unconscious, or outside direct awareness. These "losing oneself" states are often a normal development, as when intense concentration prevents one's consciously hearing conversation or noise, but an extreme dissociative state is a serious disorder, which may manifest itself as amnesia or even the assumption of other identities.

Dissociation also refers to the ability to switch from one ego state of awareness to another. For example, a patient with an eating disorder may go on a binge and describe it as a "trance," or may not be able to gauge her body image correctly.

Studies of anorectics and bulimics have shown that a sizable number have dissociated ego states in disharmony with one another, such as body image distortions or SUPERSTITIOUS THINKING.

Ego states can be activated and studied by hypnosis, revealing otherwise unexplained psychopathological behaviors: binge eating, self-induced vomiting, body image distortion, laxative abuse, self-starvation and so on. These behaviors may originate in one dissociated ego state. More often they are a result of conflict among various states; that is to say, conflicting and irreconcilable values, desires and beliefs in a patient's mind.

Torem, Moshe S. "Eating Disorders and Dissociative States." In *Eating Disorders: Effective Care and Treatment,* edited by Félix E. F. Larocca. St. Louis: Ishiyaku EuroAmerica, 1986.

distribution of body fat   The pattern of fat distribution on a person's body can have as direct a relationship to health and mortality as the total amount of body fat. For example, in women, upper-body fat may be associated with a higher risk of diabetes than lower-body fat accumulation. In both men and women, abdominal obesity is associated with an increased risk of heart disease. Thus, knowledge of body composition and fat distribution is increasingly recognized as an essential component of an overall nutritional assessment.

A relative predominance of fat in the abdominal region (called the apple shape) as well as the shoulders and neck is found more often in men and is strongly related to metabolic disturbances such as diabetes mellitus, hypertriglyceridemia and hypertension. In women, gluteal-femoral (buttocks-hip-thigh) obesity is more common, but when they do have body fat concentrated in the stomach, they have a six-times-greater chance of developing breast cancer than women with flat stomachs, according to a study conducted by Dr. David V. Schapira, associate professor of medicine at the University of South Florida College of Medicine. Researchers compared 216 women newly diagnosed with breast cancer with 432 women who were tested but did not have cancer. They found that the cancer patients had more abdominal and upper-body fat than those not diagnosed with cancer. Schapira reported that the women with fat in the stomach area had lower levels of a protein called sex hormone binding globulin, which leads to increased levels of free estrogen. Increased free estrogen levels are thought to contribute to the development of breast cancer. When the women lost weight in the abdominal region, levels of the protein increased.

In another study, conducted at Washington University School of Medicine, researchers discovered that people with beefy hips and trim waists (pear shaped) have higher levels of a protective form of cholesterol called HDL than do those who are apple shaped. This is believed to be a possible explanation of why people with fat posteriors tend to have healthier hearts than those with big bellies.

Body fat distribution has been related not only to morbidity and mortality of obesity but also to adipose tissue cellularity. That is, in abdominal obesity fat cell size is relatively enlarged, whereas in gluteal-femoral obesity the number of fat cells is increased.

While sexual differences are the most obvious influences of distribution of body fat, age is another significant factor; the body changes shape as it grows and ages. A National Institute on Aging study of 1,179 men and women aged 17 to 96 showed progressive trends toward increased upper- and central-body fat deposits with age. In women there tends to be a postmenopausal acceleration of this trend.

A Yale University study determined the degree of weight preoccupation and body dissatisfaction in 77 women between the ages of 21 and 50. Women with the greatest distribution of their fat in the hips and buttocks, relative to the abdomen and waist, were the most eating-disordered and saw attaining the "right" weight as more central to their sense of self.

Individual differences in fat distribution are largely determined by hereditary factors. Environmental factors, including diet and exercise habits, determine the extent to which individual genetic predispositions are fulfilled.

Weight loss does not guarantee that inches will be shed from desired areas. On the contrary, success as measured on the bathroom scale is often not translated into the reality of a more shapely body as visualized in the imagination. Recent studies have confirmed that some areas of the body tend to be resistant to slimming.

British researchers have documented the resistance of the thighs to weight loss regimens. Measurements of women's waists and thighs were used to compute a "fat distribution score," a ratio between abdominal and thigh circumferences. Increasing thigh size relative to waist circumference yielded a lower ratio and vice versa. Following completion of a weight reduction regimen, fat distribution scores showed little change, indicating that fat was shed proportionately from both areas of the body without altering their proportions relative to each other. This study is consistent with the experiences and frustrations of many dieters who, despite weight loss, are unable to achieve their primary goal, improvement in body shape.

A Boston study reported in the May 1991 *American Journal of Clinical Nutrition* indicates that when smokers start putting on fat, they are slightly more likely than nonsmokers to deposit it around the abdomen. Because people with abdominal obesity are more likely to develop heart disease, this finding may offer one partial explanation for smokers' higher risk of this disease.

Jensen, Michael; Haymond, Morey; Rizza, Robert; Cryer, Philip; and Miles, John. "Influence of Body Fat Distribution on Free Fatty Acid Metabolism in Obesity." *Journal of Clinical Investigation* (April 1989) 83.

Mayo-Smith, W. Hayes, C. W., Biller, B. M., Klibanski, A., et al "Body Fat Distribution Measured with CT: Correlations in Healthy Subjects, Patients with Anorexia Nervosa, and Patients with Cushing Syndrome." *Radiology* (February 1989) 170: 2.

Radke-Sharpe, Norean; Whitney-Saltiel, Deborah; Rodin, Judith. "Fat Distribution as a Risk Factor for Weight and Eating Concerns." *International Journal of Eating Disorders* 9, no. 1 (1990).

Shimokata, H., Tobin, J. D., Muller, D. C., Elahi, D., et al. "Studies in the Distribution of Body Fat: Effects of Age, Sex, and Obesity." *Journal of Gerontology* (March 1989) 44: 2.

diuretic abuse Diuretics are usually drugs, but can also be common substances such as tea, coffee and water, that help remove excess water from the body by stimulating the flow of urine. Diuretic drugs interfere with normal kidney action by changing the amount of water, potassium, sodium and waste products removed from the bloodstream. Normally, most of the potassium, sodium and water are returned to the bloodstream during the normal filtration process, but small amounts are expelled from the body along with waste products in the urine. Some diuretics reduce the amount of sodium and water taken back into the blood; others increase blood flow through the kidneys and thus the amount of water they filter and expel in the urine. They are often irresponsibly given by diet doctors so a patient can experience a quick weight loss. Any such weight loss is temporary and a consequence of the dehydrating effect.

Because diuretics are available in a wide variety of over-the-counter formulations as well as by prescription, the exact rate of diuretic use or abuse is unknown. Patients who abuse diuretics obtain them from several sources: over the counter; appropriate prescriptions for medical conditions; multiple prescriptions from two or more physicians, each unaware of the real amount of the drug the patient is using; prescriptions meant for another person; misappropriation from workplaces including nursing homes, hospitals, pharmacies and pharmaceutical distributors.

Researchers at the University of Minnesota Medical School evaluated 14 symptomatic female volunteers between the ages of 18 and 40 who used diuretics on a regular basis for nonmedical reasons. Seven (50 percent) were diagnosed as having a current or past eating disorder, and nine (64 percent) were diagnosed as having a current or past AFFECTIVE DISORDER. The results of this pilot study suggest that chronic diuretic use by young women signals the possibility of an unrecognized eating problem and/or affective disorder.

The three groups of prescription diuretics most often abused by patients with eating disorders are the thiazides, loop diuretics and potassium-sparing diuretics. Thiazides, including chlorothiazide and hydrochlorothiazide, cause depletion of potassium and other electrolytes. Adverse consequences of HYPOKALEMIA (extreme potassium depletion) include cardiac conduction defects, arrhythmias and muscular weakness or paralysis. Common symptoms include weakness, nausea, palpitations, excessive urination, excessive thirst, constipation and abdominal pain. Other potential side effects of thiazide abuse include abnormal blood levels of sodium, sugar, uric acid, fat, zinc, magnesium and calcium.

Loop diuretics include furosemide and ethacrynic acid. Excessive potassium loss and fluid depletion frequently occur, especially when used in larger-than-recommended doses. Other side effects of these agents include hyperuricemia, hypocalcemia, magnesium depletion, ototoxicity and cross-reaction in sulfa-allergic patients.

Potassium-sparing diuretics include spironolactone and triamterene. In contrast to the thiazides and loop diuretics, these agents result in a mild loss of potassium. In addition, triamterene nephrolithiasis and acute renal failure are potential adverse effects.

Most bulimic patients who misuse or abuse diuretics use over-the-counter preparations. Commonly available over-the-counter diuretics include Premesyn-PMS, Sunril Premenstrual Capsules, Midol-PMS, Odrinil, Diurex-MPR, Pamprin Menstrual Relief, Aqua-Ban, Odrinil and Diurex. Most of them contain one of three ingredients listed by the U.S. Food and Drug Administration as diuretics (Category I) effective in menstrual drug products: pamabrom, ammonium chloride and caffeine. In addition, the FDA has found that pyrilamine maleate (an antihistamine) is an appropriate adjunct to any of the Category I diuretics.

Ammonium chloride is the active diuretic ingredient in one of the most widely used over-the-counter formulations. It is considered safe in a dosage range of one to three grams daily in divided oral doses for periods of up to six days. Ammonium chloride results in formation of sodium chloride from sodium bicarbonate in the body, but the effect lasts only about four or five days. Nausea, vomiting and gastrointestinal distress are potential side effects.

CAFFEINE is considered by the FDA to be a safe and effective diuretic for over-the-counter use in doses of 100 to 200 mg every three to four hours. As a diuretic, caffeine acts by increasing the glomerular filtration rate in the kidneys. Sleeplessness is a potential side effect.

Pamabrom is considered by the FDA to be a safe and effective diuretic for relief of water accumulation during menstrual cycles. Recommended dosage is not more than 50 mg per dose and 200 mg in 24 hours.

The effects of these over-the-counter diuretics on individuals with eating disorders who may have other metabolic abnormalities owing to vomiting or LAXATIVE ABUSE can have severe consequences on renal function and fluid and electrolyte balance.

Killen, Joel; Taylor, C. Barr; Telch, Michael J.; Saylor, Keith E.; Maron, David J., and Robinson, Thomas N. "Self-induced Vomiting and Laxative and Diuretic Abuse among Teenagers." *JAMA: Journal of the American Medical Association* (March 21, 1986) 255: 11.

Mitchell, J. E.; Pomeroy, C.; Seppala, M.; Huber, M. "Diuretic Use as a Marker for Eating Problems and Affective Disorders among Women." *Journal of Clinical Psychiatry* (July 1988) 49:7.

Pomeroy, Claire; Mitchell, James E.; Seim, Harold C.; and Seppala, Marvin. "Prescription Diuretic Abuse in Patients with Bulimia Nervosa." *Journal of Family Practice* (November 1988) Vol. 27 No. 5.

doom bulimia   A term used to describe a binge-eating pattern consisting of cycles of binges and short periods of restrained eating. Binges are said to begin with "cheating" on a diet, provoking guilt and anxiety, which in turn provoke the disastrous binges. The logic of this is explained this way:

Cheating on a diet can be a very emotional affair. Even at the most rational level, there are anxieties about the struggle to get back onto the diet and about taking off the calories being eaten at that moment. This breach of discipline can be a source of profound feelings of guilt, shame and self-loathing. Such distress often contributes to eating that could be characterized as "counterregulatory" excess: the anxious state becomes a stimulus to eating. In other words, eating provokes anxiety, which provokes more eating—provoking greater anxiety and hence still more eating. The resulting long and uncontrolled eating bouts are called "doom binges." These become a regular pattern—"doom bulimia."

Furthermore, it is thought, the stress of being on a diet could itself become a stimulus for binge eating. Stress could result from the discomfort of hunger, tiredness and irritability or from non–diet-related causes. Eating would only increase stress, reinforcing anxiety as a conditioned stimulus. This could be described as confusing anxiety with hunger. (SEE BINGE EATING.)

This theory is not widely accepted.

Booth, D. A. "Culturally Controlled into Food Abuse: The Eating Disorders as Physiologically Reinforced Excessive Appetites." In *The Psychobiology of Bulimia Nervosa,* edited by K. M. Pirke, W. Vandereycken and D. Ploog. Berlin; New York: Springer-Verlag, 1988.

double-blind study   A study in which neither the researchers nor the participants know which group is the experimental group and which the control group. The purpose is to eliminate any expectations, conscious or unconscious, that might affect the outcome of the study or trial.

DSM-III (DSM-III-R)   The third and most recent edition of the *Diagnostic and Statistical Manual of Mental Disorders,* published by the American Psychiatric Association in 1980. A revised version was published in 1987 as DSM-III-R. DSM-III provides criteria for classifying psychological disorders for physicians making diagnoses and researchers compiling statistics. This manual is considered the standard for the profession.

dysfunctional behavior patterns   Abnormal, inadequate or impaired functioning. According to Polivy, Herman and Garner in *Assessment of Addictive Behaviors* (Guilford

Press, New York 1988), many of the dysfunctional behavior patterns characterizing eating-disordered patients are directly related to perceptions that perpetuate the eating disorder. Although the negative self-concept represented by the sense of worthlessness, overcompliancy, lack of trust and excessive perfectionism does not necessarily correspond to particular behavior problems, it does constrain an individual and inhibits normal interactions and relationships. The flight from maturity or femininity often creates (or exacerbates) problems with sexual behavior: patients may either avoid sex completely or act in a promiscuous but unsatisfying (and often personally distasteful) manner. The positive value perceived in symptoms such as weight loss and starvation in anorectics, binge eating and purging in bulimics and inappropriate (i.e., non–hunger-induced) eating in the obese makes it particularly difficult to substitute more acceptable behaviors.

Misperceptions about food and calories, lack of self-awareness, DICHOTOMOUS REASONING, obsession with food and eating and excessively high valuation of thinness all contribute to the chaotic eating behaviors of these patients. When patients cannot distinguish emotion from hunger, or cannot determine whether they are hungry or sated (see HUNGER and SATIETY), it becomes more likely that they will eat in response to inappropriate (e.g., emotional) internal sensations. The desire for thinness leads to DIETING, which in turn may trigger BINGE EATING. A dichotomous thinking style can promote binge-or-starve eating. Misperceptions regarding food and calories, and obsessions with food, are associated in obvious ways with disordered eating patterns.

early satiety   Bulimics who practice frequent vomiting often complain that they feel ''full'' following consumption of a relatively small amount of food, a characteristic referred to as early satiety.

eating attitudes test (EAT)   A 40-question self-test devised by Paul E. Garfinkel and David M. Garner (see GARFINKEL AND GARNER) to measure the broad range of symptoms characteristic of anorexia nervosa. A high score on the EAT does not necessarily reflect anorexia nervosa, nor does a low score invariably rule it out, since people may not respond honestly on a self-report questionnaire. However, in practice, the EAT has been shown to be quite accurate in discriminating anorectics from control subjects. It is most useful as a screening device; diagnoses of anorexia nervosa must be confirmed in clinical interviews. EAT scores can also serve as an index of anorectic patients' improvement.

Researchers in 1988 assessed eating attitudes by use of the Eating Attitudes Test in a sample of 288 young adults at Kingsborough Community College in New York City. The sample included relatively more poor and working-class persons than are found in a typical four-year college. Mean EAT scores tended to be at the high end of the range previously reported for nonclinical samples. Scores were not significantly related to socioeconomic variables. White women scored significantly higher than nonwhite women. In addition, a disproportionately high number of women from intact (as opposed to destabilized) homes scored above the EAT cutoff score.

Although no hard-and-fast conclusions can be drawn from the available data, these findings are consistent with the hypothesis that preoccupation with eating is now widely distributed across sex, race and socioeconomic status categories. They raise the possibility that viewing the quest for slimness exclusively in terms of individual psychology may have created a false picture. The preoccupation with weight of some women might represent a need for fulfillment of social needs such as enhanced status, and a sense of control of their lives. Normal female dieters may be seeking self-enhancement, while eating-disordered persons may be using the disorder to avoid facing difficulties.

Schmolling, Paul. "Eating Attitude Test Scores in Relation to Weight Socioeconomic Status, and Family Stability." *Psychological Reports* 63 (1988).

eating disorders inventory (EDI)   A 64-item self-test designed in 1983 by Garner, Olmstead and Polivy to differentiate bulimics, extreme dieters and particular subgroups of anorectic patients. The EDI evaluates an individual on a number of different subscales including drive for thinness, body dissatisfaction, sense of ineffectiveness, perfectionism, interpersonal distrust and fears of maturity—psychological and behavioral components common to anorexia and bulimia. This test was intended to augment the EAT, which focuses primarily on dieting- and eating-related symptoms. It is one of very few tests for anorexia, bulimia and bulimia nervosa that measure not only symptoms but also psychological characteristics believed to be central in these disorders. The EDI has been used experimentally to discriminate individuals with eating disorders from nonpathological weight-preoccupied women.

Welch, Garry; Hall, Anne; and Norring, Claes. "The Factor Structure of the Eating Disorder Inventory in a Patient Setting." *International Journal of Eating Disorders* (January 1988) 9: 1.

Welch, G.; Hall, A.; and Walkey, F. "The Factor Structure of the Eating Disorder Inventory." *Journal of Clinical Psychology* (January 1988). 44: 1.

eating disorders week   In 1988 the last week of April was designated Eating Disorders Awareness Week by Congress. Currently, National Eating Disorders Week is held each year during Thanksgiving week. Its sevenfold purpose:

1. To increase efforts to prevent the development of eating disorders.

2. To educate the public and professional communities regarding warning signs and appropriate interventions.
3. To increase awareness of treatment programs and support services.
4. To encourage development of healthy attitudes toward psychological and physical development, body image and self-esteem by influential individuals (i.e., parents, educators and health professionals).
5. To challenge cultural attitudes regarding thinness, perfection, achievement and expression of emotion that contribute to the increasing incidence of eating disorders.
6. To improve the ability of professionals of all disciplines to provide effective treatment and support.
7. To promote a compassionate, nonjudgmental, public understanding of eating disorders.

eating habits monitoring   Eating habits are food-related behaviors or behavior patterns. By monitoring the eating habits of eating-disordered patients, clinicians can obtain important information for the assessment and subsequent treatment of obesity and eating disorders. Methods used to measure eating behavior include patient self-monitoring, direct observation and paper-and-pencil assessment.

Self-monitoring of eating behavior involves recording such information as the type, amount and caloric value of food eaten, as well as the setting, time of day and feelings associated with eating. Although the limitations of self-monitoring strategies are evident (data may be biased and unreliable), such approaches represent a valuable therapeutic tool, providing information that is indispensable in developing comprehensive individual treatment plans. Continuous self-monitoring throughout treatment further highlights those variables that influence treatment effectiveness.

Direct observations provide data that tend to be more reliable than self-monitored data.

Some researchers observe subjects without their knowledge and rate such behaviors as amount of food chosen, number of chews, duration of meal, number of mouthfuls and amount of food uneaten. Time-sampling techniques can be incorporated into observational assessments to provide specific data such as chews per minute or calories consumed per minute (according to some researchers, a highly sensitive measure to assess treatment effectiveness). Thus far, direct observations have been employed primarily to evaluate the outcome of treatment. The potential benefits of such approaches in clinical practice are just now starting to be realized. In particular, the Eating Analysis and Treatment Schedule (EATS) has been developed for home use by nonparticipating observers. The EATS is quite useful, for it assesses actual eating behavior in the nonclinical situation in which most meals are consumed.

Questionnaires represent the third major strategy for measuring eating patterns. Two paper-and-pencil measures used by clinicians have considerable usefulness in obesity treatment and research: the Eating Patterns Questionnaire (EPQ), developed by J. P. Wollersheim in 1970, and the Revised Master Questionnaire (RMQ), developed by Straw, Straw and Craighead in 1979. The EPQ is designed to assess general patterns of eating behavior, with six factors considered: (1) Emotional and Uncontrolled Overeating, (2) Eating Response to Interpersonal Situations, (3) Eating in Isolation, (4) Eating as Reward, (5) Eating Response to Evaluative Situations, and (6) Between-Meal Eating. The EPQ is used for both clinical practice and research.

The RMQ is a refinement of the Master Questionnaire that was developed to assess eating habits. It was designed to reduce the excessive length and scale overlap of the original questionnaire. RMQ data are divided into five general categories or clusters: Hopelessness, Physical Attribution, Motivation, Stimulus Control and Energy Balance Knowledge.

Straw, R.; Straw, M. K.; and Craighead, L. "Psychometric Properties of the RMO: Cluster Analysis of an Obesity Assessment Device." Paper presented at the annual meeting of the Association for Advancement of Behavior Therapy, San Francisco, November 1979.

ectomorph   A person with a thin and skeletal or bony body type. Ectomorphs are characterized by long, thin arms and legs and a narrow trunk, conveying a rather trim, thin appearance.

Theories linking body types to emotional or psychological characteristics are not considered scientifically sound.

See also ENDOMORPH; MESOMORPH; BODY TYPES.

ego state therapy   A treatment approach applying various techniques from group and family therapy to the resolution of internal conflict in a single individual. In this therapy, the individual psyche is assumed to be made up of various parts that have different functions and constitute the whole.

Torem, Moshe S. "Eating Disorders and Dissociative States." In *Eating Disorders: Effective Care and Treatment*, edited by Félix E. F. Larocca. St. Louis: Ishiyaku EuroAmerica, 1986.

elderly, eating disorders in the   Although eating disorders are most commonly thought of as occurring during adolescence, the process of aging brings many changes that can influence such illnesses as anorexia nervosa and bulimia. After the age of 50, physical changes such as a decrease in the basal metabolic rate, a decrease in lean body mass and an increase in percentage of body fat combine with common changes in psychosocial conditions to affect nutrition. For instance, decreasing financial resources and increasing social isolation may promote the development of poor eating patterns. Favorite foods may be financially out of reach; boredom may lead to decreased interest in meals; aging people may simply lack understanding of what their bodies require. Life stresses and trauma may also have an effect on the development of eating disorders in the elderly. For example, research indicates that women who are newly grieving over the deaths of their husbands are likely to skip meals and resort to junk food.

As with adolescents, there is an increase in body fat in those over 50. Changes in the body's energy requirements may coincide with changes in daily routine due to such events as illness, relocation or retirement. If physical activity is decreased but the amount of food consumed is not, there will be a gain in weight, another common variable in already changing bodies.

Along with a decline in metabolism, the aging process brings changes in nearly all other body systems. The aging may experience changes in sight and hearing, as well as declining sensitivity to temperature, touch and taste (gustatory villae [taste buds] begin to atrophy in women in their early forties and men in their early fifties). The neurological system, especially the brain, the digestive system and the musculoskeletal system are all noticeably affected. Such physiological changes affect the body images of aging individuals, and body image is often an important variable in the initiation of dieting behaviors that may lead to eating disorders.

Clinicians at Northeastern Ohio University have reported three case histories of onset of anorexia nervosa in geriatric patients. Geriatric research has demonstrated neurotransmitter changes that may predispose the aging population to anorexia. These include a decline in norepinephrine as well as B-endorphin levels; these changes are also seen in anorexia.

Some researchers have theorized that eating disorders are becoming more common among the elderly for two reasons. First, there has been a dramatic increase in the incidence of eating disorders in the last three decades. Since at least 20 percent of patients become chronic, and not all of them shed

their illness as they age, some are likely to remain anorectic or bulimic into old age. Second, it is possible that even elderly women are beginning to succumb to the social pressures to be slim, and some may use vomiting to control their weight.

Lending credibility to the first theory, ARTHUR H. CRISP reported in the *British Journal of Psychiatry* in 1990 that an 80-year-old woman had a relapse of anorexia nervosa after being in remission for 50 years. Symptoms of the disease gradually reemerged after her husband died. Investigators considered the relapse an attempt to use a previously discovered coping strategy to keep the negative emotions of depression and grief at bay.

Giannini, A. James; Collins, James I; and Lewis, Denise. "Anorexia Nervosa in the Elderly—Case Studies." *American Journal of Psychiatry* (February 1989) 146: 2.

Kelley, J.; Trimble, M.; and Thorley, A. "Anorexia Nervosa after the Menopause." *British Journal of Psychiatry* 128 (1976).

Morley, J. E. and Silver, A. J. "Anorexia in the Elderly." *Neurobiology of Aging* (September 1988). 9: 9–16.

Price, W. A., Giannini, A. J. and Colella. "Anorexia Nervosa in the Elderly." *Journal of the American Geriatric Society* 33 (1985).

endocrine factors in obesity   The endocrine glands produce hormones that regulate the body's rate of METABOLISM, growth and sexual development and functioning. "Glands" have often been blamed by individuals for their obesity, but obesity caused by endocrine alterations are uncommon, and the increase in body weight observed with acute endocrine disease is usually limited. Hypothyroidism, adrenal hyperplasia and hypogonadism are endocrine alterations that result in modest obesity.

endomorph   A person with a body type characterized by a tendency toward roundness and substantial fat deposits. Endomorphs have wide trunks and shorter-than-average arms and legs, making them appear to be somewhat fat. People with significant endomorphy gradually fill out until late middle age, when they generally shrink a little.

Theories linking body types to emotional or psychological characteristics are not considered scientifically sound.

See also ECTOMORPH; MESOMORPH; BODY TYPES.

energy intake/expenditure in obesity

All activities of the body require energy, with all needs being met by the consumption of food (CARBOHYDRATES, PROTEINS and FATS). Energy not expended for bodily activity is stored as fat. A major question being debated by researchers is whether or not obese individuals either require or take in more energy than the nonobese.

Although previous studies had indicated that the energy intake of obese individuals is either lower than or not significantly different from those of nonobese individuals, some researchers felt that these results were inconsistent with strong evidence that total body weight is positively correlated with energy expenditure. In one study, the relationship between energy consumption and body composition was evaluated in 63 women by use of energy-intake values. It was determined that the energy needs of an obese woman are likely to be lower than that of a large, lean individual if both women weigh the same amount.

Another study demonstrated that energy expenditure over 14 days is higher in obese than in lean subjects. This demonstrated that obese subjects do not maintain their obesity because of a low energy expenditure but because of a high energy intake.

Lissner, Lauren; Habicht, Jean-Pierre; Strupp, Barbara; Levitsky, David; Haas, Jere; and Roe, Daphne. "Body Composition and Energy Intake: Do Overweight Women Overeat and Underreport?" *American Journal of Clinical Nutrition* (February 1989) 49.
Sims, E. A. "Storage and Expenditure of Energy in Obesity and Their Implications for Management." *Medical Clinics of North America* (January 1989) 73.

exercise Physical exertion for improvement or maintenance of health and fitness, as well as weight loss. Exercise alone is not usually prescribed as a weight loss method, but physical activity is a key to any weight control program. It burns CALORIES, speeds METABOLISM and helps offset the dreaded "plateau" stage in which weight loss slows or stops temporarily. (See SET-POINT THEORY.) People who exercise and diet lose more fat and less muscle than people who only diet.

Achieving a negative energy balance— that is, using up more calories than one takes in—by exercise alone has been shown to cause some weight loss. The mean weight loss achieved over a mean duration of 19 weeks, in seven studies, was 16 pounds. No long-term follow-ups are available. Although changes of exercise (energy output) and/or altered metabolic efficiency can cause weight loss when one is over- or underweight, the amount is usually not significant unless accompanied by lowered food intake.

Most studies have shown that vigorous exercisers consume more calories than sedentary individuals, but they also weigh approximately 20 percent less on average. There are no data supporting the contention that moderate activity of short duration used in weight loss programs stimulates APPETITE. In fact, for many people, moderate exercise tends to have an appetite-suppressing effect. For this reason, many experts recommend that daily exercise be performed prior to the main meal of the day.

Researchers at Mt. Sinai Hospital in New York have reported that whereas fat people burn off more calories if they eat *after* exercising, thin people burn off more if they eat *before*. The researchers believe that fat people's cells are less sensitive to insulin, the hormone that admits fuel into body cells. Intense exercise, they say, may improve the insulin sensitivity of fat people.

Studies at Stanford University comparing food intake and weight of long-distance runners (those who run approximately 40 miles per week) with those of randomly selected sedentary adults of similar age show that despite ingesting an average of 600 more calories per day (2,959 vs. 2,361), the runners weighed 25 percent less than the sedentary group, evidence strongly suggesting that exercise lowers the set point. Numerous studies have documented the observation that a program of moderate exercise reduces body fat levels while preserving or increasing lean body mass. Animal studies show that exercise produces a specific fat-burning effect and that the animals maintain the new body fat levels, demonstrating that the set point has been lowered.

The evidence establishing regular exercise as an important factor in weight control has convinced many health care professionals that one of the major causes of CREEPING OBESITY is the lack of physical activity, largely as the result of sedentary styles of life. The average American man between 35 and 45 years of age weighed six pounds more in 1980 than in 1960 (the average American woman of similar age showed an eight-pound weight increase) despite a 10 percent reduction in caloric intake over this period.

Today's emphasis on fitness and athletics has had a negative as well as positive effect on health, especially for adolescent girls. Encouraged to exercise for their looks rather than their health, girls are often told that exercise is "nature's best makeup." Researchers have found that slimness of hips is the most sought-after feature among adolescents aged 12 to 16. Dissatisfaction with hip measurement only increases during this period when hips show the most change from natural hormonal influences. Some adolescents are so intent on changing their appearance that they become obsessed with exercise.

Eating-disordered patients often use exercise as a means of purging themselves of unwanted calories—a practice that causes additional health problems, such as vitamin and mineral deficiencies that can cause damage to bones, AMENORRHEA and cardiac arrest from low potassium levels and electrolyte imbalances. Excessive exercising can become a dangerous habit and one that is difficult to break. One exercise machine maker advertises "No pain, no gain," but pain is a warning to the body that something is wrong. For anorectics and bulimics, exercise buffers some of the pain they should be feeling; they are numbing their bodies' warnings to stop their destructive behavior.

In July 1983, *Reader's Digest,* in "News from the World of Medicine," reported on University of Arizona researchers who interviewed 60 runners and found that certain mature men among them showed surprising resemblances to young women with anorexia nervosa. The men were introverted, often lonely, depressed, self-effacing and uncomfortable with the direct expression of anger. Social pressures may explain the similarities, according to the scientists. Girls often are judged by looks, and men by athletic ability. When insecure girls diet to make themselves slim, they may become anorectic; when men run to show their athletic prowess, they may become compulsive. Their behavior becomes pathological as a result of extreme psychological inflexibility, repetitive thoughts, adherence to rituals and need to control themselves and their environments.

Breaking an exercise addiction can be as difficult as overcoming an eating disorder. While the effects of anorexia can be measured on a bathroom scale, the "fitaholic's" problem is not so easily defined. Truly compulsive exercisers let their workouts dominate their existence to the detriment of family, job and social life. Obsessive runners may be taught relaxation techniques and other ways of coping with stress that can help them become less dependent on exercise for their sense of well-being.

Molé, Paul; Stern, Judith; Schultz, Cynthia; Bernauer, Edmund; and Holcomb, Bryan. "Exercise Reverses Depressed Metabolic Rate

Produced by Severe Caloric Restriction." *Medicine and Science in Sports and Exercise* 21, no. 1 (1989).

Segal, K. R.; and Pi-Sunyer, F. X. "Exercise and Obesity." *Medical Clinics of North America* (January 1989) 73.

Sussman, Vic. "Health Guide: Fitness." *U.S. News & World Report,* June 18, 1990.

Yale, J. F.; Leiter, L. A.; and Marliss, E. B. "Metabolic Responses to Intense Exercise in Lean and Obese Subjects." *Journal of Clinical Endocrinology and Metabolism* (February 1989) 68.

exposure and response prevention (ERP)   A treatment method originally used in treating phobic and obsessive-compulsive disorders, in which the patient is exposed to whatever is triggering his or her abnormal behavior, with the abnormal behavior then forcibly restrained.

In recent years, ERP has also been adapted to treatment of addictive disorders such as alcoholism and bulimia. For example, clinicians have described how a bulimic woman was made to wait increasing lengths of time between stages of the disordered behavior that culminated in vomiting. After eight weeks her vomiting, which had occurred roughly four times a day prior to treatment, ceased.

Explaining why ERP works, Rosen and Leitenberg explain in *Behavior Therapy* that "binge eating and self-induced vomiting seem linked in a vicious circle by anxiety." Eating (especially BINGE EATING) elicits the fear of weight gain; vomiting reduces it. "Once an individual has learned that vomiting following food intake leads to anxiety reduction, rational fears no longer inhibit overeating." Thus, if the end-result vomiting is delayed longer and longer after each binge-eating session, the binge eating needed to stimulate it is delayed until it no longer is needed (because the vomiting that counters it is no longer occurring). So "the driving force of this disorder may be vomiting, not binge-ing."

Rosen, J.C. and Leitenberg, H. 1982. "Bulimia Nervosa: Treatment with Exposure and Response Prevention" *Behavior Therapy* 13.

external control therapy   A form of behavior modification in which patients' responses to the consequences of their behavior are manipulated to change that behavior. Patients enter into a set of arrangements that ensure that success in a given task is followed by positive consequences and failure is followed by negative consequences. In obese patients, clinically significant weight losses, on the order of 22 pounds, have been produced using this technique.

In this therapy, an explicit agreement or contract is established between a patient and some other person (usually the therapist), specifying the targets to be attained at what times; the circumstances in which progress is to be monitored; and the consequences that will follow attainment or nonattainment of the target.

In one study, subjects agreed to deposit valuables or money with the therapist and to attend weigh-ins at scheduled intervals. Weight loss targets were agreed on. The subjects agreed that if they attended weigh-ins and achieved their targets, specified portions of their deposits would be returned to them. If they failed to attend, or failed to reach their targets, that portion would be forfeited and sent to a charity.

This method of contingency or deposit contracting has been the most widely used. Since the assumption is that the procedure will be more effective the stronger the incentives employed, fairly large monetary deposits have been used. In some programs forfeited money or valuables are sent to organizations repugnant to the patients. In others, unpleasant physical sensations are the incentive. Patients who lose weight might be fitted with snugly fitting nylon cords around their waist, sealed in position. Subsequent increases result in unpleasant sensations, effectively punishing the behaviors causing them. The New Orleans Police Force once required its overweight officers to lose five pounds each month. Failure to reach this target resulted in punishment on a sliding scale ranging from written reprimand to suspension without pay. While these contingencies were in force, the officers lost weight; when they were withdrawn, weight loss ceased.

Contingency contracting has been found to be a simple treatment procedure, capable of exerting powerful influence on patients' behavior while a contract is in force. This influence vanishes once the contract ceases, so that lost weight is frequently regained. Studies have found that when significant amounts of weight are lost through contingency contracting, about half is regained during the year after treatment ceases.

The assumption underlying the use of these techniques is that restrained eating is less likely to persist than unrestrained eating because the reinforcing satisfactions of the former are remote, and those of the latter are immediate. The imposition of external controls (though accepted voluntarily) is an attempt to reverse this natural imbalance in favor of restraint.

externality approach to obesity One of two major types of treatment for obesity (the other is the PSYCHODYNAMIC APPROACH TO OBESITY). Externality focuses on salient food-related cues in patients' environment and attempts to control their responses to them. This approach developed from experiments at Columbia University performed in 1974 by social psychologist Stanley Schachter. Schachter's group found that obese people are more likely to eat when a clock says it's mealtime or when food is put onto a plate than when their bodies signal HUNGER.

This approach assumes that what obese people need is to change their responses to these external cues, and that by allowing themselves to eat only when truly hungry, they will lose weight naturally. It has spawned a number of behavioral therapy techniques, such as putting food on smaller plates so the

amount looks larger, eating only in a particular room and so on.

Some externalists' patients have achieved remarkable results (one group lost an average of 40 pounds each in a single year), but these results have not consistently been replicated by others. Not only have patients not lost 40 pounds, they have tended to gain back what they have lost.

See also EATING HABITS MONITORING.

Schacter, S., and Rodin, J. *Obese Humans and Rats*. Potomac, Md.: Lawrence Erlbaum Associates.

Leon, G. R. "Personality and Behavioral Correlates of Obesity." In *Psychological Aspects of Obesity: A Handbook,* edited by B. B. Wolman. New York: Van Nostrand Reinhold, 1982.

Rodin, J., "The Externality Theory Today." In *Obesity,* edited by A. J. Stunkard. Philadelphia: Saunders, 1980.

F

fad diets Diets that achieve widespread, though short-lived, popularity, usually as a result of heavily promoted "best-selling" books and/or popular magazine or tabloid features.

Hardly a season goes by without at least one diet book high on the best-seller list. Some diets advocated by these books are simply variations of a basic, safe 1,000- to 2,000-calorie balanced diet. But as John A. McCurdy, Jr. explains in *Sculpturing Your Body* (Hollywood, Fla.: Frederick Fell Publishers, 1987), others may be positively dangerous, because they advocate diets that are unbalanced. Many capitalize on well-known names or places; many are accompanied by testimonials of spectacular and effortless weight loss. Fad diets generally rely on some trick to give readers the appearance of novelty. They attract faithful followings by claiming "scientific breakthroughs" such as methods to lower METABOLISM. Many tell dieters to eat only certain foods and exclude others; some even restrict the diet to two or three foods such as grapefruit or eggs. Because one can eat only so much of one food in a day, caloric intake is lowered and weight is lost. The problem is that single-food diets become boring, eventually prompting dieters to "cheat." Soon the cheating increases, dieters are back to normal eating patterns and excess weight returns . . . until another fad diet comes along.

Cheating on these diets, of course, may help to preserve dieters' health (unless they cheat with junk food, a not uncommon occurrence), since, in addition to being boring, many of these diets are nutritionally unbalanced and dangerous. If they stay on them long enough, dieters can experience irregular heartbeat, kidney stones, fatigue, nausea, dizziness, muscle loss and other serious side effects.

Fad diets can be classified into six basic types:

1. *Low carbohydrate* diets (Dr. Cooper's, Dr. Atkins', Superenergy) typically produce rapid weight loss during their first week, primarily because of dehydration. This occurs because, to compensate for reduced carbohydrate intake, the body breaks down stored sugar and protein, a process that releases water. This begins several days after the dieting starts. Because carbohydrates are not available to use as a source of energy, the body is forced to use fats instead. This leads to fatty acids being released into the blood, where they are converted to ketones. The state of "ketosis" is purported to produce appetite suppression, resulting in accelerated weight loss. In actuality, however, there is no scientific evidence that ketosis does suppress the appetite. (See KETO-GENIC DIET.)

2. *High-protein* diets (Stillman, Scarsdale, Cambridge) are based on the assumption that, since there is no storage form of protein, as there is for carbohydrate and fat, high protein intake will result in excess protein being "burned off"; in other words, some calories ingested as protein will not enter the energy balance equation and therefore, according to this theory, don't really count. Unfortunately, there is no scientific evidence to support this theory. Excess amino acids (the building blocks of proteins) are converted into glucose or fat for storage. No food can "burn" fat. Body fat is "burned" or reduced only by the body's using more energy than is supplied by food eaten.

Especially popular in the 1970s, this is the type of diet that provides a quick and substantial, but only temporary, weight loss, because fatty acids are incompletely broken down. The technical name for this process is ketosis, and it can lead to an acid and alkaline imbalance. Ketone bodies, formed when fat deposits are broken down for energy more quickly than the body can use them, must be excreted in the urine. The dieter thus loses water—and weight—in the process. But the loss is not of body fat and is quickly regained when normal eating is resumed.

3. *Low-carbohydrate, high-fat* diets (Dr. Atkins' Diet Revolution, Drinking Man's, Air Force, Mayo) hold that the ketotic state produced by increased fat consumption accelerates elimination of many "energy-rich" substances from the body. In addition, these programs induce water loss and dehydration and are usually low in certain vitamins and minerals. As these diets are generally unpleasant, they offer no hope of a permanent change in eating habits necessary for the maintenance of lower body weight. Another reason for quick weight loss with these ketogenic diets is that the body is getting energy from "lean body mass" (muscles and other organs) rather than fat. While the body must expend 3,500 calories to burn off a pound of body fat, only about 480

calories are needed to get rid of a pound of lean body mass. Balanced diets contain enough carbohydrates to provide glucose (a form of sugar), the body's basic energy source. But when carbohydrates are lacking, the body must obtain glucose from protein in muscles and major organs such as the heart.

4. *High complex carbohydrate* diets (Pritikin, Macrobiotic, Duke University Rice, F-plan) are considered more nutritionally sound. In addition to stressing consumption of unrefined CARBOHYDRATES, they allow considerable amounts of fruits as well as protein in the form of nuts, beans, peas or fish. But because of the low fat content of these dishes, they tend to be bland, unappetizing and boring. In some, the high fiber content may produce bloating and flatulence. Because of the monotony of these programs, many dieters consume less than the recommended portions and thus may experience vitamin and mineral deficiencies, particularly of calcium. The nature of these diets may promote cheating and rarely motivates dieters to make a lifelong commitment to them.

5. *Specific food* diets are based on the theory that certain foods accelerate fat breakdown. The most commonly recommended foods include grapefruit and eggs. Other substances claimed to be "fatbusters" include bananas, a combination of bananas and skim milk, apple cider vinegar, kelp, vitamin B-6 and lecithin. There is no evidence that these foods or combinations of foods accelerate fat breakdown. In addition, high fruit intake can cause diarrhea. These diets are nutritionally deficient and offer no hope of lifelong changes in eating habits.

6. *Liquid protein* diets (Optifast, NaturSlim) are said to suppress appetite. They cause dehydration and can lead to headaches, nausea, muscle weakness and even death. One extreme form of this type of diet, containing fewer than 400 calories a day, was linked to 17 deaths in 1977 and 1978. Scientists who studied the deaths found that the dieters had died of irregular heart rhythms and cardiac arrest. The Food and Drug Administration now requires warning labels on weight reduction products when more than 50 percent of the product's calories come from protein. Other VERY LOW CALORIE liquid and powdered products have appeared on the market recently with lower proportions of protein. But any diet of fewer than 800 calories a day is potentially dangerous and should be undertaken only under medical supervision.

Willis, Judith Levine. "How to Take Weight Off (and Keep It Off) without Getting Ripped Off." *FDA Consumer*, DHHS Publication No. (FDA) 89-1116, U.S. Food and Drug Administration, 1989.

fake fat   Popular name for all-natural FAT SUBSTITUTES.

family meal   A therapy technique in which an eating-disordered patient and family members eat meals together with a therapist, who helps them identify dysfunctional communication patterns within the family that perpetuate the patient's disorder. Unsubstantiated claims of dramatic recovery have been made by proponents of this technique.

Rockwell, W. J. Kenneth. "A Critique of Treatment Methods for Anorexia Nervosa." In *Eating Disorders: Effective Care and Treatment*, edited by Félix E. F. Larocca. St. Louis: Ishiyaku EuroAmerica, 1986.

family therapy   A form of GROUP THERAPY in which a therapist works with a patient and her family together; sometimes called familization therapy. Generally, a family therapy group consists of one therapist and three or more family members. In working with a family, a therapist can assess the impact of the individual's behavior on the family and observe the handling of conflicts, family roles, family decision making and communication patterns and family values. This therapy is meant to teach all members of a family how to express and fulfill their needs and change old patterns that have been mutually unsatisfactory. It can help both patients and their families bring painful emotions to the surface and understand them. The duration of family therapy varies with individual cases. Family therapy can be especially useful in treating eating disorders of adolescents and may be helpful to young adults struggling with separation from their original families.

European treatment of eating disorders, primarily anorexia nervosa, has traditionally favored family therapy, following precepts established in Italy by Mara Selvini-Palazzoli. But family therapy alone has yet to provide universally the kind of spectacular outcome that was once hoped for and publicly predicted. The current trend in most European centers treating eating disorders is, as in the United States, toward a "multidimensional" approach, with family therapy included in treatment.

Vanderlinden and Vandereycken, of the University Psychiatric Center, Kortenberg, Belgium, have suggested that neglect of the family in bulimia treatment by many therapists may be attributed to the attitude of the bulimics themselves, who tend to conceal their problem from the world. And, they add, the absence of consideration of family context in the literature of bulimia may be explained by the higher average age of bulimics than anorectics, so that many no longer live with their families.

Family Generation of Eating Disorders
Addictive diseases like eating disorders are usually identifiable as family illnesses. Families often get as sick as addicts or eating-disordered patients. Bulimics use food as a way of dealing with stress and problems of daily living, but families have no such outlet and often face the problems without knowledge, understanding or coping skills. In most cases, family members fail to recognize the unhealthy relationships and behaviors that have brought them so much discontent. They are trapped in an unhealthy family equilibrium, exacerbating and prolonging the problem.

Women with anorexia or bulimia often come from families that have difficulty with conflict and communication. Sometimes the families have long histories of conflict. As children, the patients may have experienced abuse or rejection or grown up with an alcoholic parent. Members of these families may have had difficulty communicating and recognizing one another's feelings. The parents, having perhaps grown up in such families themselves, may never have learned how to handle problems, thus experiencing frightening difficulties in their own marriages or with their children.

In the face of unresolved family conflict, daughters may focus on how they can make things better. Frequently, they feel that their parents want them to be good and not cause trouble. They may think that if they stay out of the way and do everything right, things will get better. They see their role as peacemakers. When conflict arises, they may feel they must make it better for everyone. This can lead to their discounting their own feelings and needs. Like their parents, they have not had the opportunity to learn how to deal with their emotions. They may develop eating disorders as a way to cope. On the surface, it may seem that they are able to handle things, but they still need nurturing and support.

A daughter in this situation may not feel recognized by her family as being a helpful negotiator. For a young woman with bulimia, feeding herself is a way of covering up painful feelings and giving herself the nurturing she needs. PURGING functions as a way to release tension and sometimes bury feelings.

Bulimia and anorexia are commonly found in families that are excessively protective of members' feelings. Eating-disordered individuals may have difficulty learning from mistakes because they have rarely been allowed to make any. Lack of control in their lives may compel them to start controlling their weight; their bodies are among the few things over which they feel they have any authority.

Bulimics and anorectics may also come from families that have problems expressing unpleasant emotions and strive to present themselves as "perfectly" well adjusted. Everything appears to be fine in this type of family. Under the surface are problems that no one in the family can or wants to acknowledge. A daughter, also afraid of expressing her feelings, may deal with them through food. She, like the rest of the family, has extreme difficulty admitting that they have any problems. She is very out of touch with her feelings and may have little idea why she binge eats or restricts. (See BINGE-ING; RESTRICTOR ANORECTICS.)

In one report, more than 90 percent of the eating-disordered patients described their fathers as emotionally distant. Common characteristics of the daughters were low self-esteem, confusion, loneliness, sexual fears, DEPRESSION and a general inability to master developmental tasks. With the absence of emotional support from the fathers, daughters try more to support themselves synthetically, deriving a superficial sense of self-worth from their control over their appearance and their achievement of conformity to an exaggerated ideal of beauty.

Bulimia is also often associated with dysfunctional families. In a family that must face difficult issues such as alcoholism, drug addiction, mental illness or abuse, a daughter may respond by developing an eating disorder.

After treating more than 550 cases of bulimia with family therapy, the Renrew Center in Philadelphia has seen another family type emerge. This one usually centers on the daughter. She may feel guilty about the excessive influence she has on how the family functions and about the attention she gets,

especially from her father. She turns to food to help relieve the guilt.

Family Treatment of Eating Disorders
At Renfrew, a residential facility, a family therapist is assigned to each resident. If family members have come at admission, the first family session is held that day. During treatment, five to eight sessions are usually held. Although family members are always encouraged to attend in person, some sessions may be conducted by conference phone call, to accommodate geographically distant family members. Treatment typically lasts seven to nine weeks.

Family intervention has proven very helpful, also, in treating OBESITY. In a recent study, spouses of obese patients were instructed in the behavioral principles of weight control and were told how to demonstrate good eating habits themselves, to reinforce appropriate eating behavior in their partners. Husband and wives attended sessions together and were encouraged to make a collaborative effort. Weight losses for patients with involved spouses were superior to those with uninvolved spouses and were, in fact, greater than those in any previous study.

Parents can exert an even stronger influence on their children than spouses can on each other. They have an unsurpassed degree of control over the food intake of their young children. Even among older children, the capability of parents to foster new patterns of eating behavior and discourage old ones is substantial.

"Family" can extend beyond spouses and parents to relatives, friends, neighbors and even co-workers. All or any of these represent potential allies or foes in the treatment process. Although active encouragement of failure in treatment is infrequent, subtle discouragement by others may reduce treatment effectiveness. For example, "sabotaging" spouses of obese patients have acknowledged that they feared weight loss would improve their partners' attractiveness, leading to extramarital affairs. In other couples in which both partners are obese, husbands and wives may subtly encourage each other to overeat and not to follow the treatment procedures at home, in order to help them rationalize their own poor eating habits.

Family therapy is often useful in ending this process. In it the entire family unit is designated as the "patient" and treated as a whole. As one member changes, the whole unit must change because of the need for equilibrium in the family. The goal of therapy becomes that of developing new healthy relationships to support the entire family.

Depending on their analysis of family functioning and its evolution during treatment, therapists may decide to work with whole families or meet only with separate subgroups (parents, children, with or without patients).

Brownell, Kelly D., and Stunkard, Albert J. "Behavioral Treatment of Obesity in Children." In *Childhood Obesity*. New York: Warner Books, 1986.
Ganley, Richard M. "Eating Disorders Are Family Affairs." *Renfrew Perspective*, Spring 1988.
Karpell, Merrily. "The Fear of Stepping Out of Line." *Renfrew Perspective*, Fall 1988.
Stierlin, Helm, and Weber, Gunthard. *Unlocking the Family Door: A Systemic Approach to the Understanding and Treatment of Anorexia Nervosa*. New York: Brunner/Mazel, 1989.
Vandereycken, W.; Kog, E.; and Vanderlinden, J. *The Family Approach to Eating Disorders: Assessment and Treatment of Anorexia Nervosa and Bulimia*. New York: PMA, 1989.
Vanderlinden, Johan, and Vandereycken, Walter. "Family Therapy in Bulimia Nervosa." Paper presented at the International Symposium on Eating Disorders in Adolescents and Young Adults, Jerusalem, May 26–28, 1987; reprinted in *BASH Magazine*.

famous eating-disorder patients In recent years several well-known athletes and entertainers have come forward to discuss their eating-disorder problems. The death in 1983 of KAREN CARPENTER, a popular singer, brought on by anorexia, inspired many of these women to make public their own bouts with anorexia and bulimia in the hope of influencing young people into seeking treatment. Olympic gymnast Cathy Rigby had been bulimic for four years when she retired at age 19, and her problem continued when she started her new career in sports broadcasting and commercials. She was 28 before she started getting professional help.

Ballerina Gelsey Kirkland starved herself periodically while a teenager and later learned to vomit to keep her weight down. In her autobiography, (*Dancing on My Grave*, Garden City NY: Doubleday, 1986) she talks about her pursuit of the body beautiful.

Cherry Boone O'Neill, daughter of singer Pat Boone, described her bout with anorexia in her book *Starving for Attention* (New York: Continuum, 1982). Actress and political activist Jane Fonda was bulimic for many years. Actress Ally Sheedy was both bulimic and anorectic.

John Lennon, the late Beatle, has been described by biographer Albert Goldman (*The Lives of John Lennon*, New York: William Morrow, 1988) as being anorectic for most of his adult life. Goldman says that Lennon starved himself to what he perceived as perfection. The onset of his disorder can be traced to 1965, Goldman writes, "when some fool described him in print as the 'fat Beatle.' That phrase struck such a blow to his fragile ego that the wound never healed."

fasting Abstaining from food for a period of time. During the 1960s, several clinics began to use short-term fasts to bring about rapid weight reduction. One reason they became so popular is that fasters no longer feel hungry after the first few days of starvation. However, the severe consequences of the nutritional deficiencies and extensive loss of lean body mass that characterizes clinical starvation prompted investigators to find a safer and more effective dieting treatment. As a result, VERY LOW CALORIE DIETS were developed.

Supervised fasting is one of the simplest methods of weight reduction, but it is best carried out in a medical setting because of the significant risk of complications, and even of sudden death. Risks associated with fasting include hypoglycemia and impaired glucose tolerance, KETOSIS, lactic acidosis, hyperuricemia, loss of nitrogen and lean tissue, hypoalaninemia and hair loss; loss of potassium, sodium, calcium, magnesium and phosphate; reduced kidney function, edema, anuria, hypotension, anemia, alterations in liver function, decreased serum iron binding capacity, gastrointestinal tract changes, nausea and vomiting, alterations in thyroxine metabolism and impaired serum triglyceride metabolism.

In 15 studies, the mean length of treatment was 17 weeks, with mean weight loss of 77 pounds. Few studies report follow-up, and in those that do the results are poor. Supervised fasting is a very expensive technique with poor long-term results.

Female fasting, in the manner of ANOREXIA NERVOSA, is not a new behavior. There is a long history of food-refusing behavior and appetite control by women dating from medieval times, practiced for reasons of mystical piety rather than physical vanity, as in the life of St. Catherine of Siena (1347–1380) and her imitators. A more recognizably modern version of the phenomenon became widespread in the 19th century (see FASTING GIRLS).

Benedict, Francis Gano. *A Study of Prolonged Fasting.* Washington, D.C.: Carnegie Institution of Washington, 1915; University Microfilms International, Ann Arbor, Mich. and London.

Duhamel, Denise. "Holding Fast." *American Health,* May 1990.

Graham, Janis. "Food File: Is Fasting Worth It?" *Health,* July 1991.

Segal, Marian. "A Sometime Solution to a Weighty Problem." *FDA Consumer,* April 1990.

Thompson, Trisha, and McCarthy, Laura Flynn. "The Fasting Controversy." *Harper's Bazaar,* January 1992.

fasting girls   The term used by Victorians on both sides of the Atlantic to describe cases of prolonged abstinence from food by girls or young women, in which there was uncertainty about the reasons for fasting and the intentions of the fasters. The term was used jokingly by some and disparagingly by others. Doctors generally spoke of fasting girls with skepticism. The controversy over fasting girls intensified the arguments about the relationship between mind and body that were central to the Victorian debate about religion and science. Reports of fasting girls appeared in the American press as late as 1910. Sustained food refusal was still regarded by most as a religious or supernatural phenomenon rather than a psychological disorder; it fed on a strain of religious piety and supernatural belief more common then than now. The "fasting girls" phenomenon was of widespread interest, drawing the attention of the educated and the uneducated, the elite and the ordinary. But the character of society was changing, and during this time refusal of food changed from an act of personal piety to a symptom of a disorder; physicians changed their diagnoses from anorexia mirabilis to anorexia nervosa.

Brumberg, Joan Jacobs. *Fasting Girls.* Cambridge: Harvard University Press, 1988.

fat cells   The fatty or ADIPOSE TISSUE of the body. Fat is a soft, solid, yellow, slightly greasy material that lies under the skin. When an excessive amount accumulates, it tends to build up in the thigh, hip, abdomen or neck areas. The resultant bulges are generally considered both unhealthy and unattractive. Once accumulated, these fat deposits frequently remain a permanent part of the body, as only a few people have the patience, willpower and energy to diet and exercise them away.

About 95 percent of body fat is stored in the form of triglycerides, composed of fatty acids bound to glycerol. When required for energy METABOLISM, triglycerides are broken down within fatty cells. The fatty acid component then attaches to a specific protein in the blood (lipoprotein) for transport to the muscles. Fat cells are constantly active, dispensing fat into the bloodstream for transport to the body tissues needing energy, and extracting other circulating molecules for conversion into fat to replenish the storage deposits.

Evolving research suggests that the size and number of fat cells (adipocytes) may play a role in the predisposition to obesity. Obese individuals have slightly larger and significantly more fat cells than normal-weight individuals. A greater number of fat cells is particularly characteristic of juvenile-onset obesity.

There are two important periods of development when the number of fat cells is affected: infancy (up to two years of age) and the preadolescent years (from nine to 12). A correlation is believed to exist between the number of fat cells and the rapidity of weight gain. Once fat cells have formed, they cannot be eliminated, so they must be shrunk—depleted of lipids—before an obese individual can reach normal weight. Individuals who have been obese since childhood regain lost weight more rapidly after dieting.

Once produced, fat cells do not die. When weight is lost by diminishing fat stores, existing fat cells shrink, but they are primed to manufacture and store fat more efficiently once a normal diet is resumed. This is the reason for the "yo-yo" effect of rapid weight loss and gain experienced by so many dieters (see YO-YO DIETING).

According to John A. McCurdy, Jr., the evolutionary process has favored survival of those who are able efficiently to convert food into fat for storage. Some bodies are better at storing fat than others. Stored fat is available for use as an energy source during times of food deprivation—famine, pestilence and other disasters that have often beset humanity. But in societies like ours, where food is readily available, the body seldom has an opportunity to call on its fat reserves and gradually accumulates additional fat in its storage deposits, a phenomenon sometimes called CREEPING OBESITY. When these fat reserves are used during dieting, the body naturally becomes more "fuel efficient," lowering its metabolic rate and decreasing spontaneous activity in order to conserve the fat that, in ancient times, enhanced the ability to survive.

The body can increase the amount of body fat in only two ways: by producing more fat cells, or by storing more fat in the existing fat cells. But fat cells can expand just so far and then can reach their capacity of stored fat. At one time, researchers believed that a body's number of fat cells was set by puberty. It is now known that the number of fat cells can continue to increase, doing so when existing fat cells fill to their capacity.

The body cannot eliminate existing fat cells, either through dieting or exercise; they simply shrink in size. The only way researchers have discovered to eliminate fat cells is through surgery. After years of removing fat surgically from various areas of the body, and after observing injuries in which fat tissue has been lost, doctors have determined that fat is usually not redeposited in the treated areas as long as diet and exercise are sufficient to keep the number of fat cells from increasing.

See also DISTRIBUTION OF BODY FAT; LIPOSUCTION; SET-POINT THEORY.

"Body Fat: The Hormone Factor." *Science News*, June 15, 1991.
Hirsch, J.; Fried, S. K.; Edens, N. K.; and Leibel, R. L. "The Fat Cell." *Medical Clinics of North America* 73 (January 1989).
McCurdy, John A., Jr. *Sculpturing Your Body: Diet, Exercise and Lipo (Fat) Suction.* Hollywood, Fla.: Frederick Fell Publishers, 1987.

"fat" doctors   A derisive term given by the medical profession during the 1960s to certain "reducing" doctors who, together with drug companies, created an entire industry devoted to treating obesity with "rainbow pills," various combinations of drugs (since prohibited by the Food and Drug Administration), offered in different colors, to be used at different times of day. In 1968, following the death of several patients from indiscriminate prescription of such diet pills, *Life* magazine published an exposé of these practices.

To research the exposé, a reporter, a young woman who at five feet five inches and 123 pounds had never had a weight problem, visited 10 doctors in different parts of the United States who were nationally or locally known for their easy reducing procedures. In each instance she was either put through a meaningless routine examination or just measured and weighed, and then was given varying numbers of multicolored pills. The pills contained various combinations of AMPHETAMINES, thyroid and digitalis and were prescribed with the recommendation that they be purchased at the doctors' own drug counters. A Kansas City doctor simply handed her a box of 140 pink, brown, tan and gray pills, charged her $10 and told her to return in one month. A Virginia doctor gave her 150 amphetamine-thyroid-barbiturate combination pills. And a Miami Beach doctor gave her a similar combination plus diuretics and laxatives, told her she could now eat 4,000 calories a day and lose weight, and asked her to return in a week.

There was no consensus among the fat doctors concerning diets; some advised that with these pills she could eat anything she wanted, and others offered elaborate restricted diets. The doctors also all prescribed varying degrees of exercise and liquid consumption.

With the FDA crackdown on doctors—both legitimate and fraudulent—who engage in such practices, the lucrative business of selling diet pills expanded into mail order, which is more difficult to regulate. In the late 1980s, Susan Gilbert found it flourishing. "Eat all day and still lose weight" was the headline of a typical ad published in 1987.

Bender, Arnold E. *Health or Hoax?* Buffalo, N.Y.: Prometheus Books, 1986.
Gilbert, Susan. *Medical Fakes and Frauds.* New York: Chelsea House, 1989.

fat power   A term used by advocates of a movement toward greater social acceptance for the overweight, reflecting a nationwide trend of changing attitudes. "Fat power" advocates point to the commercial success of products, services and media personalities as evidence of this shift. There are now dating services for overweight people, magazines like *Radiance* and *Big Beautiful Woman* and clothing being designed for the large-sized by such well-known names as Pierre Cardin. Among the euphemisms for obesity promoted by pro-fat groups are "size positive," "fat-positive" and "plus-sized."

See also CULTURAL INFLUENCES ON APPEARANCE.

fat recycling   Also called fat grafting; the technique of removing fat cells from one part of the body and using them in another. It is a further refinement of liposuction.

Fat recycling is a relatively new and still-evolving cosmetic surgery technique in which fat removed during liposuction can be injected into the hollows between chin and cheek, for example, during face-lifts.

See also COSMETIC SURGERY; LIPOSUCTION.

fat substitutes   Artificial fat replacement substances developed by major food processing and manufacturing companies during the late 1980s and early 1990s. SIMPLESSE (NutraSweet), a low-calorie milk-protein-and-egg-white substance, was the first all-natural substitute to win approval from the Food and Drug Administration. Initial FDA approval for Simplesse was for use only in frozen dessert products. OLESTRA, a cooking-oil replacement developed by Procter & Gamble and under review by the FDA, is, on the other hand, heat resistant and could be used in baked goods, fried foods and snacks.

According to the company, Olestra is "almost a carbon copy of regular fat, but with a molecule of sugar at its core instead of glycerine, and up to eight fatty acids attached to the core instead of customary three."

Since these two products were introduced, the fat replacement field has become quite crowded; supermarket shelves are bulging with products aimed at what is anticipated to be a billion-dollar annual market. Among these additional fat substitutes have been Stellar, made from cornstarch by A. E. Staley Manufacturing, and Slendid, made out of pectin extracted from citrus peels, developed by Hercules Inc. Procter & Gamble has developed Caprenin, a low-calorie fat that can replace cocoa butter in candy bars such as the new Milky Way II bar. Caprenin has only five calories a gram instead of the nine calories a gram in other fats. Its "secret" ingredient is behenic acid, a substance not easily metabolized by the body.

Some analysts say that the use of these low- or nonfat substitutes will revolutionize the food processing industry, dramatically increasing sales and consumption. But others feel that fat-substitute products will only take sales from existing processed food products.

The medical community has been cautious about the introduction of these fake fats. It will take some time before adequate studies are completed; to date, however, no data show that eating a fat substitute will help lower or even maintain body weight—unless overall calories are cut.

In fact, some concern is expressed that people will eat even more calories because of the fake fat. For example, a piece of fat-free cake that has 160 calories is more "fattening" than an apple that has only 65 calories and is also fat free. But nutritionists fear that a population addicted to sugar and chocolate will now feel the fat-free cake gives them an excuse to indulge.

Segal, Marian. "Fat Substitutes: A Taste of the Future?" *FDA Consumer*, December 1990.

fats One of the three main classifications of nutrients (see CARBOHYDRATES and PROTEINS), fats belong to a class of compounds known as lipids. They are derived from both animal and plant foods, but they differ chemically from each. Those originating from animal sources are saturated fats; fats from plants are usually unsaturated fats (see FATS, SATURATED; FATS, UNSATURATED). One exception is coconut oil, which is highly saturated and is widely used in food processing. Both saturated and unsaturated fats have the same caloric value, about nine calories per gram, more than twice that of carbohydrates and proteins (four calories per gram). (Some studies indicate that fat may have up to 11 calories per gram.)

Fat serves as the body's major store of energy, and METABOLISM of this substance supplies approximately 90 percent of energy requirements during prolonged EXERCISE. The higher caloric value of fat makes it a more efficiently convertible source of energy for storage than protein or carbohydrate.

The American Heart Association recommends limiting calories eaten as fat to the 20 to 30 percent range instead of the 40 to 50 percent typical of most Americans. Diets consisting of less than 20 percent fat generally lack sufficient taste and palatability for faithful adherence; much below 10 percent for a prolonged period could cause serious health problems or even death. Some fat must be included in a diet because fat serves as a carrier for several important vitamins including A, D, E and K. Very low fat diets may result in deficiency of these "fat-soluble" vitamins. Nevertheless, dedicated fat-free purists strive to eliminate all fats from their diets.

Editors of *Prevention* Magazine. *Understanding Vitamins and Minerals.* Emmaus, Pa.: Rodale Press, 1984.

McCurdy, John A., Jr. *Sculpturing Your Body: Diet, Exercise and Lipo (Fat) Suction.* Hollywood, Fla.: Frederick Fell Publishers, 1987.

fats, saturated Fats whose chemical composition includes the maximum possible quantity of hydrogen. They come primarily from animals and are often hard at room temperature. They tend to raise blood cholesterol levels. Examples of saturated fats are butter, lard, meat fat, solid shortening, palm oil, and coconut oil.

From a nutritional standpoint, some saturated fat is essential for proper growth and metabolism; a deficiency can lead to eczema and other skin disorders.

See also CHOLESTEROL; FATS; FATS, UNSATURATED.

fats, unsaturated Fats that include fatty acids whose chemical composition includes some sites on the carbon atom unoccupied by hydrogen. When many sites are vacant, they are called polyunsaturated. Unsaturated fats are capable of absorbing additional hydrogen. They are also known as free fatty acids because of their free bonds that allow them to take on more hydrogen atoms. They come from plants and are usually liquid at room temperature. Examples are vegetable oils such as corn, cottonseed, sunflower, safflower, soybean, olive and peanut. Unsaturated fats tend to lower blood cholesterol levels.

See also CHOLESTEROL; FATS; FATS, SATURATED.

fear of fat syndrome Behavior resulting from an exaggerated concern about gaining weight, not classifiable as a serious disorder such as BULIMIA or anorexia. Fear of fat syndrome is much more common than ANOREXIA NERVOSA and affects younger children.

There are both boys and girls as young as seven who experience fear of fat and on occasion diet and skip meals. They are not anorectic—they don't have an obsessive wish to be thinner—but they are obsessed with not gaining weight. This dieting before their bodies are fully formed can lead to stunted growth, a stunting of development of heart muscle and delaying of puberty. If children stop dieting, damage is usually temporary; but if they diet strenuously for more than six months, they are not likely to grow that year. Frequently this fear of fat is seen in children who are not fat to begin with.

Often the extra baby fat that appears right before puberty inspires panic dieting. Because this baby fat is not extra calories stored as fat, it does not respond well to dieting, which only increases anxiety, producing more rigorous attempts to diet. Children will frequently conceal this dieting, explaining that they are not eating dinner because they have to go somewhere, or that they ate at a friend's house or on the way home.

One study evaluated disturbed eating behaviors and attitudes among 326 adolescent girls attending an upper-middle-class parochial high school. The students reported an exaggerated concern with obesity regardless of body weight or knowledge of nutrition. Underweight, normal-weight and overweight girls were dieting to lose weight and reported frequent self-weighing. As many as 51 percent of the underweight adolescents described themselves as extremely fearful of being overweight, and 36 percent were preoccupied with body fat. The frequency of BINGE EATING and VOMITING behaviors was similar in the three weight categories. The data suggested that fear of fat and inappropriate eating behaviors are pervasive among adolescent girls regardless of body weight or nutrition knowledge.

Recent university studies of college-age women have revealed this same fear of fat syndrome. Eighty percent of the 1,335 female students in a University of Florida study said they had dieted during the past year; the average respondent was five feet five inches tall and weighed 122 pounds, well within the low-to-normal weight range. An Ohio State University study found that 67 percent of the female respondents had some kind of disordered eating pattern.

Fear of fat appears to be deeply ingrained in our society; we have cultural preoccupation with slimness. Television, magazines and even the classroom promote the goal of thinness for reasons of both beauty and health. Even medical doctors and other expert sources promote a "healthier" dietary intake. This social phenomenon not only has an impact on adult and adolescent eating habits but may also influence those of young children. Notions regarding body weight and appearance are formed very early in life. In fact, elementary school children have been shown to perceive obesity as being worse than being handicapped or disabled.

According to *U.S. News & World Report* (February 19, 1990), data compiled from a *Los Angeles Times* poll and National Center for Health statistics show that while 34 million adults in the United States *are* overweight, twice that many think they are.

See also CULTURAL INFLUENCES ON EATING DISORDERS; DIETING.

Moses, Nancy; Banilivy, Mansour-Max; and Lifshitz, Fima. "Fear of Obesity among Adolescent Girls." *Pediatrics* 83 (March 1989).

fenfluramine   A drug used in the treatment of obesity. It raises the level of SEROTONIN in the brain, which in essence tricks the mind into believing that the stomach is full. The theory behind its use is that, while not causing weight loss, it allows it by suppressing appetite. Early studies show it to be most effective on carbohydrate cravers. The most common adverse reactions to fenfluramine are drowsiness, diarrhea and dry mouth; it is also known to be potentially addictive.

Buckley, William Thomas. "The Feel-Full Pill." *Health,* January 1989.
"Dexfenfluramine." *Lancet,* Vol. 337 June 1, 1991.
Wurtman, Judith, and Wurtman, Richard. "Fenfluramine Selectively Suppresses Carbohydrate Snacking by Obese Subjects." *International Journal of Eating Disorders* 1985; 4 (April 1985).

fiber   An edible, but indigestible, part of certain foods. Fiber is important in the diet as roughage, or bulk. Fiber is found in starches, breads, vegetables and fruit.

See also DIETARY FIBER.

food addiction   Some popular writings on the subject of food have postulated the existence of a disorder they call "food addiction." Loosely construed, the concept of addiction might be said to apply to compulsive or disordered eating of certain foods, most commonly those high in sugar or starch content, but there is no scientific basis for believing that any ordinary food substance is literally physiologically addictive in the same sense as a narcotic drug. So-called food addiction is more plausibly understood as an expression of a psychological disorder, response to an unacceptably intense condition of emotional deprivation, anxiety or tension. In other words, the idea of food addiction is not medically or scientifically valid.

See also ANOREXIA NERVOSA; BODY IMAGE DISTURBANCE; BODY WRAPPING; BULIMIA NERVOSA; COMPULSIVE EATING; DEPRESSION; DIET PILLS; DIETING; FAD DIETS; FAT DOCTORS; OBESITY; PERSONALITY DISORDERS; SELFESTEEM; SOCIAL FACTORS IN OBESITY; STRESS AND EATING DISORDERS.

food allergy   A chronic condition in which there is a consistent physiological reaction to a certain food or foods. To be a true allergy, according to the American Academy of Allergy and Immunology, the condition must involve an *immunologic response* to a food protein by an allergy-specific immunoglobulin (antibody). Most food allergy symptoms are manifested on the skin (pruritus, erythema, hives, eczema, edema) or in the gastrointestinal tract (vomiting, diarrhea, abdominal pain).

Most adverse reactions to foods are nonimmunologic and therefore not allergic. Nonimmunologic responses, properly termed food intolerances, can usually be traced to toxicity, enzyme deficiencies or anaphylactoid, or pharmacologic or metabolic reactions. Headache, fatigue, muscle and joint pain and anxiety are symptoms that may be attributable to a reaction to food but not to an allergic reaction.

True allergic reactions occur most commonly in children, among whom the incidence is around 5 percent; in adults the figure is closer to 3 percent. Ninety percent of allergic reactions are caused by a relatively few foods, including milk, eggs, legumes, nuts, soy and wheat. Very severe reactions, which are called anaphylactic, are most often caused by fish, shellfish and, to a lesser extent, citrus fruits, melons, bananas, tomatoes, corn, rice and celery. Food allergy is difficult to diagnose by history and objective tests, such as skin or blood testing. It is an area of medicine in which much scientific work remains to be done, by immunologists and others.

Difficulty in diagnosis has led to a host of controversial diagnostic techniques. The most common include direct sublingual (under the tongue) or subcutaneous (under the skin) application of a suspected allergenic substance, and leukocytotic assays, in which foods are mixed with samples of patients' blood and analysis is based on the shape of the white blood cells. The trouble with the latter test is the lack of correlation between symptoms and results. Frequently a history is not recorded.

The most influential group advocating these controversial techniques, and the subsequent treatment of food allergies by avoidance of up to 300 foods, consists of the authors of popular books and articles who have made themselves widely known as "clinical ecologists" by mass media promotion. Their theories may sound plausible on TV, but all DOUBLE-BLIND, well-organized scientific studies conducted by major medical centers have shown such therapies to be no better than placebos. Many patients who have been diagnosed by these techniques are not aware that they are of questionable validity. Some

patients have underlying psychological disturbances and are misled by test results to blame food for their troubles; blame for tension fatigue syndrome, hyperactivity, schizophrenia and nonspecific neurotic and psychiatric syndromes of various kinds has been mistakenly attributed to food allergy.

Belief in this pseudoallergy theory, as it is called, is widespread; it offers a simple explanation for many complex health problems, and it has an aura of scientific rationality about it. In this way a belief system has been created that is very difficult for legitimate medical thinking to challenge. In some ways it resembles a cult. Orthodox allergists feel frustrated when treating patients who are believers, because they know that allergy is an area of medicine still lacking objective tools for diagnosis, and that is not a message patients want to hear.

It is important to point out that allergy patients may be in the care of other physicians who are too often incompletely informed about allergies and who may in effect be adding to the problem. These patients by and large do not get better, especially when there are underlying psychological disorders that go untreated.

A well-monitored elimination diet, followed by double-blind oral food challenges in a controlled setting performed by allergists, is the only method known thus far that comes close to diagnosing accurately food allergy and intolerance (and it may not be prudent when there is a history of severe allergic reaction). It takes time and is not simple. The history must record both immediate reactions—typically at 20 to 30 minutes, when the response is most acute—and later reaction in the six-to-12-hour period, which sometimes persists up to 48 hours. Knowledge of cross-reactivity with other foods and inhalants is imperative. Food-induced responses may be aggravated by viral infections, inhalant allergies or irritants, exercise or simultaneous exposure to another food to which a lesser sensitivity exists.

Food allergies can be deceptive and may sometimes be mistaken for pollen allergies. For example, tearing or reddening of the eyes may be caused by an allergy to wheat or by an allergy to cat hairs.

Food allergies can cause excessive urination, urinary tract infections, prostate disorders, gynecological problems, swollen eyelids, irregular heartbeat, high blood pressure, muscle aches and pains, chest pains, abdominal spasms or swelling. But the most common symptoms are fatigue and sleeplessness. Often experienced at its worst in the morning, food allergy fatigue can be accompanied by general weakness, drowsiness and a sensation of heavy limbs.

Many inherited allergies start in childhood. There have been recorded cases of sensitivity to milk, fruit, vegetables and fish that reach back two or three generations. In addition, too much exposure to one kind of food at one time may overwhelm the immune system and trigger the allergic process. The most common cause of allergy, other than heredity, is lack of variety in the diet. Food allergies also may begin after serious health problems or major psychological stress.

Depending on the interaction between allergens, symptoms can continue from seven to 10 days, sometimes longer, as is often seen with wheat. It takes four days for food to pass through the gastrointestinal tract—longer if the patient does not have a normal pattern of bowel movements. Frequent exposure to the same food can cause the patient to carry four or five doses spaced at different intervals along the gastrointestinal tract, thus prolonging the reaction.

Anderson, J. "Introduction to Food Allergy, Science and Reason." *Allergy Proceedings* 7, no. 6 (1986).
Brody, Jane. "Food Allergies: A Growing Controversy." *New York Times Magazine,* April 29, 1990.
Ferguson, Anne. "Food Sensitivity or Self-Deception?" *New England Journal of Medicine* 323: 7 (August 16, 1990).
Hunter, J. O. "Food Allergy—or Enterometabolic Disorder?" *Lancet,* August 24, 1991.
Linkford, Patricia, and Katsantonis, George. "Food Allergies Exist but You Probably Don't Have One." *BASH Magazine,* December 1989.

forced feeding Feeding accomplished through invasive tubes in the nose or by a new process called total parenteral nutrition.

Forced feeding is the most dramatic treatment for anorexia. In severe cases, in which body weight falls to dangerous levels, parents and physicians may decide to admit an anorectic to a hospital for forced feeding on the grounds that it will prevent her death and restore her to a mental state that will make meaningful therapeutic interaction possible. In these critical cases physicians recommend "renourishment" or "refeeding" because they believe that the biological effects of starvation create a psychological prison from which patients cannot escape. In this view, the anorectic must gain a certain amount of weight before she can progress in psychotherapy or make rational decisions about treatment.

See also HYPERALIMENTATION.

fraudulent products With so many people striving to lose weight and dealing with FEAR OF FAT SYNDROME, it is little wonder that unscrupulous promoters prey on those looking for "miracle" cures. The NATIONAL ASSOCIATION TO AID FAT ACCEPTANCE (NAAFA) takes an active interest in the battle against health frauds, including weight loss scams, and maintains a membership in the National Council Against Health Fraud.

One example reported in the *NAAFA Newsletter* was the widely promoted "Fat Magnet" diet pill that became the target of action by the U.S. Postal Service. Placing a temporary restraining order on mail received by the Beverly Hills company promoting this product, the Postal Service alleged that the solicitations contained such false representations as "The substance in the Fat Magnet

can attract, bind, and flush out body fat.''
In March 1990, NAAFA reported that the
Federal Trade Commission had frozen the
assets of Allied International, manufacturer
of the ''Fat Magnet.'' The U.S. District
Court was to hear the case, based on false
and misleading advertising. Advertisements
for the product claimed that the pills ''break
into thousands of particles, each acting like
a tiny magnet, attracting and trapping many
times its size in undigested fat particles . . .
then, all the trapped fat and calories are
naturally flushed out of the body'' (*NAAFA
Newsletter*, March 1990). The FTC asked
for an injunction to force the firm to cease
sales and to issue $5 million in refunds. On
April 11, 1991, the FTC announced that the
manufacturer had agreed to establish an es-
crow fund for consumer redress.

Another example was Dream-Away and
Advanced Dream-Away, the manufacturer
of which was ordered to pay $1.1 million in
refunds to consumers who bought their products. Promoters claimed that, by simply taking their pills, one could lose weight while
sleeping.

The Food and Drug Administration reports that one out of six people uses a fraudulent product in the course of a year. On the
FDA's top 10 list of health frauds are instant
weight loss schemes, often advertised in
magazines or newspapers. This makes weight
loss pretty much a wide-open market, according to FDA staffers, who cannot check
or control every item being offered.

Another group of products being watched
by both the FDA and the Better Business
Bureau are anti-CELLULITE products, which
proliferate during bathing suit season. Many
of these ''cures'' are imports from France,
where consumer protection is less stringent.
Even the better-known cosmetics companies
have recently been risking federal regulators'
ire by entering the $20 million anti-cellulite
market. The FDA's primary concern is
whether marketers claim their products conceal or actually eliminate this fat (which
would classify them as drugs). In 1987 the

FDA filed complaints against 23 cosmetics
companies for unapproved products that make
such claims. Since then, an additional 50
have been filed. Thus far, no product has
received FDA approval to claim it will actually eliminate cellulite.

Darnton, Nina. ''The Battle of the Bulges.''
 Newsweek, March 2, 1992.
Diamond, S. J. ''Public Is Aware of Diet Fraud.''
 Los Angeles Times, November 1, 1991.
Toufexis, Anastasia. ''Fountain of Youth in a
 Jar.'' *Time*, October 14, 1991.

free fatty acids   Free fatty acids (FFA)
in the blood originate from the release of
ADIPOSE TISSUE triglycerides. They represent
virtually the only route by which these fat
stores can be transferred to nonfat tissue for
net loss via oxidation. Free fatty acid metabolism in obesity has therefore been the
subject of many studies over the last 30
years. Unfortunately, conflicting conclusions regarding several aspects of FFA metabolism have appeared, including the
antilipolytic (lipolysis: the chemical breakdown of fat) effectiveness of insulin in obesity, the relationship of FFA release to the
amount of body fat and the lipolytic responsiveness of obese individuals to catecholamines (secretions).

To determine whether differences in DIS-
TRIBUTION OF BODY FAT result in specific
abnormalities of free fatty acid metabolism,
researchers conducted studies of women of
varying body fat distribution. They concluded that the basal release of FFA from
adipose tissue to meet lean body mass energy
needs is greater in upper-body obese women
than lower-body obese or nonobese women.
The net lipolytic response to epinephrine (a
hormone that acts as a stimulant to several
metabolic processes) is reduced in upper-
body obese women compared with lower-
body obese and nonobese women. Their
results may explain many of the conflicting
reports in the literature regarding FFA metabolism in human obesity and emphasize
the need to characterize the type of obesity

being studied before investigations of FFA metabolism in humans.

G

gallstones Stonelike masses that form in the gallbladder. Gallstones form when cholesterol crystallizes after mixing with acids from the liver. Their cause is unknown, although there is evidence of a connection between gallstones and obesity. Lean women have a better chance of avoiding gallstones; obese men and women trying to lose weight may be more likely to develop them, especially if they resort to severe forms of dieting, since fasting reduces the amount of other acids in the body that dissolve cholesterol. Those are the findings of separate studies that strengthen the association between weight and gallstones.

Even a woman who is moderately overweight—15 to 20 pounds—doubles her risk of developing gallstones, and her risk increases as she puts on more weight, according to a study by the Brigham and Women's Hospital in Boston. A woman who is 75 to 100 pounds overweight is approximately six times more likely to develop gallstones than a woman of normal weight.

Obese people trying to lose weight through extreme and often unhealthy measures such as extended FASTING or caloric restriction may be putting themselves at risk for developing gallstones, according to a University of California at San Francisco study. Thirteen of 51 obese male dieters (25.5 percent) who consumed no more than 500 calories a day for eight weeks developed cholesterol gallstones, and three had a buildup of cholesterol that leads to formation of the stones, the study showed. None of the 26 nondieting controls developed gallstones.

The University of Texas Health Science Center studied 1,202 Mexican Americans and 908 non-Hispanic whites from 1979 to 1982. They selected Mexican Americans for this study of the role of obesity and body fat distribution in gallbladder disease specifically because, statistically, Mexican Americans have a higher incidence of gallbladder disease and also have greater overall adiposity and an unfavorable body fat distribution (upper-body and central adiposity) relative to non-Hispanic whites. Their findings showed central body fat distribution to be a risk factor for clinical gallbladder disease in women, independent of age, ethnic group and overall adiposity.

Bankhead, Charles D. "Plummeting Pounds Gain Blame." *Medical World News*, July 1990.

Haffner, Steven; Diehl, Andrew; Stern, Michael; and Hazuda, Helen. "Central Adiposity and Gallbladder Disease in Americans." *American Journal of Epidemiology* 129 (March 1989).

Maclure, Malcolm; Hayes, K. C.; et al. "Weight, Diet, and the Risk of Symptomatic Gallstones in Middle-Aged Women." *New England Journal of Medicine* 321: 9 (August 31, 1989).

Sichieri, Rosely; Everhart, James; and Roth, Harold. "A Prospective Study of Hospitalization with Gallstone Disease among Women: Role of Dietary Factors, Fasting Period, and Dieting." *American Journal of Public Health* 81: 7 (July 1991).

Garfinkel and Garner Paul E. Garfinkel, M.D. (b. 1946), and David M. Garner, Ph.D. (b. 1947), collaborators in the research and treatment of eating disorders. Garfinkel is psychiatrist-in-chief at Toronto General Hospital and professor of psychiatry at the University of Toronto. Garner is a professor of psychiatry at Michigan State University and the director of research for the Eating Disorders Program there. They developed the widely used EATING ATTITUDES TEST.

Their principal works include *Anorexia Nervosa: A Multidimensional Perspective* (New York: Brunner/Mazel, 1982); *Handbook of Psychotherapy for Anorexia Nervosa and Bulimia* (New York: Guilford Press, 1985); and *The Role of Drug Treatments for*

Eating Disorders (New York: Brunner/Mazel, 1987).

gastric bubble   A compacted plastic balloon inserted into the stomach via a large tube and inflated with air. When the tube is removed, the gastric bubble remains free-floating in the stomach to control appetite. The principle behind it is that limiting the stomach's capacity to store food will force the patient to eat smaller meals. Unlike STOMACH STAPLING, which works on the same principle, there is no risk from surgery, and the balloon can be removed, while stapling is permanent. The procedure has been called a "quick-fix . . . for a generation into instant gratification."

Typically, the operation is performed on an outpatient basis. It takes about 45 minutes for a physician to insert the balloon through a patient's mouth and esophagus, position it in the stomach and inflate it, to about the size of a small frozen-juice can. The patient then spends five days on a liquid diet while becoming accustomed to the balloon. One patient lost 15 pounds in the first two weeks, but once her appetite returned, the pounds came off more slowly.

In testing on animals prior to its use in humans, the stomach adapted to the presence of the balloon by expanding and doubling in weight. There was also an increase in its acid-producing capacity, which could lead to ulcers. In actual use in 70 patients over a period of six months, Lloyd Garren, developer of the balloon, reported that five ulcers resulted. In another study conducted by D. M. Kruss and A. P. Livak of the Hines, Illinois, Veteran's Hospital, patients experienced nausea and diarrhea for two days after insertion, 13 percent of the patients developed ulcers and many other patients reported less severe side effects. In this study patients attained only small, transient weight loss.

The bubble was very popular in the mid-1980s, with 80 to 100 a month being sold by the manufacturer at $165 to $400 each.

One death from complications was reported after 20,000 procedures. However, skepticism on the part of gastroenterologists' professional groups meant that the balloon continued to be regarded primarily as a research device. A flurry of bad publicity and doctors' complaints, mostly about complications and poor results, led the manufacturers to tighten their recommendations, and in 1985 the U.S. Food and Drug Administration recommendation was increased to 100 percent over ideal body weight (it had been approved originally for anyone 25 percent or more overweight), eliminating its use by people without life-threatening conditions, for cosmetic reasons. There was an immediate and sharp drop in demand.

According to a report published in the *Miami Herald*, the manufacturer of the gastric bubble removed the device from the market in 1988 in response to a study conducted at Georgetown University, which concluded that it was ineffective and unsafe. In this study, 90 patients, all described as "very much overweight," were divided into three groups. Some actually had the bubble inserted, and others went through a mock procedure. Real or mock insertion and removal procedures were performed during the course of the study. Neither the patients nor their personal doctors knew whether bubbles were in place at any given time. All patients were given the same low-calorie diet and BEHAVIOR MODIFICATION procedures to follow. The results: all patients, with or without the bubbles, had the same weight loss success rate, but the patients with the bubbles suffered unpleasant side effects not reported by nonbubble patients.

There has been no definitive research done on weight gain or loss after the balloon has been removed.

Barkin, J. S.; Reiner, D. K.; Goldberg, R. I.; Phillips, R. S. "Effects of Gastric Bubble Implant on Weight Change with or without Compliance with a Behavior Modification Program." *American Journal of Gastroenterology* 83: 9 (September 1988).

Kramer, F. M.; Stunkard, A. J.; Spiegel, T. A.; Deren, J. J. et al. "Limited Weight Losses with a Gastric Balloon." *Archives of Internal Medicine* 149 (February 1989).

Zamula, Evelyn. "Stomach 'Bubble': Diet Device Not without Risks." *FDA Consumer,* April 1987.

gastric partition procedures Operations designed to simplify gastric BYPASS SURGERY and to eliminate some of the problems associated with bypass operations. In general, gastric partitioning operations have not quite matched weight loss results associated with gastric bypass operations.

See also GASTRIC RESTRICTION PROCEDURES; STOMACH STAPLING.

gastric restriction procedures Operations used to reduce the volume of food ingested. They have replaced operations aimed at creating malabsorption (by causing food to pass through the digestive tract too quickly for nutrients to be absorbed) in the treatment of patients with morbid (life-threatening) obesity. To be effective, they require patients to accept the premise of eating less. They are not recommended for patients who are food or cola addicts or alcoholics. All forms of gastric restriction operations fail in a certain category of patients who overeat the food provided in a liquid diet and in those who eat continuously; these patients find that they can consume as many milk shakes as they want as long as they drink them slowly, and consequently, they do not lose weight. Gastric restriction procedures include gastric BYPASS SURGERY, gastric partition, and STOMACH STAPLING.

Edward Mason, a pioneer in the field of gastric restriction operations, divided the stomach so that a small pouch was formed, through which the food passed. The small size of the pouch and the small exit from it significantly decrease the amount of food that can be consumed at one sitting. His design was altered in the late 1970s by J. F. Alden, who partitioned the stomach rather

than dividing it. (See GASTRIC PARTITION PROCEDURES.)

Gastric bypass operations can be done with low operative morbidity and mortality and result in a significant postoperative weight loss. Patients undergoing this operation do not experience the problems associated with JEJUNOILEAL BYPASS. These operations can cause a 38 percent weight loss within 12 months, and long-term experience suggests that weight loss is maintained for as long as five years in these patients. Complications include gastric outlet obstruction, vomiting, dumping syndrome (sweating and weakness after eating, associated with rapid emptying of stomach contents into small intestine), gastric leaks, and wound infections. Based on the Diagnostic and Therapeutic Technology Assessment report conducted by an American Medical Association scientific panel, such gastric bypass surgery is slightly preferred over GASTROPLASTY in terms of safety but is still considered experimental by more than a dozen of the 38 panel members and unacceptable by five of them.

In 1991, a National Institutes of Health panel reversed an earlier negative view on surgical procedures for treating severe obesity as newer procedures with fewer complications have been developed.

Pollnar, Fran. "Obesity Surgery Regaining Favor." *Medical World News,* May 1991.

"Psychosocial Effects of Gastric Reduction Surgery for Obesity." *International Journal of Obesity* Vol. 6 (June 1982).

gastroplasty An operation in which the stomach is sectioned; the term encompasses all procedures that divide the stomach into an upper and lower gastric pouch with a stapling device but that do not divide the upper and lower gastric remnants. A modification of gastric BYPASS SURGERY, gastroplasty has not been universally adopted, since patients have not been shown to lose an adequate amount of weight. While not considered quite as safe as the gastric bypass, its effectiveness received comparable marks in a report by the American Medical Association.

In Great Britain, according to Owen, Abraham and Kark, gastric reduction procedures have been shown to produce impressive short-term results in the treatment of morbid obesity. Introduced in 1982, vertical banded gastroplasty or one of its modifications is the most widely used technique and has the fewest reported complications of any surgical weight loss procedure. These stomach operations have almost superseded small intestinal bypass operations, which cause disabling metabolic disturbances. Earlier methods of gastroplasty failed largely because of pouch enlargement and inappropriate dietary supervision.

The original method consisted of a horizontally stapled or sutured pouch with a loop drainage. This was a highly technical procedure, which included all the usual risks of cutting into the stomach and intestines. Next a horizontally stapled pouch with central or lateral drainage was developed, which entailed much simpler technique. Weight loss was unsatisfactory in the majority of cases, however, and the method was abandoned. Failures related directly to varying pouch sizes and resultant pouch distension.

Some food intolerances are common after gastroplasty, especially for red meat, bread and fruit. Constipation is also common, because of the inability to take DIETARY FIBER. Vomiting frequently follows gastric restriction surgery until patients learn to eat smaller amounts. Rapid early weight loss results from the VERY LOW CALORIE (VLC) DIETS that patients are forced to stay on, and it is important that patients do not approach near-starvation calorie levels—hence the need for close supervision by dietitians to avoid the hazards of excess lean tissue loss and to attain a slow, sustained weight loss over nine to 12 months, with stabilization thereafter.

There is no long-term information available on pouch size after five to 10 years.

The very small initial pouch size provides a long time lag before any expansion takes place. By that time, it is hoped, diet and eating habit modifications should be firmly established.

Hocking, M. P.; Kelly, K. A.; and Calloway, C. W. "Vertical Gastroplasty for Morbid Obesity: Clinical Experience." *Mayo Clinic Procedures* 61 (1986).

Makarewicz, P. A.; Freeman, J. B. and Burchett, H. "Vertical Banded Gastroplasty: Assessment of Efficacy." *Surgery* 98 (1985).

Owen, E. R. T. C.; Abraham R.; and Kark, A. E. "Gastroplasty for Morbid Obesity: Technique, Complications and Results in Sixty Cases." *British Journal of Surgery* 76 (February 1989).

genetic factors in eating disorders

There is evidence that eating disorders run in families. Females are particularly vulnerable, and there have been a number of reports of identical twins both developing anorexia nervosa. In some cases, imitative behavior may be a factor. Comparisons of families of anorectics and bulimics with families without eating disorders have found some differences: families of bulimics report more hostile interactions; families of anorectics are as warm and supportive of their children as nondisordered families but have more marital problems. Some mental health specialists theorize that anorectic children serve as "lightning rods" for families who cannot face or resolve their problems. However, most evidence is capable of other explanations, so until more scientifically controlled studies are carried out, a genetic factor in generating eating disorders must remain speculative.

A 1982 study showed that the parents of bulimic and anorectic subjects tended to have particular personality characteristics. Fathers of bulimics were more impulsive and mothers were more depressed, and both reported more dissatisfaction with family relationships than the parents of restrictor anorectics. There was also greater incidence of affective disorder reported in the families of bulimic anorectics.

See also AFFECTIVE DISORDERS AND EATING DISORDERS.

Schepank, H. "Genetic Determinants in Anorexia Nervosa: Results of Twin Studies." *Psychosomatic Medicine Psychoanalysis* 37 (3) (1991).

Strober, Michael. "Family-Genetic Studies of Eating Disorders." *Journal of Clinical Psychiatry* 52: 10 (suppl.) (October 1991).

genetic factors in obesity   Obesity often follows family lines, and evidence from twin studies and other family studies, although not completely consistent, have for some time implied inheritance.

Recent studies have shown that biochemical differences between obese people and those of normal weight are most likely genetic in origin. A Danish study showed that adopted children, as adults, were much more like their biological parents than their adoptive parents in body weight. In this study, adoptees separated from their natural parents very early in life were compared with their biological full and half siblings reared by their natural parents. The adoptees represented groups categorized as thin, medium weight, overweight or obese. Weight and height were obtained for 115 full siblings of 57 adoptees and for 850 half siblings of 341 adoptees. In full siblings, body mass index (weight in comparison with height) similarities significantly increased with weight of the adoptees. The half siblings showed a steady but weaker increase in similarities across the four weight groups of adoptees. There was no significant correlation among sex of the adoptees, sex of the siblings or (for the half siblings) sex of the common parent. In contrast with the findings for half siblings and natural parents, there was a striking, significant increase in body mass index similarities between full siblings of overweight and obese adoptees. Researchers

concluded that the degree of obesity in adults in the same environment appears to be influenced by genetic factors independent of sex, which may include polygenic (deriving from the cumulative action of several genes) as well as major (single) gene effects on obesity.

In another study of identical twins, siblings and nonrelatives, weight gain in response to consumption of excess calories seemed to run in families. Because of these and similar studies, more students of obesity are now looking at metabolism as a biochemical phenomenon that is derived from inherited traits. Some feel that people might differ genetically in fat-cell receptors, some of which promote the breakdown of fat and others, fat accumulation. There may also be an inherited difference in the ability to generate body heat from food, which uses up some of the calories a person consumes. A Swiss study showed that women who had been obese since childhood generated significantly less body heat from a meal than did women of normal weight. Even after weight loss, the obese women showed a deficit in heat production.

In a Canadian study, reported on in 1990, Laval University researchers studied 12 pairs of twins, all thin young men. The twins spent 120 days in a closed section of a dormitory and were fed 1,000 more calories a day than they needed to maintain their weight. One pair of twins gained only nine and a half pounds from the extra 84,000 calories, while another gained 29 pounds. Of the sets of twins that gained the most, one pair gained it more in the abdominal area, and another pair gained more in the buttocks and thighs. Although there were marked differences between the sets of twins, each brother gained almost identically to his twin. The twins who gained the least added more muscle than fat; those who gained the most added more fat than muscle. Conclusions drawn were that genetic factors are likely involved in adaptations to overfeeding, variations in weight gain, fat distribution, tendency to store energy as fat or lean tissue and the various determinants of how energy is metabolized.

In another twin study reported in 1990, University of Pennsylvania researchers studied 93 pairs of identical twins who were reared apart, 154 pairs of identical twins reared together, 218 pairs of fraternal twins reared apart and 208 pairs of fraternal twins reared together. They found that the identical twins had almost identical body mass indices, whether they were reared apart or together. Fraternal twins, on the other hand, showed more differences even if they were reared together.

While these studies have centered on adult obesity, researchers have also pointed to a number of genetic factors that predispose children to obesity. Their parents' own weight is one. In the United States, only 3 to 7 percent of parents with normal weight have obese children. But in families in which one parent is obese, 40 percent of the children are obese; if both parents are obese, 80 percent of the children are obese. This is true only of natural children, not of adopted or foster children.

Another genetic factor is inherited body type. Endomorphic (heavy and rounded) and mesomorphic (husky and muscular) body types increases the likelihood of obesity.

Still another genetic factor is the activity level with which an infant is born. Sixty-two percent of the calories consumed by an infant are used for growth, resting metabolism and defecation; 38 percent are available for physical activity. Extremely thin infants move more and eat more than normal babies, and extensively fat ones move less and eat less. The fatter the baby, the less active it is. This low rate of activity causes a positive energy balance—more calories are consumed than are used up in activity—which is what causes the fat accumulation. This tendency to inactivity stays with obese children.

Bouchard, C. "Genetic Factors in Obesity." *Medical Clinics of North America* 73 (1) (January 1989).

"Heritability of Weight Gain and Obesity" (letters). *New England Journal of Medicine*, 323: 15 October 11, 1990.

Sorenson, Thorkild A.; Price, R. Arlen; Stunkard, Albert J.; and Schulsinger, Fini. "Genetics of Obesity in Adult Adoptees and Their Biological Siblings." *British Medical Journal* 298 (January 14, 1989).

geophagia   A condition in which the patient eats chalk or earth or clay; a type of PICA (the desire to eat inedible substances). After surveying the literature, Isolde Prince concluded that in many cultures geophagia is a common, acceptable, benign practice without psychological implications. In fact, geophagia occurring among nutritionally deprived populations is looked at differently than pica in the Western world, where nutrition is much more likely to be at a satisfactory level.

Although still subject to considerable debate, in nutritionally deprived populations geophagia probably fulfills nutritional needs for elements important for growth and development. These nutritional factors are particularly important during childhood and pregnancy. The main debatable point is whether clay eating provides elements such as iron, zinc and calcium and is a significant treatment for anemia, or whether clays remove these elements from food and give rise to anemia.

An important paradox in the geophagia literature is that even though populations consume earth in significant quantities with impunity, for some individuals earth eating is pathological and even lethal. It has been proposed that this paradox can be resolved by attributing the malignant form to the co-occurrence of sickle-cell anemia. In this interpretation, the malignant *cachexia africana* and perhaps *pobough lang* are not caused by earth eating, but earth eating is an attempt at cure by those who are suffering from a severe, often lethal, hereditary anemia.

Prince, Isolde. "Pica and Geophagia in Cross-Cultural Perspective." *Transcultural Psychiatric Research Review* 26 (1989).

Rudavsky, Shari. "Dirt Eaters of the World, Unite." *Omni*, March 1989.

gloom bulimia Compulsive overeating during times of sadness. Low self-esteem or a helpless reaction to perceived failure or loneliness might be sedated by the absorption of energy, or countered by the sensory pleasures of eating. As a result, gloom could replace depletion as the conditioned or occasioning stimulus for overeating. Memory experiments have provided evidence that sad and happy moods can serve as internal cues.

Excessive eating as a conditioned response to sadness in gloom bulimia can be described as a confusion between HUNGER and the depressed mood. Mood ratings do not consistently change in either direction during BINGE EATING, although anxiety (and sometimes sadness) is often reduced by vomiting immediately after the binge.

Booth, D.A. "Culturally Controlled into Food Abuse: The Eating Disorders as Physiologically Reinforced Excessive Appetites." In *The Psycho Biology of Bulimia Nervosa*, edited by K. M. Pirke, W. Vandereycken and D. Ploog. Berlin and New York: Springer-Verlag, 1988.

gonads obesity Obesity caused by hypogonadism (abnormally low functioning of the gonads, with consequences for growth and development); it is marked by a concentration of fat tissue in the pelvic and breast regions. Other features may include poor beard growth in men, decreased growth of pubic hair and lack of development of the genitalia. Many obese females with this disease have mild hirsutism, irregular menses or AMENORRHEA. Young obese girls sometimes have premature or early menarche (first menstrual period in puberty).

grazing A word used to describe the practice of eating six or more small meals throughout the day, on the assumption that this will better lead to weight loss than the traditional three meals. Researchers remain divided in the debate; some studies have shown that "grazers" lose more weight than traditional eaters; in others the "grazers" have *gained* weight; in still others, there was no difference between the two groups.

"Grazing and Weight Loss." University of California, *Berkeley Wellness Letter*, February 1990.

Gregory, Dick (1932–) An entertainer, comedian and former fat man whose weight plummeted when he fasted as a protest against the Vietnam War and in favor of civil rights for blacks. Since that time he has repeatedly taken under his care massively obese persons to encourage them to lose weight on his BAHAMIAN DIET program using his own diet powder. Although he has treated these patients for free at his Bahamian facility, his exploitation of their plight on national talk shows and in print media to promote his products has stirred controversy in the medical profession and among activist groups such as the National Association to Aid Fat Acceptance. Allegations have also been made by former patients regarding the conditions and qualifications of the staff at another facility Gregory operates in Florida.

See also LIQUID FORMULAS.

group therapy A form of psychotherapy in which discussion takes place among a therapist and a number of patients rather than between a therapist and a single individual. According to the American Medical Association Encyclopedia of Medicine,

Interaction among members of the group is thought to be therapeutic and for certain problems is considered to be more effective than the traditional patient-therapist relationship. The group may range in number from three to forty people, but eight to ten people is the usual size. Members meet for an hour or more once or twice a week to discuss their problems openly with one another under the guidance of a therapist.

Since 1980, group therapy has become a common form of treatment for both anorexia and bulimia. Group treatment and support groups provide an arena for demystifying the eating disorder, diminishing feelings of isolation and secrecy, fostering realistic goal setting, sharing successful techniques, expressing feelings and obtaining feedback. PSYCHOTHERAPY groups are most effective in the treatment of bulimia. They may be open-ended or have a time limit, membership may be closed or participants may join at any time and the duration and frequency of sessions may vary. The focus is on individual dynamics and group process.

Belgian researchers studied the progress of 53 eating-disordered patients during inpatient group treatment by comparing the changes in perception of each patient by the patients themselves, the other group members and the therapeutic team. Remarkable differences were found among these judgments. Patients tend to deny problems or to evaluate their progress rather optimistically, while fellow patients and staff members are all more skeptical in their evaluations. The research team concluded that the evaluation procedure may have more value as a therapeutic tool than as an assessment method.

Although group therapy is now frequently used as a component of eating-disorders treatments, subsequent outcome studies indicate that its effectiveness remains problematic.

One school of thought holds that group therapy is a good model for understanding female development issues. The theory behind this is that women are generally socialized to function cooperatively in groups and that therefore the social dynamics of group therapy mimic or parallel the processes of female socialization. Because the majority of eating-disorder patients are fe-

male, it is possible that the success of group therapy for such patients may be related to this.

A setting such as that found in group therapy or a self-help group provides eating-disordered women a social format in which they can express opinions differing from the social consensus yet remain a part of the group (and the larger culture). As group members feel increasingly confident expressing thoughts and concerns that do not support thinness as an ideal, they are practicing skills of autonomy within a framework of social relationships and minimizing their fear of rejection and isolation.

Many issues can thus be explored in group sessions, from "what if" questions to actual experiences ("What happened to you when you quit purging?"). Group therapy can also help an individual to initiate serious treatment. Many patients have a difficult time beginning individual psychotherapy but may be less defensive and resistant to recovery in a group setting. A patient may accept confrontation from peers in a group more readily and in a more positive light than from a therapist.

Group therapy does not, however, represent a panacea. Many eating-disorder patients will deny that they have problems or will deny any feelings about their condition. This can keep them from developing the openness toward the group that is essential to allow the group to function fully. The group format helps decrease this resistance to trust, but there is no guarantee of success.

Goodner, Sherry. "Group Therapy for Eating Disorders." *BASH Magazine*, 1987.

Piazza, Eugene U., and Steiner-Adair, Catherine. "Recent Trends in Group Therapy for Anorexia Nervosa and Bulimia. In *Eating Disorders: Effective Care and Treatment*, edited by Félix E. F. Larocca. St. Louis: Ishiyaku EuroAmerica, 1986.

growth hormone in obesity Growth hormone is a substance secreted in the anterior lobe of the pituitary gland that directly influences protein, carbohydrate and fat ME-TABOLISM and controls the rate of skeletal and visceral growth. Compared with normal-weight subjects, obese subjects have impaired growth hormone secretion. Their plasma growth hormone responses to provocative stimuli, such as insulin-induced hypoglycemia, L-dopa, arginine infusion, glucagen, exercise, opioid administration and sleep, are blunted. The deranged growth hormone regulation is related to obesity itself, and in obese subjects who lost weight, growth hormone secretion becomes normal promptly. Conversely, overfed lean subjects have a weight-related impairment in growth hormone secretion.

Cordido, Fernando; Casanueva, Felipe F.; and Dieguez, Carlos. "Cholinergic Receptor Activation by Pyridostigmine Restores Growth Hormone (GH) Responsiveness to GH-Releasing Hormone Administration in Obese Subjects." *Journal of Clinical Endocrinology and Metabolism* 68, no. 2 (1989).

Gull, Sir William Withey (1816–1890)
An eminent London physician of the 19th century who was one of the first to use the term "anorexia nervosa." He worked and lived for many years at Guy's Hospital in London and treated Queen Victoria and her family. Gull described anorexia nervosa as a disease distinct from starvation among the insane and unrelated to organic diseases such as tuberculosis, diabetes or cancer. Most important, he observed that this disorder specifically affected young women between the ages of 16 and 23.

H

HCG A hormone (human chorionic gonadotropin) extracted from the urine of pregnant women, used in treating obesity. It is typically administered daily by injection.

The rationale for this treatment is that weight change during pregnancy is likely to be long lasting; therefore, by mimicking pregnancy and simultaneously inducing weight loss, a permanent change may be accomplished. In the mid-1930s, injections of HCG did seem to help reduce accumulations of fat on hips, buttocks and thighs that make boys with Froelich's syndrome look like girls. The hormone was described as seeming to "melt away" this fat. With the "melting" fat as a major source of nourishment, the boys were able to survive on only 500 calories a day. Thus, although HCG alone did not reduce weight, it did make drastic calorie curtailment possible. Follow-up studies, however, have not demonstrated that HCG patients stay thin any longer than patients in other programs.

Because there had been no scientifically adequate controlled clinical studies to establish the safety and effectiveness of HCG in the treatment of obesity, the U.S. Food and Drug Administration (FDA) in 1974 began requiring that HCG carry a warning label: "There is no substantial evidence that it increases weight loss beyond that resulting from caloric restriction, that it causes a more attractive or 'normal' distribution of fat, or that it decreases the hunger and discomfort associated with calorie-restricted diets." In 1975, the FDA declared HCG ineffective.

Clinicians who agree with the FDA's findings caution that in addition to patients' having to suffer through repeated injections of HCG, any benefits appearing to come from it are actually attributable to the strict low-calorie, high-protein diet (and diuretic pills) usually prescribed along with the shots.

This treatment is no longer in use by the medical profession.

Barrett, Stephen, and Knight, Gilda. *The Health Robbers*. Philadelphia: George F. Stickley, 1976.
Bradley, Patrick. "Human Chorionic Gonadotrophin: A New Role?" *Obesity/Bariatric Medicine* 8, no. 2 (1979).

Haag, Jessie. *Consumer Health: Products and Services.* Philadelphia: Lea & Febiger, 1976.

Singer, Steve. "When They Start Telling You It's Easy to Lose Weight." *Today's Health,* November 1972.

Weintraub, Michael, and Bray, George. "Drug Treatment of Obesity." *Medical Clinics of North America: Obesity* 73 (1) (January 1989).

hidden hunger   A phenomenon in which messages between the brain and stomach are in error so that conscious feelings of HUNGER do not in any way correspond to actual bodily needs. Because they do not know when they really are hungry, it is difficult for overweight people, in whom this phenomenon occurs, to control their eating.

homosexuality and eating disorders When psychiatrist JOEL YAGER of the University of California, Los Angeles found that nearly 50 percent of the men who enter treatment for anorexia nervosa describe themselves as homosexual, he questioned whether there might be a link between homosexuality and anorexia or bulimia. In a comparison study he conducted of homosexual with primarily heterosexual males, the gay men were more fearful of being fat and were more likely to feel fat despite others' perceptions. They also reported a higher incidence of BINGE EATING and PURGING. The homosexual men also scored higher on the EATING DISORDERS INVENTORY scales for drive for thinness, INTEROCEPTIVE DISTURBANCE, BULIMIA, body dissatisfaction, maturity fears and ineffectiveness.

Yager also found that gay men had a different body image preference. While heterosexual men preferred a more muscular or "macho" physique, they preferred being slender. Yager speculated that homosexual men may be more likely to develop eating disorders because of this concern with slim bodies, a traditionally feminine attitude.

This speculation is just that; it is not established fact.

Hudson, Walter (1945–1991) Because of his immense bulk (nearly 1,200 pounds), Walter Hudson was bedridden in his Long Island home for some time. Indeed, at age 42 he had not been out of his home for 27 years, when, in 1987, he achieved sudden notoriety. When he became wedged in a door frame and had to be cut out by the local fire department, his story became news. DICK GREGORY publicly adopted him as a "cause," but after several months of dieting, when Hudson refused to leave his home for Gregory's weight loss facility in the Bahamas, Gregory withdrew his support.

Hudson next became a spokesperson for a commercial diet product, which Gregory then sued, claiming that Hudson's television commercial "deceptively misleads viewers into believing that Hudson lost his weight through [it] rather than through use of [Gregory's] products."

In commercials, Hudson claimed to have lost more than 900 pounds; in 1989 he weighed 520. He later formed his own company to sell clothing for large-size men, women and children. He died in 1991, apparently of heart failure.

hunger   An urge to eat prompted by an immediate physical need for food. In healthy people, hunger and APPETITE usually coincide. Opportunities to eat, however, may arouse appetite even in the absence of real hunger, and some experiences can be so unsettling or traumatic that they can cause loss of appetite even in the presence of hunger.

Some researchers have distinguished two kinds of hunger: stomach hunger and mouth hunger. Stomach, or physiological, hunger derives from the physiological need to refuel. Compulsive eaters rarely experience it; they eat from mouth hunger. Mouth, or psychological, hunger has nothing to do with sustaining life. Mouth-hungry people eat "just because it's there," "because you have to put something into your mouth," "because it tastes good," "because it looks so deli-

cious,'' ''because it's time for breakfast/
lunch/dinner,'' ''because someone went to
the trouble to prepare it,'' ''because it would
be a shame to throw it away,'' ''because I
feel lonely/anxious/depressed'' or ''because
I feel happy/excited/like celebrating.'' Mouth
hunger is what you feel pulling you toward
the refrigerator as soon as you sit down to
work or what compels you to leave your
house at 11:30 P.M. in search of an all-night
ice cream stand. Mouth hunger is what continues to send spoon after spoon of ice cream
to your mouth long after you've begun to
feel ill. Mouth hunger is the hunger we
attempt to control with diets.

HILDE BRUCH emphasized that the inability to recognize hunger is a trait that is of
fundamental significance for the development of severe eating disturbances. Bruch
also noted that obese children are routinely
fed when they cry for reasons other than
hunger. Consequently, their ''real'' hunger
is responded to inappropriately, with under-
or overfeeding. Eventually, these children's
ability to differentiate accurately between
hunger and emotional states becomes undermined. Emotional distress is confused with
hunger, and these potentially obese children
may overeat in response to virtually any
internal arousal state. As obese adults, they
suffer from a deficit in hunger awareness.
Studies have shown that obese subjects are
relatively insensitive to stimuli typically associated with hunger and do not usually eat
more in response to hunger cues.

Bruch, Hilde. *Eating Disorders: Obesity, An-
orexia Nervosa, and the Person Within.* New
York: Basic Books, 1973.
Hirschmann, Jane R., and Munter, Carol H.
Overcoming Overeating, Reading, Mass.: Ad-
dison-Wesley, 1988.

hyperactivity Increased or excessive activity. The term commonly refers to manifestations of disturbed behavior, mostly in
children, characterized by constant movement, distraction, impulsiveness, inability to
concentrate and aggressiveness. It is also

characteristic of anorectics; many are usually
active, with a tendency to exercise even
when emaciated. Some rarely stay still; even
when confined to bed, they have been known
to perform isometric exercises under the
blankets. This preoccupation with physical
fitness is closely related to the consuming
desire for thinness. The apparently unusual
capacity for physical exertion is not evidence
of special physical toughness; it is an indicator of a determination to be active despite
the actual state of physical health. Sometimes anorectics will push themselves to the
point of collapse, causing them finally to
seek or be taken for medical treatment.
Physical overactivity can also serve to dis-
tract attention from hunger.

HILDE BRUCH wrote that hyperactivity is
rarely complained of, or even mentioned, by
the parents of anorectics but that it will be
found with great regularity if looked for.
Hyperactivity usually develops before the
noneating phase. It may take many forms.
Sometimes an existing interest in athletics
and sports becomes intensified. Sometimes
anorectics may engage in activities that seem
to be aimless, walking for miles, doing chin-
ning and bending exercises, refusing to sit
down or literally running around in circles.
Some may roam around at night, too restless
to sleep, or they will do housework, cooking
and cleaning by the hour. They themselves
do not feel that they exercise too much, and
parents do not notice or are not alarmed.
Anorectics, and their parents, can therefore
deny hyperactivity.

The relationship between hyperactivity and
disordered eating has been corroborated via
animal research. One of the common findings in animal studies of the effect of restricting food intake is an increase in
restlessness and spontaneous motion. When
rats are placed on a limited feeding schedule,
they increase the number of times they spin
their exercise wheels. After a few days of
increased activity, however, adult rats will
alter their cycles so that most of their activity
occurs during the hour or two before feed-

ing, and the total number of revolutions of the wheels per day will be somewhat lower than during times when they are feeding at their own pleasure. Prepubertal rats, on the other hand, do not adjust their activity in this way and will literally run themselves to death if feeding is not increased. This suggests that the heightened energy output that frequently accompanies dieting may be biologically determined.

Bruch, Hilde. *Eating Disorders: Obesity, Anorexia Nervosa, and the Person Within.* New York: Basic Books, 1973.

Casper, Regina C. "Hypothalamic Dysfunction and Symptoms of Anorexia Nervosa." *Psychiatric Clinics of North America* 7(2) (June 1984).

Kron, L., Katz, J. L., and Gorsynski G. "Hyperactivity in Anorexia Nervosa: A Fundamental Clinical Feature." *Comprehensive Psychiatry* 1978: 5 (May 1978).

hyperalimentation   Intravenous feeding. It involves the infusion of a protein solution made up of hydrolysate, glucose, electrolytes, minerals and vitamins at a constant rate through a catheter that has been surgically placed in a major blood vessel such as the subclavian or jugular vein. Helpful in the treatment of anorexia nervosa, it avoids the arguments about FORCED FEEDING. While it prevents patients' surreptitiously disposing of food, vomiting and other tricks, inventive anorectics find ways of interfering with the flow; they even manage to turn the machinery off. But by bringing about a rapid correction of poor nutrition, hyperalimentation makes patients more accessible to psychotherapy. Hyperalimentation is considered to be a drastic treatment measure and is regarded negatively by many who cite possible infections and overhydration, as well as unwise control over patients who are already struggling to escape feelings of powerlessness.

hypercellularity   The condition of having too many cells.

It appears that the number of fat cells in the body cannot be decreased. However, during periods of rapid growth, a proliferation of cells can be slowed or stopped. Thus it is believed that changing nutrition at the proper time may modify the rate of cell development. This is especially important in treating obesity-prone children.

See also FAT CELLS.

hypergymnasia   A term used by Adel Eldahmy, medical director of the Long Beach (California) Eating Disorders Clinic, to describe the excessive exercising an increasing number of bulimic patients turn to once they have stopped PURGING. Instead of vomiting or using laxatives, they go to a gym seven days a week, two or three hours a day, to burn off calories. They've been scared sufficiently to stop purging, but they don't see anything wrong with exercising until they're dangerously dehydrated.

See also EXERCISE; HYPERACTIVITY.

hyperplastic obesity   A severe, lifelong type of obesity that is anatomically generalized (not concentrated in any area or areas of the body) and resistant to therapy. It is further characterized by an increased number of fat cells of normal or of increased size.

See also HYPERTROPHIC OBESITY.

hypertension   Chronic high blood pressure (excessive pressure of the blood against the arterial walls); usually defined as a condition in which resting systolic pressure is consistently greater than 160 mm of mercury and diastolic pressure is over 90 mm.

Because a number of studies have demonstrated that blood pressure falls during periods of caloric restriction, weight reduction is an accepted treatment for hypertension. Some clinicians, however, have failed to detect significant blood pressure lowering in cases of substantial weight loss. In clinical studies in which obese rats were fed, fasted and refed, blood pressure did not correlate directly with varying body weight but appeared instead to be regulated by nutritional conditions. These findings conflict with the traditional view that weight loss or gain per se triggers changes in blood pressure.

In these studies, repeated cycles of weight loss and gain induced hypertension in the obese rats. Because there is also evidence that humans develop hypertension during rapid regaining of weight, some clinicians suggest that more emphasis should be placed on long-term maintenance of weight loss in obese hypertensive patients, since caloric restriction may actually exacerbate hypertension if followed by rapid regaining of weight.

Hypertension tends to occur in patients with greater lean body mass and thus greater weight, but these people are not necessarily fatter than those people with normal blood pressure.

Ernsberger, Paul, and Nelson, Douglas. "Refeeding Hypertension in Dietary Obesity." *American Journal of Physiology* 254 Jan 1988; 254 (1 Pt 2).

Hamilton, C. L. "Problems of Refeeding after Starvation in the Rat." *Annals of New York Academy of Science* 157: 1004–17, 15 May 69 Cit. no. 4202116 (1969).

Szepsi, B.; Vegors, R.; Michaelis, D. E.; and DeMony, J. M. "Long-Term Effects of Starvation-Refeeding in the Rat." *Nutritional Metabolism* 19 (1975).

hypertrophic obesity   Adult-onset obesity. It is more amenable to therapy than childhood obesity or obesity caused by or associated with a pathological condition. Physiologically, it is characterized by the increased size, but not number, of fat cells.

See also HYPERPLASTIC OBESITY.

hypnotherapy   The use of hypnosis in the treatment of psychological disorders. It is intended to help patients remember and come to terms with disturbing memories or emotions that they have repressed from consciousness.

According to the American Medical Association, scientific studies regarding the ef-

fectiveness of hypnotherapy are lacking. Hypnosis has been used effectively as part of a therapeutic strategy for anorexia nervosa. Hypnotherapeutic intervention is most effective when symptoms such as hyperactivity, distorted body image, feelings of inadequacy and perfectionistic tendencies are present. It may also help patients to overcome resistance to therapy.

Hypnotic suggestion has been used to increase patients' awareness of hunger by associating it with the pleasure of eating. Hypnoanalysis has been used for uncovering psychodynamic conflicts behind anorectic symptoms. A combination of behavior therapy and hypnosis has been used to associate food and appetite with pleasant memories and to help patients ventilate feelings of aggression and hostility.

Gross, Meir. "Use of Hypnosis in Eating Disorders." In *Eating Disorders,* edited by Félix E. F. Larocca. San Francisco: Jossey-Bass, 1986.

hypokalemia   A potassium deficiency often resulting from chronic vomiting because of the loss of salt, minerals and other nutrients. It commonly results in cardiac dysrhythmia (lack of rhythm) and, if severe, may lead to sudden death. When accompanying malnutrition, hypokalemia also adversely affects the renal and gastrointestinal systems. Hypokalemia also results in specific injury to the kidney tubules, affecting their ability to concentrate urine. The resulting clinical manifestations are frequent urination and increased thirst. Its effects on the gastrointestinal system include gastric fullness, regurgitation of food, heartburn, constipation and exacerbation of external hemorrhoids.

hypothalamic disease   A disease, trauma or tumor that affects the APPETITE center located in the hypothalamus (a part of the brain controlling functions of the autonomic nervous system), resulting in obesity. Individuals suffering from this condition usually have an insatiable appetite, eating compulsively day and night. Their obesity advances relentlessly, and eventually they become massive in size. In some instances there is a decrease in normal brain function.

Patients diagnosed as having hypothalamic disease often have a history of brain damage caused by trauma or inflammation. Such cases show a generalized type of obesity with no areas of the body being spared. Excess ADIPOSE TISSUE tends to concentrate in the face and neck region as well as the upper arms, upper legs and pelvis. In men there may be a retraction of the testes, and in young women development of secondary sexual characteristics may be delayed. Diagnosis is based on these physical findings, as well as on brain scans and thyroid function tests. The prescribed treatment for this disease is weight reduction as well as treatment of intracerebral lesions. Early death may result from extreme obesity and complications of stasis pneumonia or septicemia from infected skin sites.

Frawley, Thomas F. "Obesity and the Endocrine System." *Psychiatric Clinics of North America* 7: 2 (June 1984).

Powley, T. L., and Keesey, R. "Relationships of Body Weight to the Lateral Hypothalamic Feeding Syndrome." *Journal of Comparative Physiological Psychology* 70 (1970).

I

iatrogenesis in eating disorders   The origin of a medical condition in the "attitude or activity of a physician" (Miller and Keane). An iatrogenic disorder is an abnormal mental or physical condition produced inadvertently as a result of treatment by a physician for some other disorder.

In the treatment of eating disorders, various practices and mistakes in treatment can result in iatrogenic disorders:

- Failure to attend to food and weight issues in PSYCHOTHERAPY. A study of normal volunteers has shown that semistarvation can produce an overall dampening of emotions or lead to the experience of severe DEPRESSION, ANXIETY, mood changes, feelings of inadequacy and social withdrawal. Semistarvation is responsible for food preoccupations, radically altered eating habits, and BINGE EATING in some individuals.

  Recognizing the effect of starvation on food intake behavior, then, could decrease iatrogenesis. David Garner (see GARFINKEL AND GARNER) has recommended that any proposed treatment model be aimed at breaking the self-perpetuating cycle of emotions, diet and behavior by taking this cycle into account when regulating the quantity and quality of food intake.

- Establishment of unrealistic goals in treatment. Although arriving at an ideal normal weight for a patient is difficult, iatrogenesis occurs when the goal weight established is so low as virtually to preclude recovery. For example, a bulimic patient may have a higher-than-average set point (see SET-POINT THEORY), and therefore her weight goal should be higher than that on a standard height/weight chart. Most bulimic patients have weights greater than those of the average population, and between a third and a half have weight consistent with obesity. Garner has noted that "a significant proportion of bulimic patients choose a 'desired weight' which is consistent with anorexia nervosa and those who prefer a more statistically normal weight may be no less unrealistic if they have a biological propensity for obesity."

- Inappropriate application of BEHAVIOR MODIFICATION techniques grounded in insensitivity to a particular patient's responses.

  For example, if coercion or punishment is used to encourage or discourage an eating behavior, the patient may eat to avoid the negative reinforcement and then purge—thus developing bulimia. The difference between successful and unsuccessful treatment depends on the way the program is applied; too-rigid application may only perpetuate, or complicate, the disorder.

• Unnecessary TUBE FEEDING. The greatest problems associated with tube feeding derive from its use as a punishment. In a psychologically vulnerable patient, this may cause confusion about bodily functions, confirm an already existing sense of worthlessness or cause mistrust; it may also lead to physiological complications.

• Inappropriate treatment with medication. Five different types of medication are sometimes misused: diuretics, laxatives, emetics, thyroxine and "diet pills." Misuse of drugs serves to aggravate eating disorders as well as distort diagnosis.

The danger of iatrogenic effects also exists in the abstinence and addiction models of bulimia. For example, OVEREATERS ANONYMOUS (a group whose practices are based on those of Alcoholics Anonymous) views bulimia as a progressive and lifelong illness, controllable only by abstinence from the "addictive" substance. But abstaining from food is much more difficult than abstaining from alcohol. Several main principles of Overeaters Anonymous could be iatrogenic for the bulimic patient:

• The belief that overweight or obesity is the result of "compulsive overeating." Most studies of the obese indicate that they do not eat more than individuals of normal weight. People who are compulsive overeaters are also compulsive dieters and may be responding to a sense of hunger in their bodies. This sense of hunger could be responsible for the food preoccupations and cravings that are often reported.

• The idea that bulimics are suffering from a "progressive illness which cannot be cured, only arrested." Bulimic patients can be treated successfully and cured.

• The principle of controlling overeating through abstinence from "the addiction."

This principle encourages DICHOTOMOUS REASONING in a bulimic patient, with the bulimic patient adopting a self-defeating "all-or-nothing" attitude.

• Participation in self-help and support groups. Association with others who have an eating disorder may foster a group identity pleasurable or satisfying to a patient. Difficulty can develop in relinquishing a support group and moving beyond the "sick role" into greater recovery. The association of several popular stars with eating disorders has also somewhat glamorized them. The goals of a self-help group should be to provide mutual support without reinforcing the disorder.

Goodner, Sherry. "Summary of St. Louis BASH Meeting, May 18, 1985" including a presentation by Dr. David Garner of the Departments of Psychiatry, University of Toronto.

Miller Benjamin, and Keane, Clare Brackman. *Encyclopedia and Dictionary of Medicine and Nursing.* Philadelphia: W. B. Saunders, 1972.

ice The slang term for an appetite-suppressing drug sold illegally on the streets, which is 98 percent pure crystal methamphetamine. It is as addictive and dangerous as crack cocaine. *USA Today* reported on December 26, 1989, that "ice" was at that time being used by dieters in Hawaii and California and had spread as far east as Oklahoma. Experts said most users are women, some of them using it for weight loss. Although it does cause weight loss for a short time, addiction and toxic problems soon set in. Ice can be smoked, snorted or injected; is domestically produced; is comparable in price to crack; and gives the user a high—and suppresses appetite—for up to 14 hours. A crack high lasts an average of 15 minutes.

Kelley, Jack. " 'Ice Age' May Dwarf Crack Crisis." *USA Today,* December 26, 1989.

imipramine The first true ANTIDEPRESSANT, in use since the 1950s under the commercial name Tofranil. A tricyclic antidepressant, it has been used by millions of people and has an established record of long-term safety. Imipramine has few side effects, among them dry mouth, light-headedness on standing up (which usually disappears after a week or two) and sleepiness. It has been used successfully in the treatment of bulimia, with patients receiving it reducing their binge frequency about 75 percent.

infant obesity   The incidence of obesity in infants has not been determined, but it appears to be increasing. Recent studies suggest that two trends in infant feeding may account for some of this increase—the trend toward bottle feeding rather than breast feeding, and the trend toward earlier introduction of solids. Whether bottle feeding contributes to the development of obesity is controversial. Most available evidence indicates that breast feeding does not prevent obesity, but it may help prevent overfeeding. Although infants are able to take solids at very early ages without apparent harm, they receive no desirable nutrients that cannot be provided by milk formula. Instead, such feedings usually result in the ingestion of more calories and protein than are required for optimum growth.

It is generally recommended that obese infants not be made to lose weight but that their weight be controlled. An obese infant's rate of weight gain should be slowed to parallel his or her linear growth. Recommended is a limitation of 50 to 55 calories per pound of body weight per day during the first six months of life, and 41 to 46 calories per pound of body weight per day from six to 12 months of age. Substituting skim milk for formula is not recommended, but water may be offered periodically in its place. Researchers believe that thirst is often mistaken for hunger.

A number of studies have claimed that rapidity of weight gain in infancy is a better guide to the risk of being overweight at the age of six or eight than is the weight of the parents. For example, in one study, adults whose obesity appeared to have begun in infancy had a higher number of fat cells than a group of equally fat adults whose obesity was of more recent origin. In addition, psychological problems encountered in attempting to lose weight have been more pronounced in patients with early-onset obesity. An infant who becomes obese usually remains obese as an adolescent and as an adult.

Researchers at the University of Edinburgh investigated the learning experiences involved in HUNGER and SATIETY in early infancy, and their relation to eventual obesity and other eating disorders. Findings appeared to contradict an earlier theory that there might exist a critical period in early development when the number of FAT CELLS becomes fixed and predisposes a fat infant to become a fat child and ultimately a fat adult.

Collipp, Platon J., ed. *Childhood Obesity.* New York: Warner Books, 1986.
Wright, Peter. "Mothers' Assessment of Hunger in Relation to Meal Size in Breastfed Infants." *Journal of Reproductive and Infant Psychology* 5 (1987).
Wright, Peter. "Development of Feeding Behaviour in Early Infancy: Implications for Obesity." *Health Bulletin* 39 (1981).

insomnia   Chronic inability to sleep, or consistent interruption of sleep by periods of wakefulness. Insomnia is not a disease but may be a symptom of many diseases. Bulimics frequently report troubled sleep patterns and insomnia and use BINGE EATING as a kind of sleeping pill. Sleep disturbance is a regular complication of starvation. Insomnia, especially premature early morning awakening, affects many anorectics and depressed people.

insurance   Treatment for eating disorders is frequently either not covered or only partially covered by hospitalization policies. In *Simon v. Blue Cross and Blue Shield of Greater New York,* a New York State appeals court in 1988 held that hospitalization of a person for anorexia nervosa is medical, not psychiatric, care and therefore is not subject to insurance policy limitations on psychiatric coverage. The physician who examined the patient at the time of her first hospitalization asserted that because of rapid weight loss the patient was "emaciated, malnourished, dehydrated, and hypotensive. She required immediate medical treatment for these conditions."

This case is covered in *Hospital and Community Psychiatry*, June 1989, page 662; reprinted in *BASH Magazine*, August 1989, page 223.

International Journal of Eating Disorders A journal founded in 1981 to foster and publish research on anorexia nervosa, bulimia, obesity and other atypical patterns of eating behavior and body weight regulation.

interoceptive disturbance An inability to identify accurately internal sensations such as HUNGER, SATIETY, fatigue, cold and sexual feelings. HILDE BRUCH suggested that both anorexia nervosa and juvenile obesity are fundamentally related to this disturbed awareness. Anorectic patients often describe extreme confusion about their bodily sensations; sometimes they appear devoid of thoughts and feelings reflecting personal experiences. Rarely can they focus on and accurately describe their emotional and physical states.

ipecac A dried root of the plant ipecacuanha grown in Brazil. It is the source of emetine, a powdered white alkaloid emetic used to induce vomiting and the active ingredient in ipecac syrup, abused by some eating-disordered patients.

Ipecac syrup is sold over the counter in the United States in 30cc bottles, equivalent to 21 mg of emetine base. The long persistence of emetine in the body is the basis for cumulative toxicity. The effects of emetine toxicosis are gastrointestinal, neuromuscular

and cardiovascular. Gastrointestinal symptoms include diarrhea, nausea, vomiting and dysphagia (difficulty in swallowing). The neuromuscular manifestations include weakness, aching, tenderness and stiffness of muscles, especially those of the neck and the extremities. There have been case reports of myopathies, including fatal cardiomyopathy, associated with the use of ipecac syrup. The most serious toxic effects are cardiovascular and include hypotension, precordial path, tachycardia and dyspnea. It is estimated that an accumulated dose of 1.25 grams of emetine base can produce death in an adult. The drug is used commonly in emergency situations involving overdoses.

The AMERICAN ANOREXIA/BULIMIA ASSOCIATION (AABA) has lobbied the U.S. Food and Drug Administration against over-the-counter sales of ipecac. Because of the wide availability of the drug and its speedy emetic action, ipecac was abused, according to AABA sources, by an estimated 30,000 young women in 1987.

Friedman, Enrique J. "Death from Ipecac Intoxication in a Patient with Anorexia Nervosa." *American Journal of Psychiatry* 141, no. 5 (1984); reprinted in *BASH Newsletter*, August 1984.

J

Janet, Pierre (1859–1947) A French psychiatrist and researcher specializing in the study of hysteria. He was the first to describe in modern medical terms the symptoms of BULIMIA. In his book *Les Obsessions et la psychasthenie* (1903), he wrote about a young women who developed compulsive eating binges, many of them in secret.

jaw wiring Wiring the jaws together to prevent the eating of solid foods and allowing only liquid nutrition directly restricts calorie intake. Weight reduction usually occurs during this time; as much as 70 and 80 pounds have been lost when jaws have been left wired for long periods of time. However, much of this is regained once they are unwired. Some patients find the conspicuousness and the claustrophobic qualities of jaw wiring to be rather unpleasant.

This procedure has been used primarily to help compulsive eaters. Once a week the braces are loosened so the teeth can be brushed.

jejunocolonic bypass An intestinal bypass procedure developed in the 1960s that was intended to aid weight loss; it is no longer performed, however, because of detrimental side effects (severe diarrhea, uncontrolled weight loss, malnutrition, liver dysfunction) during the postoperative months. Patients did lose much weight, but as side effects worsened, surgeons had to reconnect their intestines. Subsequently, all lost weight was regained. Regained weight proved that the bypass was the cause of weight reduction, however, and this experience provided the impetus for continued investigation into surgical weight control.

See also BYPASS SURGERY.

jejunoileal bypass The most frequently performed small intestine bypass operation in the treatment of patients with morbid obesity, until it was replaced by gastric bypass in the late 1970s. Is is effective in producing weight loss (an average of 100 pounds five years after surgery), but side effects and complications are substantial.

After jejunoileal bypass, patients lose approximately one-third of their weight within the first year. Weight loss is thought to be due principally to malabsorption of nu-

trients, caused by diarrhea, which occurs in all patients following this operation. Most patients develop complications after jejunoileal bypass, many of which are severe. There is a 30 to 40 percent rehospitalization rate within the first year after surgery.

Of the many complications following jejunoileal bypass, one of the most serious is the insidious development of hepatic fibrosis and cirrhosis in up to 10 percent of cases. As a consequence, this operation has now fallen out of favor except in rare and selected cases. Many patients remain, however, with intact and apparently successful bypasses. Even 10 years after bypass, persistent abnormalities of hepatic morphology are evident in most patients.

Because overeating is still possible after this procedure, it does not necessarily lead to a life-style conducive to long-term success of weight reduction. But the psychosocial consequences of weight loss include improved mood, self-esteem, interpersonal and vocational effectiveness, body image and activity, all of which encourage the patient to maintain his or her success.

Blackburn, George, and Bistrian, Bruce. "Surgical Techniques for the Treatment of Adolescent Obesity." In *Childhood Obesity,* edited by Platon J. Collipp. New York: Warner Books, 1986.

Boon, A. P.; Thompson, H.; and Baddeley, R. M. "Use of Histological Examination to Assess Ultrastructure of Liver in Patients with Long Standing Jejunoileal Bypass for Morbid Obesity." *Journal of Clinical Pathology* 41 (December 1988).

Powers, Pauline S., and Rosemurgy, Alexander. "Current Treatment of Obesity." In *Eating Disorders: Effective Care and Treatment,* edited by Félix E. F. Larocca. St. Louis: Ishiyaku EuroAmerica, 1986.

Yetiv, Jack Z., *Popular Nutritional Practices: A Scientific Appraisal.* Toledo, Ohio: Popular Medicine Press, 1986.

K

ketogenic diet A diet that produces elevated levels of acetone or ketone bodies, accompanied by mild acidosis or ketoacidosis. In this kind of diet the ratio of calories derived from fat to those from carbohydrates is three or four to one.

The combustion of fatty acids in the bloodstream produces ketones, which eventually are broken down into carbon dioxide and water by the liver and other tissues of the body. Under abnormal conditions such as diabetes mellitus, starvation or a diet composed almost entirely of fat, the breakdown of fatty acids may be halted at the ketone stage, causing increasing levels of ketone bodies in the blood and body tissues. Ketones are powerful appetite suppressants that account for the loss of HUNGER occurring on the second day of any rigorous fast.

Ketone-producing diets have been around for more than 100 years. William Harvey, an English surgeon, first experimented with high-protein, low-carbohydrate, ketone-producing diets in the mid-1800s. The diet he developed is generally known as the Banting Diet (see BANTING, WILLIAM), after an early patient of Harvey's who was so delighted by the effects of the doctor's weight loss program that he published a pamphlet in praise of it. Since that time versions of the Banting Diet, with minor modifications, have appeared at regular intervals: as the Pennington or Dupont Diet in 1953, the Air Force Diet in 1960, the Drinking Man's Diet in 1965 and the Stillman and Atkins diets in the 1970s.

Elevated levels of ketones are potentially dangerous (see KETOSIS).

ketosis A condition in which excessive amounts of ketones accumulate in the body. Ketones are chemicals the body makes when there is not enough glucose in the blood and it must break down fat for its energy. When this occurs, fatty acids are released into the blood; these fatty acids are then converted to ketones. Ketones can poison and even kill body cells. Ketones that build up in the body for a long time can lead to serious illness and coma. Symptoms include a "fruity" odor to the breath, loss of appetite, nausea, vomiting and abdominal pain. Ketosis can be diagnosed by a test to detect ketones in the urine. FASTING can cause ketosis. Treatment in this case is a gradual reintroduction of a nutritious diet.

Ketosis also occurs in uncontrolled diabetes mellitus, because carbohydrates are not properly utilized. In these cases, it is treated with either diet change or insulin.

kleptomania A psychological compulsion to steal. Kleptomania in the form of shoplifting is a bulimia-associated symptom affecting many bulimic patients. This stealing is invariably compulsive, and the patients experience the same guilt feelings as they do when binge eating. Other than food or laxatives stolen for the purpose of binge eating or purging, bulimics rarely steal to get something they cannot afford to buy. This symptom occurs even in persons who have no history of shoplifting prior to the onset of bulimia. Patients have been known to feel so guilty after stealing something that they attempt surreptitiously to return it the next day, only to find themselves compulsively stealing something else.

An increasing number of shoplifting bulimics are entering therapy through the courts, as an alternative to prosecution or sentencing. In fact, some therapists see shoplifting as, in effect, a cry for help.

L

Lasègue, Charles (1816–1883) A French psychiatrist who was one of the first to publish a detailed description of anorexia nervosa. In 1873 he described the disorder as a variant of hysteria. While his contemporary, the Englishman SIR WILLIAM WITHEY GULL, concentrated on the medical aspects of anorexia, Lasègue emphasized its psychological aspects. He confirmed what Gull had suggested, that anorectic women came from families willing and able to spend emotional and financial resources on them. He was the first physician to suggest that refusal of food constitutes a form of conflict between a maturing girl and her parents.

Last Chance Diet   A fad diet prominent in 1976, when the *Last Chance Diet Book* became a best-seller and led to the widespread use of liquid protein products without medical supervision. These products provided 300–400 calories per day in the form of collagen hydrolysate, a protein low in biological value. Some 100,000 people had used these products by the end of 1977, and 60 deaths had been reported to the Centers for Disease Control. Seventeen of these were attributed to the diet; in the next year the Food and Drug Administration issued warnings about it.

See also FAD DIETS.

laxative abuse   Misuse of laxatives is a fairly common problem among bulimic women, and laxatives appear to be the type of drug most commonly abused by anorectic patients. This misuse usually involves the ingestion of many times the amounts recommended by the manufacturer.

Researchers have found that patients who use self-induced VOMITING for weight control tend to eat significantly more during binges yet weigh less than those who use laxatives, suggesting that laxative abuse is relatively ineffective for this purpose and that dietary restraint is responsible for any weight loss among laxative abusers. One study found that the weight loss experienced by patients following ingestion of laxatives resulted from temporary fluid loss; the amount

of caloric absorption prevented by laxative use was minimal.

Laxatives containing stimulant compounds are favored by those with eating disorders because these agents will reliably produce a watery diarrhea fairly promptly, and a sense of weight loss, if sufficient amounts are ingested. Most laxative abuse is practiced independently, but laxatives are often prescribed by diet doctors in an effort to speed food through the intestines so nutrients are not absorbed and turned to fat.

Complications of laxative abuse include:

- *Constipation*   These drugs produce a reflex hypofunctioning (decreased functioning) of the colon, resulting in constipation. Constipation becomes a particular problem during laxative withdrawal.
- *Cathartic Colon*   Patients who have taken stimulant-type laxatives for long periods of time can develop permanent dysfunctioning of the colon, accompanied by radiographic and microscopic changes in the bowel.
- *Bleeding*   Chronic recurrent use of stimulant-type laxatives can result in gastrointestinal bleeding and hidden or obvious blood loss.
- *Dehydration*   Stimulant-type laxatives promote fluid loss through the intestine, which can result in volume depletion and lead to a secondary hyperaldosteronism, a condition caused by secretion of excessive amounts of the electrolyte-regulating hormone aldosterone by the adrenal cortex; this in turn results in reflex peripheral edema (swelling), which is a particular problem during laxative withdrawal. This reflex fluid retention can be quite dramatic.
- *Electrolyte Abnormalities*   Laxative-induced diarrhea markedly elevates the electrolyte content of the feces. HYPOKALEMIA and acidosis may result.
- Other medical complications that have been described include the development of steatorrhea (excessive fat in the feces) and protein-losing gastroenteropathy (disease

of the digestive tract), pancreatic dysfunction, osteomalacia (softening of bone) pseudofractures, hypocalcemia (reduction of calcium in the blood) and hypomagnesemia (abnormally low level of magnesium in the blood).

In California, laxative sales restrictions are being debated by legislators. It is thought by many that some restrictions should be placed on the sale of over-the-counter laxatives because thousands of young women are overdosing on laxatives in their quest for weight loss.

Bankhead, Charles D. "Myths Fueling Widespread Abuse of OTC Laxatives." *Medical World News,* January 8, 1990.
Moriarty, K. J., and Silk, D. B. "Laxative Abuse." *Digestive Diseases* 6 (1988).
Willard, S. G.; Winstead, D. K.; Anding, R.; and Dudley, P. "Laxative Abuse in Eating Disorders." *Psychiatric Medicine* 7 (1989).

lipoprotein lipase   An enzyme that aids in the storage of body fat. Studies have shown that obese people may have difficulty achieving a normal level of lipoprotein lipase. A University of Colorado study reported that obese people, in comparison with people of normal weight, produce too much of the enzyme and that even after weight loss their enzyme activity had not fully returned to normal.

Levels of lipoprotein lipase in ADIPOSE TISSUES affect the maintenance of fat-cell size, body weight and obesity. Genetic and diet-induced obesity have been found to be associated with increases in lipoprotein lipase levels in the adipose tissue of humans and rodents after overnight fasting. Progressive increases in body mass index in humans are associated with increases in adipose tissue lipoprotein lipase. Most evidence suggests that an increase in levels of lipoprotein lipase in adipose tissue preserves rather than causes obesity.

One study found that people who had maintained a large weight loss for eight or more years still produced too much of the enzyme. But as soon as those obese people who have lost weight start regaining it, their enzyme level drops.

Eckel, Robert H. "Lipoprotein Lipase." *New England Journal of Medicine* 320: 16 (April 20, 1989).

liposuction   A surgical procedure pioneered in Europe in the 1970s to remove localized deposits of excess fat; also called lipoplasty or lipectomy. The surgeon inserts a long, thin, hollow blunt-edged tube called a cannula through a quarter-inch incision. This tube is attached via another hollow tube to a machine with a powerful vacuum apparatus that sucks out subcutaneous (beneath the skin) fat. The collecting tube is transparent, allowing the surgeon to see the tissue being removed. Liposuction has been referred to as "maid service for your fat: The surgeon vacuums the areas you didn't have the time or energy to clean up yourself." Though controversial, it is becoming an increasingly common type of cosmetic surgery today.

Giorgio Fischer, a surgeon in Rome, was the first to devise an instrument to remove fat by suction and the first to perform liposuction surgery. The original procedure removed fat almost totally from the suctioned area, creating a large cavity that filled with body fluids. Because the skin overlying it did not shrink correspondingly, the procedure left an unsatisfactory result.

To combat this problem, Yves-Gérard Illouz, a French surgeon, devised a method for dissecting fat with a blunt tube (cannula) that removed fat in a regular series of tunnels created sequentially by probing the fat deposit to be treated. In this new procedure, both the adjacent fat and the small blood vessels running through the area remained intact, allowing continuous contact between the skin and the underlying tissue. This helped the skin to shrink slowly and regularly over the newly contoured area, with less likelihood of developing ripples and depressions. Keeping original blood vessels in the area helped fluids that leak into it during the postoperative period to be more easily absorbed into the body. This shortened the prolonged wound drainage that characterized earlier suction procedures.

Liposuction was developed to remove from a healthy, normal-weight person localized genetically derived fat deposits that do not respond to diet or exercise. It is not intended to be a treatment for obesity. The most frequently treated areas include the hips and thighs and the abdomen. Liposuction can also be done on the neck, face, arms and legs.

Results Typically, according to Dr. Thomas Gant, a plastic surgeon in Edmonds, Washington, from one to two pounds is removed during a single liposuction. Taking out more than four pounds can result in fluid shifts, which can cause shock. Not all fat is removed from a location. The surgeon leaves some fat cells behind because fat cells grow and shrink, depending on nutrition and the age of the patient. Removing all the fat cells would result in a disproportionately flat area.

Not everyone achieves satisfactory results, mainly because there is no control over how the skin will contract over suctioned areas. Some patients end up with "dents" and more uneven skin and sagging than they had before surgery. Others have dropped two full clothing sizes.

Liposuction surgery differs from fat loss through dieting and exercise. When fat is lost in those ways, FAT CELLS become smaller, though their number throughout the body remains constant. These "starved" fat cells send messages to the brain indicating their depleted state, stimulating HUNGER. When they receive extra CALORIES, these cells once again store fat for future needs. Liposuction, in contrast, actually removes fat cells from the treated area. These are not replaced unless there is a subsequent weight gain large enough to fill the remaining cells to their capacity. For this reason, patients who have undergone liposuction surgery must monitor

their caloric intake to maintain positive results. It should be noted that reaccumulated fat is not necessarily deposited in the same locations that have been suctioned. This new fat generally tends to spread itself evenly throughout the body.

Liposuction also removes fat from specific, targeted areas, but diet and exercise may reduce nonpreferred areas while leaving other areas virtually intact. Women with large thighs, for instance, are often frustrated by the persistence of this phenomenon even when their diet and exercise regimes lead to virtual emaciation of their faces and upper bodies. And men with "spare tires" around their middles are often unable to eliminate them entirely by dieting despite considerable weight loss.

Limitations Liposuction surgery is not the ultimate answer to dieters' prayers, though. The procedure does have distinct limitations.

Good skin tone is important for continued success, because once fat is removed, the skin must shrink to fit a new contour. Assuming that prolonged accumulation and drainage of body fluids does not occur, skin that is sufficiently elastic will heal without dimples, dents or ripples. But skin that has lost its elasticity may not contract as rapidly or satisfactorily.

Liposuction can be performed under local or general anesthesia. At the present time, the surgery is commonly performed on an outpatient basis in an office surgical suite or ambulatory surgical facility. However, medical opinions differ about whether the procedure should be done in an office or in a hospital. Dr. Pierre F. Fournier, a past president of the International Academy of Cosmetic Surgery, has stated that "anyone who is going to have a large amount of fat removed should be operated on in a hospital and observed overnight. Such patients will probably need intravenous fluids and may need blood transfusions."

Liposuction surgery is a body-contouring operation, not a weight loss procedure. Only small amounts of fat in terms of weight, one-half to two pounds, are actually removed during an operation, and this fat is considerably lighter than the solutions administered intravenously during the surgery. It is not uncommon for a patient actually to observe a weight gain of several pounds in the first few days following surgery because of this fluid replacement. But the kidneys rapidly eliminate excess fluid, and body weight soon returns to its preoperative level. Most patients with small to moderate fat bulges lose only a few pounds but may drop two to three clothing sizes. Many patients, however, report continuing weight loss for several months following liposuction, stabilizing at a loss of five to 10 pounds.

In 1988, a nationwide survey compared public attitudes about plastic surgery then with those of 1981 and found that 48 percent approved of it for themselves or others, a 50 percent increase from seven years earlier. The growing acceptance reflects people's increasing willingness to use plastic surgery to bring their bodies into conformity with their ideal body images. Besides liposuction, other procedures that have been performed increasingly often include ABDOMINOPLASTY (the tummy tuck), up 215 percent between 1981 and 1988. According to the Foundation for Facial Surgery, liposuction was the most frequently performed cosmetic surgery procedure in 1989, with 367,000 operations.

Complications Early reports of problems, including loss of limbs and a dozen deaths, led to investigations of liposuction procedures by the American Society of Plastic and Reconstructive Surgeons. In 1987 the society issued a report stating that "suction-assisted lipectomy is normally safe and effective" when performed by a properly trained, experienced surgeon with board certification in plastic surgery and a proven track record of success in liposuction. Legally, any surgeon can perform liposuction. This fact was brought out during a 1989 hearing held by the U.S. House of Representatives Small Business Committee's Subcommittee on Regulation and Business Opportunities. Chairman Ron Wydan (D-

Oregon) concluded that a liposuction surgeon "can buy $4,000 worth of equipment on Monday morning, do two procedures in the afternoon and make money all day Tuesday," even if he or she lacks accreditation.

But proponents of liposuction cite its safety record. John McCurdy, Jr. wrote that a compilation of more than 5,000 cases performed through 1983 showed only six complications, most minor (loss of skin and limbs was blamed on untreated infection; deaths occurred when liposuction was performed along with other surgery, or by unqualified surgeons).

Liposuction is major surgery and, as such, carries all the inherent risks, including potential problems with anesthesia, infection, discomfort, recovery time, side effects, complications and, of course, high cost. Minor complications associated with liposuction can include bruising, swelling and local sensory changes. Some complications can be permanent, such as bodily lumps, craters, asymmetry and permanent creases and furrows where the fat is removed. If the suction occurs too close to the skin's surface, it may tug at the skin tissue, causing it to ripple. The worst complications are excessive bleeding and loss of body fluids. Patients who have large amounts of fat removed (two liters or more) run the risk of shock if fluids are not adequately replenished during the surgery.

Bleeding is the most common complication following liposuction surgery. All patients undergoing surgery lose blood to some extent; this bleeding normally causes some bruising. Bleeding excessive enough to require transfusion is extremely rare during liposuction, but it has occurred. Surgeons blame such occurrences on patients who are "bleeders" but were not recognized as such prior to surgery, or on patients who have taken aspirin prior to surgery.

As with any procedure involving incisions in the skin, liposuction does leave scars. Usually these are small, about one-quarter inch, and are camouflaged by placement within natural skin lines. However, surgeons caution that persons predisposed to "over-active" scars need to discuss this problem with their doctor prior to surgery.

Early complaints of dents, depressions and skin waviness were blamed on the uneven removal of fat during liposuction. Today's specialists claim to have solved most of the problem by leaving a pad of fat on the undersurface of the skin and confining fat removal to deeper areas. Most surgeons now use smaller cannulas to make smaller, more numerous tunnels through the fat. This results in a smoother, more even shrinkage of skin over the suctioned area. The most troublesome area is the inner thigh, where skin does not contract as well as skin in other areas.

When uneven contours do exist after swelling has gone down, a second liposuction procedure is usually performed under local anesthesia. Surgeons say it is far easier to remove small amounts of excess fat than to fill in depressions caused by excessive fat removal.

Cost of liposuction surgery can range between $1,000 and $5,000 depending on the length and complexity of the procedure. Liposuction is not covered by most insurance plans because it is considered elective.

In early 1990, Thomas Dressel, a surgeon who performs liposuction in Minnesota, announced that he had become the first to use a laser during liposuction surgery. He claimed that cutting fat via laser before sucking it out of the body minimizes bleeding. The laser also seals blood vessels in tissue left behind. But other surgeons have expressed concern that using a laser would significantly and unnecessarily lengthen the procedure without any added benefit for the patient.

Heber, David; Gant, Thomas; Cline, Carolyn; Roper, Pamela; and Biggs, Thomas. "Fat Surgery: What Liposuction Can and Can't Do for You; The Nuts and Bolts of Liposuction; Is Liposuction for You?" *Shape*, April 1988.

Lillis, Patrick J., and Coleman, William P., III, ed. "Liposuction." *Dermatologic Clinics* 8: 3 (July 1990).

McCurdy, John A., Jr. *Sculpturing Your Body: Diet, Exercise and Lipo (Fat) Suction.* Hollywood, Fla.: Frederick Fell Publishers, 1987.

Montgomery, Sy. "Vacuuming the Fat Away." *Working Woman*, May 1988.

liquid formulas   A number of commercial diet supplement drinks promoted since the 1970s, the earliest and most highly publicized of which was Robert Linn's "Pro-linn," described as "a formula composed of all the amino acids needed to form a protein molecule." Such liquids have been used by hospitals for years to feed seriously ill patients. Once Linn's formula was published, other brands, such as Winmill, Gro-Lean, Ran-Tein, T-Amino, LPP, E.M.F., Pro-Fast, Nu-Trim/20 and Multi-Protein Slim, appeared.

The first liquid protein supplements were withdrawn when the Centers for Disease Control attributed 60 deaths to their use. The protein in these early supplements was collagen based; their inadequate amino acid composition led to dangerous loss of lean muscle mass, including heart muscle. In addition, these early diets did not provide adequate potassium, which may have resulted in serious disturbances of heart rhythm.

Then, during the mid-1980s, a new generation of liquid protein diets was developed. Made from high-quality protein, with adequate vitamins, minerals and electrolytes to maintain health, some of them are even intended for use in programs of medical monitoring, nutrition education, behavior modification, exercise and support groups sponsored by the manufacturers. Three widely used programs are Optifast (Sandoz Nutrition), Medifast (Jason Pharmaceuticals) and Ultrafast (National Center for Nutrition). In November 1988 these reformatted liquid protein diet programs received a commercial boost when the popular TV talk-show host Oprah Winfrey revealed that the loss of nearly 70 pounds that she had experienced was the result of following the Optifast liquid diet program.

Formula diets come in dry form as mixtures of essential nutrients; water must be
added before use. Prepared in two to six
servings, most of these diets provide milk
or egg (not vegetable) protein and varying
proportions of carbohydrate and fat. The
addition of carbohydrate decreases ketosis,
hyperuricemia, electrolyte depletion and
loss of lean tissue proteins. Fat improves
palatability and provides essential fatty
acids.

Users who stay with the program usually
lose four to 10 pounds during the first week
of the formula diet and two to five pounds
per week thereafter. Twelve-week programs
usually result in a loss of 22 to 33 pounds.
One study evaluated 4,026 morbidly obese
patients who showed interest in the Optifast
diet program. Ten percent failed to join or
did not meet entry criteria; one-fourth of
those remaining left the program within the
first three weeks; among the 2,717 remaining
patients, one-third reached the desired weight
during treatment, but fewer than half of these
remained within 10 pounds of that weight
when examined 18 months later. In other
words, 80 to 90 percent of patients who
wanted to lose weight were ultimately unsuccessful.

These programs are recommended only
for those people who are at least 30 percent
or 50 pounds above desired body weight.
Liquid diets may cause gingivitis and other
dental problems, along with the normal adverse effects of rapid weight loss. According
to the Federal Trade Commission (FTC),
these programs require professional supervision because there is evidence that patients
on liquid diets risk developing gallstones.
Also to be considered are the high costs
(generally between $1,400 and $2,800), time
needed for medical monitoring and group
support, and social restrictions when dinner-
time comes. Episodes of sudden death
(sometimes associated with myocardial abnormalities) like those that occurred with
older liquid protein preparations have not
been reported with current diet formulas.

However, even these new liquid formulas
have come under attack. In October 1991
the FTC charged marketers of Optifast 70,
Medifast 70 and Ultrafast with making deceptive claims that their programs are safe
and effective over the long term. As a result,
liquid formula diet promoters must back up
their claims of weight loss with more substantial studies over a longer duration.

See also DIETING; FAD DIETS.

"Contraction Seen in Weight Loss Market." *Food
    Institute Report,* November 30, 1991.
Nicholas, Patricia, and Dwyer, Johanna. "Diets
    for Weight Reduction: Nutritional Considera-
    tions." In *Handbook of Eating Disorders,* ed-
    ited by Kelly D. Brownell and John P. Foreyt.
    New York: Basic Books, 1986.
Saddler, Jeanne. "FTC Targets Thin Claims of
    Liquid Diets." *Wall Street Journal,* October
    17, 1991.
Wadden, T. A.; Stunkard, A. J.; and Brownell,
    K. D. "Very Low Calorie Diets: Their Effi-
    cacy, Safety, and Future." *Annals of Internal
    Medicine* 99 (1983).
Yetiv, Jack. *Popular Nutritional Practices: A
    Scientific Appraisal.* Toledo, Ohio: Popular
    Medicine Press, 1986.

M

major affective disorder The name
given to a group of psychiatric disorders of
which the two principal members are manic-
depressive illness (bipolar disorder) and major DEPRESSION. Major affective disorders
are biologically based illnesses with strong
hereditary components, for which specific,
effective treatments are available.

Harrison Pope and James I. Hudson, in
their book *New Hope for Binge Eaters,* suggest that both anorexia and bulimia are var-
iants of a major affective disorder. Evidence
for this includes reports of depression in
anorexia and bulimia patients before the onset of symptoms of the eating disorder; persistence of depressive symptoms in anorexia

nervosa after weight recovery; a positive family history of a major affective disorder in anorectic and bulimic patients; positive biological indicators of depression in anorexia and bulimia (i.e., positive dexamethasone suppression and TRH stimulation tests); and positive treatment outcomes for patients on antidepressant medications.

Stephen C. Woods and Deborah J. Brief acknowledged this theory in "Physiological Factors" (*Assessment of Addictive Behaviors*, edited by Dennis M. Donovan and G. Alan Marlett), but they cautioned that not all patients with eating disorders respond to ANTIDEPRESSANTS, and many recover without the use of antidepressant medication. They add that current research does not support the notion that all patients with eating disorders are suffering from a major affective disorder, or that antidepressants should be prescribed in all cases.

Laessle et al. assessed DSM-III lifetime diagnoses in 52 patients with a lifetime history of anorexia or bulimia by means of a standardized diagnostic interview. It was found that 44.2 percent had a lifetime diagnosis of DSM-III major affective disorder, with abstaining anorectics having a lower rate of depression than bulimics. In the great majority of cases, the onset of affective disorder postdated onset of the eating disorder by at least one year. In patients whose eating disorder was in remission, the rate of depressive symptoms was lower than in those in the acute stage of their illnesses. These findings, combined with recent studies of biological changes in eating disorders and psychological theories of depression, caused the researchers to suggest that in most cases in which the two conditions are associated, depression is secondary to the eating disorder. A full report on the study appeared in the December 1987 *British Journal of Psychiatry*.

Then in 1989, a study reported in the November *American Journal of Psychiatry* showed that rates of major affective disorder in relatives of bulimic patients, who themselves had no history of major affective disorders, were higher than in relatives of CONTROL GROUP subjects.

male anorectics   Boys and men do develop anorexia nervosa, but much less commonly than girls and young women. It is believed by many experts in the field that this condition may be more common in males than it seems to be but not readily recognized by doctors because of its reputation as a female disorder. Recent estimates are that 5 to 10 percent of all cases occur in males. Based on the number of those who seek treatment, experts estimate that at a minimum, several hundred thousand men are affected by eating disorders.

Studies of male anorectics tend to agree that in general the behavior of males resembles closely that of their female counterparts, with a few exceptions. One is that males who become anorectic tend to do so on average at an earlier age than females. In addition, relatively more males come from working-class homes. Some studies have found that a family history of anorexia nervosa is particularly common in male cases. The anorectic male tends to be massively obese before becoming emaciated. Finally, there is an impression that male anorectics respond to treatment less well and may be more likely to become chronic or drop out of treatment programs.

HILDE BRUCH says that male anorexia "occurs in youngsters who seemingly were doing well but whose accomplishments were a facade, an expression of compliance, and not of self-initiated and self-directed goals. In their desperate struggle to become 'somebody' and to establish a sense of differentiated identity, they become overambitious, hyperactive, and perfectionistic."

Arnold E. Andersen, associate professor of psychiatry at the Johns Hopkins School of Medicine, reported at the BASH VII International Conference on Eating and Mood Disorders that 76 males had presented themselves for consultation or treatment to the

Johns Hopkins Eating and Weight Disorders Clinic over approximately 10 years. This was almost exactly 10 percent of the patients seen there.

According to Dr. Andersen, males and females were similar in many ways, all meeting the essential DSM-III-R diagnostic criteria of self-induced starvation and morbid fear of fatness. Males did differ from females, however, in a number of ways: in contrast to women who in general felt fat prior to dieting, men on the average actually were obese. More than 50 percent of them were medically obese, usually mildly to moderately.

Men were seldom as concerned about clothing size or weight as females. Instead, they were intensely concerned with body shape. This has been confirmed in independent studies comparing the relative frequency of occurrence of articles, advertisements and the like on dieting and change of shape in magazines read primarily by men and those read primarily by women. Men more than women attempted to change body size and shape by way of athletic activities. Finally, men more often dieted in order to avoid medical consequences of overweight, such as heart disease.

Families of boys aged nine to 12 who develop anorexia are often described as psychologically disturbed or distressed, with the child having an unsatisfactory relationship with both parents.

Most males with anorexia begin weight loss during adolescence. These boys are more often mildly to moderately obese before onset than girls who become ill at the same age. Many, but not all, adolescent boys with anorexia show confusion about sexual identity. In personality tests they present a spectrum of disorders from perfectionistic and obsessive to borderline personalities not capable of maintaining stable relationships, and display rapid and inappropriate mood changes.

Restrictive male anorectics (see RESTRICTOR ANORECTICS) show complete impotence and absence of sexual activity and interest. When they regain weight, they experience a gradual return of normal sexual feeling.

Fichter and Daser (1987), in a report on 42 anorectic males, while noting that systematic studies of psychosexual development and gender identity in anorexia are lacking, hypothesize that atypical gender-role behavior in boys and male adolescents may be associated with an increased risk of developing anorexia or bulimia. Their results showed that in 31 percent of cases of primary anorexia nervosa the father was absent from the family.

Because few suspect eating disorders among teenage boys and men, the problems often go undiagnosed and untreated for many years. When finally recognized, the disorders are often far advanced and that much more difficult to treat.

Andersen, Arnold E. "Anorectic Behavior Isn't Quite the Same in Males." *BASH Magazine*, July 1989.

———. "Anorexia and Bulimia in Adolescent Males." *Pediatric Annals* 13, no. 12 (1984).

Andersen, Arnold E., and Mickalide, Angela D. "Anorexia Nervosa in the Male: An Underdiagnosed Disorder." *Psychosomatics* 24 (December 1983).

Beumont, P. J. V.; Beardwood, C. J.; and Russell, G. F. M. "The Occurrence of the Syndrome of Anorexia Nervosa in Male Subjects." *Psychological Medicine* 2 (February 1972).

Fichter, M. M.; Daser, C. "Symptomatology, Psychosexual Development and Gender Identity in 42 Anorexic Males." *Psychological Medicine* 17(2) (May 1987).

male bulimics   Occasional BINGE EATING on high-calorie, easily ingested foods may be done by as many as 30 percent of male college students, according to studies. The percentage of males meeting the DSM-III criteria for BULIMIA NERVOSA, however, is less than 5 percent. In one report, male students reporting to a university psychiatric clinic represented 10 percent of patients diagnosed as bulimic.

The figures could be artificially low. In tests, men have freely acknowledged "frequent consumption of large quantities of food at times other than during meals"; unlike women, however, they tended not to label this behavior as binge eating.

Generally, men have been found to be more comfortable with their weight and perceive less pressure to be thin than women. However, for male bodybuilders, long-distance runners and homosexuals, emphasis on body and physical appearance approaches the levels seen generally in women in our culture and puts these men at higher risk for developing eating disorders.

A past history of obesity is another risk factor for males. Obese young males, being a minority in our society, are often targets of cruel verbal and physical taunting. They might easily become preoccupied with their body and their physical appearance.

In some bulimia studies, the rare men with the diagnosis of bulimia nervosa all had a history of dieting from their mid- or late teens; indeed, this was all they had in common—only some had been anorectic, only some obese.

According to Root, Fallon and Friedrich in *Bulimia: A Systems Approach to Treatment*, "it appears more difficult for the male bulimic to seek help, perhaps because the socialization of men discourages help-seeking and because bulimia has been described as a 'woman's problem.'"

malnutrition   Poor nourishment resulting from improper diet or from some defect in metabolism that prevents the body from digesting or absorbing food properly. Extreme malnutrition may lead to starvation.

Eating disorders sometimes result in malnutrition. While intentional malnutrition is the hallmark of anorexia nervosa, it represents a significant medical complication of bulimia in 20 percent of cases. Principal manifestations of malnutrition involve five body organ systems: endocrine (amenorrhea and estrogen deficiency), cardiovascular (lowered blood pressure and reduced heart rate), neuromuscular (osteoporosis), renal (kidney stones and renal failure) and gastrointestinal (gastritis and decreased acid secretion).

marriage and anorectics   Some women marry while anorectic, even though they are likely to be infertile. The anorectic will often choose a partner who suits her as the kind of person she has become rather than as she was before becoming anorectic. For instance, the husband may be quiet and sexually undemanding, or alternatively superficially glamorous but privately wary of personal or sexual involvement. The marriage may be stable while the wife remains anorectic, but it will often be strained and tested if and when a process of recovery begins.

marriage and bulimics   Many bulimics vow to give up BINGE EATING and PURGING once they are married, hoping that marriage itself will magically transform their lives. Researcher Marlene Boskind-White has found that this does happen for some, but others resume their habit in secret, feeling more guilty and ashamed than ever. Bulimics have been known to keep their behavior a total secret from their husbands for as long as 15 years. But the deception often destroys a marriage. Some husbands conclude that their wives must be carrying on affairs because of their exaggerated sense of privacy. When they finally do find out that it's "only" an eating problem, they are relieved and often don't realize that it is even more significant than the affair they had suspected.

Boskind-White, Marlene, and White, William C. *Bulimarexia*. New York: W. W. Norton, 1983.

mass media influence on eating disorders   In a report published in *Journal of School Health* (August 1988), M. Elizabeth

Collins of Indiana University stated that children and adults are exposed to more than 5,260 commercial "attractiveness" messages per year, including 1,850 that deal directly with beauty. The report concluded that many viewers, particularly children, accept as real what appears on television, with concepts of attractiveness consequently going unchallenged. Constant ads implying that individuals must make up and make over to look acceptable eventually may undermine the self-confidence of adolescents struggling for identity. Today's adolescents have been exposed to extreme thinness as a standard of attractiveness since they were children. They may strive for the bodily "perfection" depicted in the media, believing that they are somehow inadequate in comparison with the ideal and would be acceptable if only they could lose more weight.

A review of studies examining children's selections of television characters as behavioral models identified physical strength and activity level as significant predictors of character identification for boys; physical attractiveness was found the most important determinant of character identification for girls.

While the report stopped short of blaming the media for actually causing women to be dissatisfied with their bodies, and admitted that it is impossible to calculate the relative importance of the media compared with other sources of messages about attractiveness, it did assert that "mass media must be considered a contributor to the thoughts, desires, and, possibly, self-concepts of individuals."

Other researchers have made similar statements about mass media: that enormous pressure to be thin is exerted in subtle but aggressive ways through programs and advertisements in which thin people prosper and the obese are ridiculed; that the media, in their many forms, are among those agencies and groups prospering directly or indirectly from selling images of slenderness; and that the current ideal of extreme thinness

most likely began with advertising images of women.

Researchers have called for the mass media "to refrain from suggesting that interpersonal and intrapsychic problems are solvable through the vehicle of controlling what we eat or how much we weigh" (Collins, quoting J. L. Katz in the *International Journal of Eating Disorders* 4 [1985]).

menstrual dysfunction Abnormal functioning of the menstrual cycle in females. Menstrual dysfunction is a common condition accompanying ANOREXIA NERVOSA and BULIMIA NERVOSA. Early studies emphasized the role of weight loss and lean/fat ratio in AMENORRHEA. But later studies conducted at the University of Rochester Medical Center, Rochester, New York to determine the incidence of menstrual abnormalities in a group of women with abnormal eating attitudes but without obvious eating disorder symptons found that 93.4 percent (compared with 15.0 percent of the CONTROL GROUP) reported an abnormal menstrual history. These data suggest that menstrual dysfunction often occurs in women with abnormal eating behavior but without weight loss or diagnosable eating pathology.

Kreipe, R. E.; Strauss, J.; Hodgman, C. H.; and Ryan, R. M. "Menstrual Cycle Abnormalities and Subclinical Eating Disorders: A Preliminary Report." *Psychosomatic Medicine* (January–February 1989). 51:1

menus for dieters Research has indicated that the order in which a person eats different foods during a meal can help him reach SATIETY at strategic moments and maintain a feeling of fullness for a longer period of time. Starchy or sugary foods contribute substantially after 10–20 minutes and continue as long as glucose is being absorbed rapidly. Thus, to be satisfying, a main meal should start with potatoes, pasta, rice or bread, and even sugars in sauces and dressings, to the extent that such items can be included in a nutritionally balanced reduced-calorie diet. While soups are customarily a first course, because of their low concentration of CARBOHYDRATES they may not "spoil" the appetite at the right time later in a meal. But they may be useful to dieters as a main course, because their low average calorie density and slowly digesting particles will help to slow the rate of gastric emptying after the meal. Thus, such foods may spread out satiety, helping to fight the temptation to snack or take the next meal early.

Gibbs, J., and Smith, G. P. "The Neuroendocrinology of Postprandial Satiety." *Frontiers in Neuroendocrinology* (August 1984). Vol. 8
Woods, Stephen C., et al. "Peptides and the Control of Meal Size." *Diabetologia* 20 (1981).

mesomorph A person whose body type is square and muscular. Mesomorphs have an athletic physique characterized by a broad trunk and shoulders with well-proportioned muscular arms and legs.

Theories linking body types to emotional or psychological characteristics are not considered scientifically sound.

See also ECTOMORPH; ENDOMORPH; BODY TYPES.

metabolism The sum of all chemical and physical processes by which the body transforms food and keeps itself alive. Metabolism is a two-phase process: catabolic and anabolic. In the catabolic, or destructive, phase, the body breaks down foods into simpler chemical substances. During this process, energy is released in the form of heat. The anabolic, or constructive, phase uses these substances to create new cells or mend damage.

The rate of metabolism can be increased by exercise; by elevated body temperature (as in a high fever), which can more than double the metabolic rate; by hormonal activity, such as that of thyroxine, insulin and epinephrine; and by specific dynamic action

that occurs following the ingestion of a meal. Reduction of caloric intake, on the other hand, will lower the rate of metabolism. Studies with animals have shown that the rate may drop during starvation to 60 percent of prestarvation levels. The lower the normal metabolic rate, the more, and the more quickly, it drops in response to caloric restriction.

Obese patients with the lowest metabolic rates prior to a diet lose the least amount of weight. It has been estimated that a dieter can expect to lose an average of 40 grams (1.5 ounces) per day for the first month if calories are cut from 2,000 to 1,500 per day. During the second month, expected weight loss would be half that amount—20 grams per day; during the third month, 10 grams per day; after that, no loss at all. Such evidence indicates that the metabolism adapts to caloric restriction by becoming more efficient.

To assess potential long-term effects of weight loss on resting metabolic rate (RMR) (the minimum rate necessary to keep the body functioning while at rest), the RMRs of seven obese women were measured before weight loss, during a PROTEIN-SPARING MODIFIED FAST and for two months after, while at a stable reduced weight. Body composition was also determined at each interval. RMR significantly decreased 22 percent with initiation of the modified fast. RMR values during the modified fast and during the maintenance diet at stable reduced weight were not different, and all were significantly lower than the prediet RMR. Loss of lean tissue could not account for the decrease because changes in RMR per unit of fat-free mass paralleled the total RMR reduction. A sustained decrease in RMR accompanied weight loss and persisted for eight weeks or more despite increased caloric consumption and body weight stabilization.

The effects on body weight of these adaptive changes in metabolism are especially dramatic after a diet is over. Starvation studies of animals show that, if calories during the refeeding period are restricted in proportion to the weight loss during fasting, the rate of weight gain is a direct function of the amount of weight lost; the greater the amount of weight lost during fasting, the greater the weight gain per calorie eaten during refeeding. In one study, rats starved to 20 percent below normal weight gained 29.6 grams during a period of refeeding while eating less food than controls, which gained only 1.6 grams. This represents an 18-fold increase in metabolic efficiency.

In a study of genetically obese mice, specially constructed cages allowed genetically normal mice to control the amount of food eaten by the obese mice. Even when the obese mice received a mere two-thirds what the normal mice ate, they still gained weight more rapidly. These animals metabolized food more efficiently to store more food. Low levels of physical activity did not account for these results, because during this time the normal mice spent much of their time sleeping, waking up only when they felt like eating. Meanwhile, the obese mice paced nervously waiting for the sound of the normal mice hitting the lever signaling their next meal.

Two studies released in early 1988 provided the strongest evidence yet that metabolism and genetics, not just eating behavior, determine who will become obese and who won't (see GENETIC FACTORS IN OBESITY). The research found that people who become overweight tend to burn fewer calories than those who don't, either because they use food calories more efficiently or because they're less active. Both studies suggest that "normal" weight for obese people may be quite different from normal for thin people. One study in Cambridge, England focused on infants, and another, in Arizona, focused on adult Pima Indians, long the subject of obesity research because most Pima adults are overweight.

The British study examined infants of either very thin or very fat mothers. Half the babies of fat mothers were overweight by the time they were a year old. But even at three months they were burning 20.7 percent fewer calories than the others even though they weren't yet overweight and weren't eating any more.

The Arizona study found that adults with slower metabolisms, burning 200 calories a day below the average for the group, were four times as likely to gain 16 pounds in the next two years as adults with fast metabolism. Once the heavy adults gained this weight, their metabolisms readjusted and were no longer slow, implying that their bodies were essentially "trying" to achieve a higher weight.

In another part of the study, the researchers found that adults who gained more than 22 pounds over the following four years were burning an average of 87 calories a day less than people who didn't gain that much. The study also showed that slow metabolism ran in families.

In a Canadian study, researchers studied the responses of lean and obese subjects to a short period of intense exercise. The lean subjects had marked changes in circulating concentrations of lactate, pyruvate, FFA (FREE FATTY ACIDS) and catecholamines, consistent with the need for rapid mobilization, uptake and utilization of carbohydrate and fat-derived fuels. The responses of the obese subjects differed in respect to absolute levels of glucose, insulin, FFA, glycerol and epinephrine. The postexercise hyperglycemic (high blood sugar), hyperinsulinemic (high insulin-deficiency) state was more intense in the obese subjects and associated with higher plasma FFA (free fatty acids in the blood) and blood sugar levels in them, suggesting that after exercise, as in many other situations, obese subjects have insulin resistance. (When cells do not receive insulin from the blood as a result of high blood sugar levels, hunger continues even after eating.)

A University of California team studied the effects of caloric restriction and exercise on resting metabolic rate (RMR) in five obese people. Subjects consumed a 500-

calorie-a-day diet for four weeks, with the subjects remaining sedentary during the first two weeks and then exercising 30 minutes daily during the last two weeks of caloric restriction. After two weeks of dieting, RMR decreased to approximately 87 percent of the predieting control value. Over the last two weeks of dieting with the addition of daily exercise, the fall in RMR was reversed as it returned to the predieting level.

In two studies of the relationship of resting metabolic rate in lean and obese children, researchers assessed differences in metabolic rate as a function of child weight and of the relation between child and parent weight. In both studies obese children had higher metabolic rates than lean children. Weight accounted for between 72 and 78 percent of the variance. Including parental weight did not improve the prediction of resting metabolic rate. After six months of treatment, obese children decreased the proportion by which they were overweight, but lean children showed no change. Resting metabolic rate in both groups remained unchanged after six months. These results indicate that the resting metabolic rate is higher in obese than in lean children and that changes in proportion of excess weight that result solely from increases in height do not decrease resting metabolic rate over six months. Taking parent weight into account does not improve the prediction of child resting metabolic rate.

The National Research Council estimates that the caloric requirements for maintenance of weight in the United States have declined approximately 10 percent over the last decade or so.

In a 1989 news item, *Insight* magazine reported that new studies "seem to show that a metabolic difference may be the precursor to psychological problems that lead to such eating disorders as bulimia and anorexia nervosa." The article cited a recent study conducted at the Western Psychiatric Institute and Clinic in Pittsburgh, which found that recovering bulimics needed only 10 calories per pound of body weight daily to maintain their normal weight. That is less than 73 percent of the 13.8 daily calories per pound that the average woman needed. Anorectics who had returned to a normal weight needed about 60 percent more calories than the average female to maintain their healthy weight.

Although, a disrupted metabolism and other physical changes resulting from an eating disorder could trigger changes in the body's need for calories, Walter Kaye, director of the inpatient eating disorder clinic at Western Psychiatric, said that an inborn difference in metabolism could explain some people's vulnerability to eating disorders and why posttreatment relapse rates are so high.

Eliott, D. L.; Goldberg, L.; Kuehl, K. S.; and Bennett, W. M. "Sustained Depression of the Resting Metabolic Rate after Massive Weight Loss." *American Journal of Clinical Nutrition* 49:1 (January 1989).

Epstein, L. H.; Wing, R. R.; Fernstrom, M. H.; et al. "Resting Metabolism Rate in Lean and Obese Children: Relationship to Child and Parent Weight and Percent-Overweight Change." *American Journal of Clinical Nutrition* 49:2 (February 1989).

Hammer, R. L.; Barrier, C. A.; Roundy, E. S.; Bradford, J. M.; and Fisher, A. G. "Calorie-restricted Low-Fat Diet and Exercise in Obese Women." *American Journal of Clinical Nutrition* 49:1 (January 1989).

Molé, Paul L.; Stern, J. S.; Schultz, C. L.; Bernauer, E. M.; and Holcomb, B. J. "Exercise Reverses Depressed Metabolic Rate Produced by Severe Caloric Restriction." *Medicine and Science in Sports and Exercise* 21:1 (February 1989).

"New Studies Link Fatness, Metabolism and Heredity." *NAAFA Newsletter*, March 1988.

Soares, M. J., et al. "Day-to-Day Variations in Basal Metabolic Rates and Energy Intakes of Human Subjects." *European Journal of Clinical Nutrition* Vol. 43, No. 7 (July 1989).

Vansant, G., et al. "Short and Long Term Effects of a Very Low Calorie Diet on Resting Metabolic Rate and Body Composition." *International Journal of Obesity*, 1989 suppl.

Weingarten, H. P.; Hendler, R.; and Rodin, J. "Metabolism and Endocrine Secretion in Response to a Test Meal in Normal-Weight Women.'' *Psychosomatic Medicine* 50:3 (May-June 1988).

Yale, Jean-François; Leiter, Lawrence A.; and Marliss, Errol B. "Metabolic Responses to Intense Exercise in Lean and Obese Subjects." *Journal of Clinical Endocrinology and Metabolism* 68, No. 2 (1989).

metoclopramide   A drug that increases the speed with which fluid and food pass from the stomach; it is often used prior to surgery. Metoclopramide has been prescribed to relieve the bloating complained of by many ANOREXIA NERVOSA patients after meals. However, the use of metoclopramide has been associated with significant depression and with hormonal changes, limiting its potential use in treating anorexia nervosa.

movement therapy   A psychotherapeutic treatment method based on the premise that the way we move is intrinsically connected to our thoughts and feelings. Dance, as spontaneous body movement, has been used almost from the beginning of history to express feelings and attitudes. The American Dance Therapy Association defines movement/dance therapy as "the psychotherapeutic use of movement to further the physical and emotional integration of the individual." It is a technique that uses nonverbal interaction between people as the primary means for accomplishing therapeutic goals.

As described by RENFREW CENTER movement therapist Ziona Brotleit,

The relationship established between patients and therapists by sharing a movement activity supports and enables behavioral change. The movement therapist helps patients learn about themselves from the way in which they move and assists them in bringing about desired changes.

The tendency of women with eating disorders to block their emotions and to fear loss of control is seen in blocked, split, rigid and restricted movement styles. Their self-esteem problems are demonstrated primarily in significant body image distortions. They seem to lack healthy boundaries in relationships and have either a rigid or an unclear sense of their kinesphere (personal body space). They tend to use more gestural than postural movements and lack the natural fluidity of movement.

At the end of movement therapy, eating disordered patients seem more comfortable watching themselves in the mirror and their body image is less distorted and more acceptable to them. They generally seem more self-accepting and sure of themselves.

Brotleit, Ziona. "Moving Forward." *Renfrew Perspective*, Summer 1989.

Silk, Geraldine. "Creative Movement for People Who Are Developmentally Disabled." *Journal of Physical Education* Vol. 60, No. 9 (November 1989).

Stark, Arlynne. "American Dance Therapy Association, a Kinesthetic Approach." *Dance Magazine*, November 1987.

Stern, Ricky. "Many Ways to Grow: Creative Art Therapies." *Pediatric Annals* 18:10 (October 1989).

multicompulsive   Having more than one compulsion simultaneously. Ten percent of bulimics are reported to display compulsive behavior in other areas, such as alcohol, drugs, stealing and sex. Multicompulsive behavior is very difficult to treat.

Bulimics and anorectics sometimes become involved with drugs such as cocaine, methamphetamine, CAFFEINE and over-the-counter DIET PILLS as they learn about and experiment with their appetite-suppressing qualities. As their eating disorders worsen, substances such as alcohol, marijuana, barbiturates and so on become an enticing anodyne for painful reality.

Eating-disordered women may actually convince themselves that their substance abuse in some way helps lessen the severity of their eating disorders. But in reality, substance abuse tends only to exacerbate their effects. For example, a bulimic woman who also abuses cocaine will extol the drug's tendency to offset food binges and decrease her appetite. Upon further discussion, however, she will be less enthusiastic about addressing her BINGE EATING and PURGING as she copes with the DEPRESSION and despair that set in after the cocaine has worn off. An eating-disordered marijuana abuser may insist that her use of the drug is not a problem, emphasizing its relaxing effect. But she may neglect to mention the subsequent "killer munchies" that trigger marathon binges.

Eating-disordered women may be particularly vulnerable to substance abuse when they are attempting to break away from bulimic or anorectic behavior. As uncomfortable feelings and memories begin to surface, they may seek intoxication as a means to numb their feelings without resorting to compulsive behavior toward food. Richard L. Pyle, a clinician with the Department of Psychiatry of the University of Minnesota, reports that at least 2 percent of the women coming to his clinic for evaluation are currently abusing alcohol and that one in five has had previous treatment for chemical dependency.

Bulimic women who abuse alcohol present special problems. Perhaps the most significant problem is the high frequency of SUICIDE attempts. In one study, 32 percent of bulimic women who had a history of alcohol abuse reported suicide attempts, compared with none by non–alcohol-abusing bulimics and 26 percent by a third group of bulimic women with a history of major depression. In addition, bulimic women who had a history of chemical dependency had an older age of onset; significantly more DIURETIC ABUSE and LAXATIVE ABUSE; worse functioning in social, financial and work areas; a higher incidence of stealing both before and after the onset of their eating disorder; and, more often, a history of previous inpatient treatment for bulimia (56 percent versus 4 percent).

Daily substance abuse produces sufficient loss of control that outpatient treatment of bulimia nervosa is often unsuccessful. In-patient care may be required to treat the chemical dependency, either concurrently with or preceding outpatient care for bulimia nervosa. Many clinicians also believe that a history of substance abuse in bulimia nervosa is associated with negative treatment outcome.

However, a two- to five-year follow-up study by Dr. Pyle's clinic indicated that, after treatment in an intensive outpatient group psychotherapy program, 24 patients who had a history of chemical abuse did as well as 65 who did not. In both groups 67 percent of the patients were symptom free at follow-up, and 25 percent were virtually unchanged. Only one of the 24 women with a history of chemical dependency required chemical dependency treatment during the follow-up, which averaged three and a half years, and three of 65 bulimic women without a history of chemical abuse required chemical dependency treatment. Therefore, Dr. Pyle summarized, a history of chemical abuse does not necessarily influence outcome negatively; and following successful treatment, patients with a history of alcohol abuse are no more at risk for chemical dependency than those with no history of alcohol abuse.

Doctors are also reporting a new trend of girls and young women using highly addictive cocaine and crack to lose weight. Drug dealers even promote these drugs with weight loss in mind, telling girls as young as 10 that boys like only thin girls and that crack (or cocaine) will help them lose weight. Crack, which is cheaper, is used mainly by poorer users, whereas cocaine is the drug of choice for the wealthier. Crack and cocaine suppress HUNGER by stimulating the central nervous system. Users feel no need to eat or sleep.

Mitchell, James E.; Pyle, Richard L.; et al. "A 2–5 Year Follow-up Study of Patients Treated for Bulimia." *International Journal of Eating Disorders* Vol. 8, No. 2 (March 1989).

Morrison, Beckie. "Learning to Overcome Addictions." *Renfrew Perspective*, Winter 1989.

Pyle, Richard L. "The Subtle, Puzzling Affinity of Drugs and Bulimia." *BASH Magazine,* September 1989.

music   Slow music reduces APPETITE, according to Johns Hopkins University research reported in 1991 in *McCall's, Tufts University Diet and Nutrition Letter* and *Small Business Reports.* Researchers counted the number of bites people took during meals while listening to music. Subjects who listened to no music took 3.9 bites per minute, with a third asking for second helpings. Those who listened to lively music ate an average of 5.1 bites per minute, with almost half requesting second helpings. But subjects listening to soothing flute instrumentals ate only 3.2 bites per minute, and none requested seconds. Most of the slow-music diners left about a quarter of the food on their plates and said they were full. They also had fewer digestive complaints and said their food tasted better. Researchers speculated that heightened taste occurred because chewing forces air from the throat to the nose, allowing the nose to smell the food. Because odor is an important element in the sense of taste, slower chewing gives a heightened sense of flavor.

See also EATING HABITS MONITORING; TASTE.

N

NAAFA (National Association to Advance Fat Acceptance)   Formerly known as the National Association to Aid Fat Americans, this nonprofit, tax-exempt organization formed in 1969 seeks to increase the happiness and well-being of fat people.

Its basic purposes are to assist the large number of people regarded by the medical profession as "persistently or incurably overweight" to adapt to themselves and in-

crease their self-confidence; to promote social tolerance toward fat people; to serve as a forum in which important problems affecting heavy people can be openly discussed; to disseminate knowledge pertaining to the sociological, psychological, medical and physiological aspects of obesity; and to sponsor research concerning these aspects of obesity. NAAFA is concerned with the general issues of fat people's lives, such as job discrimination, individual psychological problems and difficulties with respect to social acceptance and mobility. Its goal is to remedy these difficulties rather than to make members leaner. Its monthly publication is the *NAAFA Newsletter.*

neurogenic binge eating   A pattern of binge eating seeming to result from a neurological problem, extensively studied during the 1970s.

Researchers speculated that an epilepsy like seizure may cause some binge eating. They concluded provisionally that two categories of BULIMIA should be distinguished: psychogenic (psychologically caused) and neurogenic (neurologically caused) binge eating.

The overwhelming majority of bulimics are psychogenic bingers. Bulimics who binge eat as a result of anger and frustration and claim that they "can't help it" may be out of control, but they usually come to understand that they are using food to ease psychological pain.

Neurogenic binge eating is an entirely different experience, one that resembles a sudden possession or an eating seizure. The victim may be going about her business and suddenly be overwhelmed by an intense, insatiable desire to eat. She feels as if not she herself but forces outside her were making her eat—episodically, unpredictably and uncontrollably. She feels disoriented and strangely unlike herself during her binge, as if in an altered state of consciousness, and if she sleeps afterward, she is likely to be confused momentarily when she awakens.

The original researchers suspected that this mysterious disorder may have been an electrical disturbance in the brain similar to epilepsy, because patients stopped binge eating while taking Dilantin, an anticonvulsant drug.

These patients are described as generally in good physical health and may be underweight, normal weight or overweight. However, unlike other binge eaters, they experience an "aura" prior to bingeing (flashes of light, unusual smells, increased tension or fear); perceptual disturbances (feelings of depersonalization) while bingeing; occurrence afterward of a phenomenon of a kind typical of postconvulsive states (extended sleep, loss of consciousness, confusion, memory loss, loss of bladder control); rage attacks (temper tantrums, headaches, dizziness, stomachaches or nausea and a numbness or tingling in the upper or lower extremities); and neurological "soft signs," such as occurrence during a binge of an abnormal electroencephalographic (EEG) pattern, more typically seen in drowsiness or sleep. However, James E. Mitchell, in "Medical and Physiological Aspects of Bulimia" in *Handbook of Eating Disorders,* notes that "this pattern is also present in some normal subjects. The question of EEG abnormalities in bulimia deserves further study."

Although Rau and Green report a positive treatment outcome for patients with neurological signs and a weight deviation of greater or less than 25 percent from normal body weight, other studies have reported less-promising results with anticonvulsants.

Mitchell, James E. "Bulimia: Medical and Physiological Aspects." In *Handbook of Eating Disorders,* edited by Kelly D. Brownell and John P. Foreyt. New York: Basic Books, 1986.

Rau, J., and Green, R. "Neurological Factors Affecting Binge Eating: Body over Mind." In *The Binge-Purge Syndrome: Diagnosis, Treatment, and Research,* edited by R. Hawkins, W. Fremouw and P. Clement. New York: Springer, 1984.

neurotransmitters   Chemicals that transmit electrical impulses or "messages" from one neuron (nerve cell) to another or to a muscle cell.

Much scientific study has been directed at key chemical messengers in the brain that play a major role in regulating hormone production. Researchers have found anorectics and bulimics to have abnormal levels of certain neurotransmitters. For example, low levels of the neurotransmitter SEROTONIN are linked to bulimia, as well as the mood disorders, depression and impulsive behavior associated with bulimia. Low serotonin levels may contribute to bulimics' binge eating of food high in carbohydrates.

In anorexia, lower-than-normal levels of beta-endorphin, a natural brain opiate, and of the neurotransmitter norepinephrine are found in the spinal fluid. Because the norepinephrine levels are low in anorectic patients who have regained weight, it is possible that this neurotransmitter abnormality precedes weight loss and may, in fact, indicate a genetic connection to the eating disorder. But the same biochemical condition also could result from anorectics' starvation practices.

Fava, Maurizio; Copeland, Paul M.; Schweiger, Ulrich; and Herzog, David B. "Neurochemical Abnormalities of Anorexia Nervosa and Bulimia Nervosa." *American Journal of Psychiatry* 146:8 (August 1989).

nicotine   A potent oily alkaloid found in the tobacco plant; it is also the most addictive drug used in the United States. In *Sculpturing Your Body: Diet, Exercise and Lipo (Fat) Suction,* John A. McCurdy says,

Nicotine appears to lower the set-point. In spite of the observation that cigarette smokers eat as many as 200 calories per day more than nonsmokers, they are usually slimmer than nonsmokers. Most people gain weight, an average of ten to fifteen pounds, when they stop smoking, a consequence of elevation of the set-point. Health professionals agree, however, that the hazards of smoking far outweigh the possible risks of accumulating more body fat as a consequence of set-point elevation after one stops smoking.

Among those hazards are chronic bronchitis, emphysema, heart disease, high blood pressure and stroke, blood clots in the heart or brain, lung cancer and miscarriages.

See also SET-POINT THEORY.

night eating syndrome   The name given by Albert J. Stunkard in 1959 to an eating pattern in which an obese person succeeds in keeping his eating-disordered behavior under control during the day, in the interest of normal functioning, but is unable to resist it at night when alone. HILDE BRUCH described such a patient:

She was quite efficient in her work, although her severe obesity became increasingly a handicap. When she was alone at night, the tension and anxiety became unbearable. "I think then that I am ravenously hungry and I do my utmost not to eat. My body becomes stiff in my effort to control my hunger. If I want to have any rest at all, I've got to get up and eat. Then I go to sleep like a newborn baby." Patients with Night Eating Syndrome are unable to adhere to any dietary regimen as long as their problems and conflicts are unresolved, or as long as they remain in an anxiety- and rage-provoking environment. They can reduce without difficulty in a hospital but will regain as soon as they return to the old setting.

Bruch, Hilde. *Eating Disorders: Obesity, Anorexia Nervosa, and the Power Within.* New York: Basic Books, 1973.

novelties   Commercial items, usually useless for any practical purpose, designed to appear useful or amusing. Some novelties are devices contrived to be taken seriously by people interested in losing weight or becoming trim, for instance, by appearing capable of reshaping a person's body while he or she remains completely passive. Such items are sold in health food stores, drugstores, special clinics and salons, as well as through the mail.

A few of these, like "appetite-suppressing" eyeglasses with colored lenses that are supposed to project an image to the retina that dampens the desire to eat, are or border on the ridiculous. Yet hundreds, even thousands, of overweight people allow their unhappiness with their condition to override their common sense and are duped by such products regularly.

One weight reduction novelty, BODY WRAPPING, was invented in France. Areas of the body to be reduced are smeared with a cream, which may contain such ingredients as sea salt, herbs and cod liver oil, and wrapped in special bandages or garments. The intent is to "melt" or "burn" fat, especially CELLULITE, right off the body. The creams, gels, wraps, belts and sweatsuits are said to reduce body dimensions by removing fluids—that is, the user sweats it off. This is a very temporary loss because the fluid is regained when the person eats or drinks. Moreover, rapid and excessive fluid loss is potentially dangerous because it can cause severe dehydration and chemical imbalance. The U.S. Food and Drug Administration has taken legal action against several promoters of these products for making unsubstantiated weight loss claims.

Other French techniques for fighting cellulite are more aggressive, and some are potentially dangerous. Machines massage a woman's legs with powerful jets of air or administer a barrage of "fat-dispersing" injections.

A reducing machine that delivers slight electrical shocks to selected muscles, causing them to contract and supposedly do the client some good, has achieved some degree of popularity. A 35-minute session with the machine is supposed to be equivalent to 1,500 push-ups or sit-ups without the unpleasant aches and pains required from such strenuous exercise.

The electrical muscle stimulator has legitimate uses in physical therapy but is useless for weight loss or figure firming. Claims that stimulation from these devices has the figure-toning effect of as many as 3,000 sit-ups, for example, are without any scientific basis. Further, these devices, often promoted through mail order for home use, can be dangerous if not handled correctly. There have been reports of electrical shocks and burns, and the devices can be particularly hazardous to pregnant women and to people with heart problems, pacemakers or epilepsy.

Hillel Schwartz believes that the popularity of these novelties lies in the "key word" for American dieting: secrecy. He says that although dieters want to have others notice weight loss, most do not want others to know they are dieting. Thus, such implements of fat destruction as girdles, corsets and wooden roller belts (the forerunners of today's vibrating machines) became popular because they could be hidden under the dieter's clothing.

Schwartz, Hillel. *Never Satisfied: A Cultural History of Diets, Fantasies and Fat.* New York: Free Press, 1986.

Willis, Judith Levine. "How to Take Weight Off (and Keep It Off) without Getting Ripped Off." *FDA Consumer,* Food and Drug Administration, DHHS Publication No. 89-1116.

nutrients   Substances in food necessary for life. They include carbohydrates, fats, proteins, vitamins, minerals and water. Carbohydrates, fats and proteins provide energy, and vitamins and minerals are essential for the METABOLISM that uses this energy. Water, composing 60 percent of our total body weight, provides the medium in which chemical reactions take place.

nutrition   The combination of processes by which the body takes in and uses the foods necessary for maintenance, energy, growth and renewal. It includes digestion and METABOLISM.

nutritional counseling   Frequently recommended in the treatment of eating disorders. As physicians Michele Siegel and Judith Brisman and Margot Weinshel explain in

their book *Surviving an Eating Disorder,* "Some people with eating disorders have extremely chaotic eating patterns or have not eaten a 'meal' in years. Nutritionists, who are trained to assess nutritional imbalances and develop dietary programs, can help recovering clients correct nutritional deficits and develop healthy eating habits, perhaps for the first time." The authors say that counseling is most successful after binge eating, purging or starving behaviors have decreased, when food is no longer used as a coping mechanism and eating is a response to physiological, not psychological, hungers.

Professor P. J. V. Beumont, presenting a paper on "Dietary Advice" at the BASH VII International Conference in April 1989, agreed that nutritional counseling is an important component of the treatment of all bulimic patients and is usually essential if therapy is to be effective. He gave the following reasons why nutritional guidance is so important:

- Eating behavior is often so erratic in bulimics that patients need to regain control of their habits before they become involved in other forms of treatment such as PSYCHOTHERAPY.
- Bulimics view their problem as one of overeating and do not understand that gorging is a response to prior restrained eating practices.
- Bulimics have many fears and misconceptions about food and weight control that need to be identified and corrected. (They firmly believe that if they eat regular meals or high-energy foods, they will inevitably get fat.)
- Bulimic patients have had disordered eating habits for so long that they need to learn to recognize when they are hungry and when they are satisfied.

Sometimes nutritional counseling is recommended in order to provide an appropriate diet. But a diet is not always the answer to an eating disorder. Many eating-disordered people are actually experts on diet and nutrition. They know what they should be eating. Eating disturbances are not due to lack of knowledge or information but to the psychological disorders that keep people from using them. Thus nutritional counseling works best, some experts feel, after psychological treatment has progressed.

Beumont, P. J. V. "Diet Guide for Bulimics." *BASH Magazine,* June 1989.

Siegel, Michele; Brisman, Judith; and Weinshel, Margot. *Surviving an Eating Disorder.* New York: Harper & Row, 1988.

O

obesity Body weight in excess of biological needs; excessive fatness.

Moderate obesity is 20 or 30 percent to 100 percent above ideal body weight. Moderately obese persons are more likely to develop hypertension or diabetes mellitus than nonobese or slightly obese persons.

Morbid obesity is 100 percent or more above ideal body weight, and is life-threatening. Conditions associated with morbid obesity include coronary heart disease, hypertension, cardiorespiratory dysfunction, thromboembolic disease, diabetes mellitus, hepatobiliary diseases, osteoarthritis, Pickwickian syndrome, increased operative risks, uterine, fibroid and endometrial cancer, edema of the lower extremities, renal disease, skin problems, susceptibility to infection and psychosocial incapacity.

Although 24 percent of American men and 27 percent of American women between the ages of 20 and 24 are obese, according to the National Institutes of Health (NIH) criteria, more than 90 percent of these obese individuals are only mildly so.

Assessment and Measurement An NIH panel in 1985 defined obesity as an excess of body fat, frequently resulting in a significant impairment of health. The panel found that health risks increased with increasing weight and suggested that a level of 20

percent or more above desirable body weight is associated with sufficient risk to justify clinical intervention. Others have suggested that a 30 percent level of overweight should be the criterion for clinical obesity, because some research indicates that the risk is not truly significant below that level.

In terms of body composition, young men up to age 27 with more than 20 percent body fat, men 28–50 with greater than 30 percent, young women with greater than 30 percent and women 28–50 with greater than 37 percent body fat are considered "overfat" or obese and should consider beginning a program for reducing body fat percentage.

The NIH panel on obesity, noting the limitations of standard height and weight tables (the most commonly used of which is published by the Metropolitan Life Insurance Corporation), recommended a measurement termed the body mass index (BMI) as a standard for the determination of obesity. The BMI is calculated by dividing body weight (in kilograms) by the square of height (in meters) (BMI = weight divided by height squared). Body mass index is a useful measure in clinical practice because it is easily understood and allows comparison with standard research data. However, like other standard measurements, it cannot by itself provide an adequate assessment of weight loss. A 20-pound weight loss has a different significance for a 150-pound person than for a 300-pound person. Moreover, because muscle tissue is heavier than ADIPOSE TISSUE, reductions in absolute weight may not directly correspond with decreases in body fat resulting from exercise programs. Percentage over ideal weight is perhaps a better measurement for weight loss, because it takes into account both height and weight. This measurement, however, does not represent a totally adequate measure for comparing results across studies.

Excess fat accumulation is associated with increased FAT CELL size; in extremely obese individuals, the number of fat cells is also increased. In the simplest terms, obesity is an imbalance between intake of food and expenditure of energy. The excess taken in is stored in fat deposits, resulting in an increase in body weight.

Possible Causes Why this imbalance occurs remains uncertain. Although genetic influences appear to be the most likely factor in explaining a tendency toward obesity, the precise trigger for its development is unknown. As a result, there is a variety of methods for treating obesity, with results that also vary.

Until recently, obesity was considered to be caused simply by eating too much, as a result of psychological problems with food: using food to deal with DEPRESSION, anxiety, boredom, even happiness. The prevailing theory was that to lose weight an obese person needed only to eat less. Recent studies have shown, however, that tendency to overweight is biological rather than psychological or diet driven. Some studies have shown that thin people, as a group, tend to eat more than obese people. People with identical diet and exercise programs may become, or remain, fat or thin. The difference is now believed to be genetic.

Other research has demonstrated that obesity tends to occur in families. One large study, which collected data from approximately 10,000 individuals, revealed that hereditary factors accounted for 11 percent of the variance in the incidence of obesity, and family environment for 35 percent.

Jeffrey, Dawson and Wilson wrote that metabolic determinants of obesity have gained increasing attention from researchers. In a year's time, they explain, the average person of normal weight consumes more than one million calories, but there is little variation in body weight because a comparable number of calories is used in bodily maintenance and activity. Taking in 10 percent more calories or expending 10 percent less energy would lead to a 30-pound weight gain within a year. Researchers conclude that in normal-weight individuals, body weight is regulated with extraordinary accuracy. Moreover, research suggests that the hypothalamus is directly linked to weight regulation, containing a feeding center that controls appetite and SATIETY and maintains body weight. Some studies have shown that, rather than causing obesity, metabolic and endocrinological anomalies actually result from it.

Jeffrey et al. also list social learning processes as playing a major etiological role in most cases of obesity:

A social learning theory of obesity is based on the concept of energy balance and the assumption that our eating and physical activity habits, good or bad, are mostly acquired patterns of behavior. Thus, social learning theory specifically focuses on the acquisition and maintenance of behaviors that result from environmental factors. This conceptualization has clear implications in the assessment and subsequent treatment of an eating disorder.

Rodin et al. stated in *Medical Clinics of North America* (January 1989) that the role of psychological variables in the etiology of obesity is still not fully understood. The etiologic significance of many factors once thought to be important—lack of impulse control, inability to delay gratification, or faulty eating habits—has not been supported by experimental evidence. Other factors, depression and dysphoria, for example, appear to be consequences rather than causes of obesity, although they may serve to maintain and intensify weight-related problems. Dieting in response to weight concerns appears, perversely, to be implicated in increasing overweight. Response to food cues in the environment may also play a causal role in some cases of obesity.

Emotional Overeating Some people, when they are nervous, tense, angry, frustrated or upset, often indulge in overeating because food has become an emotional outlet for them. It acts as a sedative, giving them a feeling of well-being and security. Overindulgence in food helps to control the emotional stress they experience. Many of these people show signs of other exaggerated oral activity, such as excessive talking, laughing, giggling or nail biting.

Physicians have categorized four major types of emotional overeating:

• Overeating as a response to tension, anger, upset, loneliness or boredom.
• Overeating as a substitute gratification for lack of sex or love, or when faced with an intolerable life situation such as the hostility of a parent or spouse.
• Overeating due to addiction to food. (See BINGE EATING, COMPULSIVE EATING and CRAVING.)
• Overeating as a symptom of an underlying depression and hysteria.

HILDE BRUCH believed that obesity is an essential and desirable state for a considerable number of emotional overeaters. These people use their excessive fat like a security blanket—as a protective barrier against the world. For these people, loss of weight is fraught with psychological danger and may result in serious psychological consequences.

Risk Factors   Obesity is the most common chronic medical condition in America today and affects all age groups, according to the National Center for Health Statistics. For example, one-year-old children today typically weigh 50 percent more than one-year-old children of a generation ago. The center reports that 40 percent of American women and 32 percent of American men aged 40–49 tip the scales at 20 percent above desirable weight.

Additional data from the National Health and Nutrition Examination Survey show that 34 million adult Americans are overweight, 12.4 percent of whom are severely overweight (7.2 percent of women, 4.9 percent of men). Obesity is directly or indirectly associated with disorders that account for approximately 20 percent of all deaths.

According to data provided by the National Center for Health Statistics:

• Women are more likely to be obese than men, regardless of age, although recent findings suggest that this may be changing.

• Obesity is more prevalent in lower socio-economic groups, particularly among females.
• Rural populations tend to be more overweight than urban populations.
• Blacks, as a group, are more likely to be obese than whites.
• Americans, as a group, have become heavier during this century.

Several conditions are recognized as placing an individual at risk for developing obesity:

Heredity   Recent studies have confirmed previous findings that heredity is involved in the development of obesity. Doctors and scientists have examined different families and found that obesity is more common in some than in others. Some researchers have gone so far as to call "family" the most important risk factor for obesity, citing a 1965 study that found that 80 percent of the children of two obese parents will be obese, 40 percent of the children of one obese parent will be obese and 10 percent of the children of two lean parents will be obese. In foster families with overweight parents, the natural children tend to be more overweight than the foster children.

A "biological clock" factor refers to genetic characteristics that influence adolescent growth and amount of body fat. Throughout childhood, the obese as a group develop faster not only with respect to weight and height but also in terms of overall size, skeletal and dental maturation. This is particularly evident among those obese from infancy. This lends support to the notion that the growth of ADIPOSE TISSUE is not completely independent of the growth and maturation of other tissues, and that each may influence the other.

Morphology of Fat Tissue   In general, those adults with a childhood history of obesity display the most marked degree of adipose tissue hyperplasia (abnormally high number of cells), and obese children begin to differ significantly with respect to size and number of fat cells as early as age two. In nonobese children, fat cell size and number increase during the prepubescent and adolescent periods, after remaining relatively stable from the age of two. In contrast, massively obese children have achieved adult cell size by age two, and after that time they show a constant increase in cell numbers.

Early Dietary Excess   There is evidence that fat cell size expands in the first 12 months of life and fat cell number increases up to 12 to 18 months of age. Using various weight-based indices, some researchers have attributed obesity to infant feeding practices.

Family Environment   Theories based on family-centered learning emphasize the psychosocial interactions in the social environment of the family as important factors in the development of obesity. In some cases this may involve major disruptive events, such as long separation from the mother or an overly protective family environment, but these causes are considered much less common than a family disinclination to physical activity and exercise, or a social, emotional and physical environment within the family that favors overindulgence. Family eating habits are often blamed for childhood obesity.

Social Learning Theory   There is reason to suspect that, at least for adult-onset obesity, factors involving social learning after the early years within the family are very much involved. The effectiveness or frequency of attempts to lose weight is thought to vary, especially by social class, even as early as adolescence. Social learning also influences knowledge of weight control techniques and of nutrition.

Psychological Time Bomb Theory   Theories of obesity as resulting from neuroticism or excessive emotional reaction to adolescent stress have been largely ruled out by recent studies. The evidence for them is considered less convincing than that for more sociologically and culturally oriented explanations. However, numerous studies suggest that obese

people, once they have become obese, may develop psychological symptoms and that these may become particularly apparent during weight reduction efforts. They are especially pronounced among those with an earlier age of onset and a greater degree of obesity. Such individuals are generally very sensitive about their condition. Because obese adolescents are discriminated against both in employment and in high-ranking college admissions, it has been suggested that these social selection factors, felt most strongly in late adolescence, tend to encourage obese adolescents into social environments more permissive of obesity; thus they become even fatter.

Affluent Sedentary Society   In our highly mechanized, automated society, most people expend little energy in muscular work. Children and adolescents are more sedentary than formerly, and energy output is even lower among adults. The obese are generally less active than others. The widespread availability of palatable, cheap (and commercially promoted) foodstuffs is another characteristic of the affluent society in Western countries today. Given such abundance, food and eating not only may be used to satisfy physiological needs but also are readily available means for coping with various emotional states. Food cues in the physical and electronic environment also favor overindulgence if the propensity for it is there. Recent studies emphasize the importance of the social environment in these respects.

Health Complications   Many studies have found that obesity either contributes to or is associated with a number of diseases, including diabetes, high blood pressure, coronary heart disease, complications of pregnancy, osteoarthritis and some cancers and infections. Scientists also report that obesity may foretell certain diseases, such as breast and uterine cancer. As pounds are added, more cells divide, increasing the odds that they will divide abnormally and develop into tumors. Animal studies show that eating fewer calories reduces colon and breast cancer risk regardless of dietary fat levels. Cancer risk was also reduced in rats that ate as much as they wanted but maintained lean body mass with exercise.

Severe childhood obesity increases the risk of a number of diseases. An immediate danger is deformation of the spine or the long bones of the limbs. These changes in the skeletal system may be particularly pronounced if obesity is accompanied by vitamin D and calcium deficiency.

A low hemoglobin blood count is quite common in obese children, making them more susceptible to tonsilitis and respiratory infections and prolonging their duration. Obese children also tend to have significantly higher levels of glucose, cholesterol and triglycerides, putting them more at risk for developing atherosclerosis (vascular fat deposits), which can lead to heart attacks and strokes.

Several studies have shown that the risk of liver and kidney damage from surgical anesthesia with halogenated anesthetic agents is greater than normal for patients who are obese.

Women with a high concentration of abdominal fat seem to be at higher risk for diabetes mellitus, cardiovascular disease, mental disorders and psychosomatic disease than other women, according to a study of 1,492 Swedish women. Findings of this study were reported in *Appetite* 12 (1989).

Benefits of Obesity Not all clinicians subscribe to the supposition that all obesity is harmful. There have been critics of prevailing views on obesity for nearly 40 years, some asserting that obesity is more of an aesthetic and moral problem than one of physical health. Some researchers have even proposed that there may be advantages, medical and other, to being fat.

One detailed study of the effects of weight on mortality followed nearly the entire population of Norway for 10 years after an initial physical examination. Optimal life expectancy occurred at weights 10 to 30 percent above actuarial standards. Weights slightly less than standard were far more hazardous than those slightly more.

The fact that obese persons have a normal life expectancy presents a paradox, since the incidence of a number of serious risk factors is increased in obesity. Paul Ernsberger, a biomedical researcher at Cornell University Medical School and a leading proponent of the theory that obesity is not necessarily hazardous, suggests that the solution to this puzzle is that there are advantages as well as disadvantages to being heavy. He states that obese persons are less likely to develop cancer, citing numerous studies. The obese, he says, are also protected against infectious diseases, chronic obstructive pulmonary disease, osteoporosis, mitral valve prolapse, intermittent claudication, renovascular hypertension, eclampsia, premature birth, anemia, diabetes Type I, peptic ulcer, scoliosis and suicide. These health benefits of obesity might potentially offset its hazards.

Obesity is also associated with improved survival in several diseases. Ernsberger states that heavy persons with hypertension, diabetes Type II and hyperlipidemia have a more favorable prognosis than thin people with these same ailments. Obese hypertensives have been shown to outlive lean hypertensives in 15 separate controlled studies.

Although hypertension, diabetes and hyperlipidemia have reduced complications and mortality in heavy persons, this does not mean these conditions are benign in obesity, nor does it mean that diabetics and hypertensives should be encouraged to gain weight, since this may worsen their condition. However, Ernsberger suggests that the threat to the health and longevity of fat people posed by diabetes and hypertension may be overestimated, owing to the failure to take into account the ameliorating influence of obesity on these conditions.

Janet Polivy of the University of Toronto and Toronto General Hospital, who has researched obesity and eating disorders for 15 years, stresses that it is unclear whether obesity is a ''problem'' in any but the social sense. She says the so-called health hazards of obesity have been grossly overstated. While medical disorders do result from excessive body weight, many of the diseases blamed on overweight are not a simple result of excess weight per se. More often, they are caused by overeating, by large and rapid weight fluctuations and possibly most often by dieting. Specifically, she cites heart attacks usually blamed on obesity, but actually caused by diet pills and inadequate diets.

Researchers at the University of Nebraska Medical Center analyzed 8,428 adult hospital admissions and reported their findings in the May 1988 *Journal of Gerontology*. Obesity was associated with higher mortality only when subjects were 100 percent or more overweight; being at or below ideal weight was usually associated with increased mortality. The lowest mortality occurred at moderate overweight. Underweight seemed to be a more important predictor of mortality than overweight in older hospitalized subjects.

Psychological Effects   Not all medical professionals believe that childhood psychological problems are at the root of adult obesity. In his book *The Dieter's Dilemma,* William Bennett suggests that although there are people who overeat in a desperate attempt to handle inner conflicts, they are probably a small fraction of fat people. In fact, he says, fat people as a group are mentally quite healthy, considering what they must put up with. They are not more neurotic than thin people and, in some ways, less so, since they have maintained their mental health through decades of well-intentioned but ineffective efforts to explain and ''improve'' them.

Yet Jeffrey, Dawson and Wilson, in *Assessment of Addictive Behaviors,* say,

> Unpleasant affective responses and overeating commonly occur together. Negative feelings such as anger, resentment, anxiety, or loneliness, when handled by eating, lead to contin-

ued obesity and to the development and maintenance of maladaptive behavior. Thus, some individuals learn to use food to escape from tension or boredom or to assuage pain or depression. On the other hand, food and overeating also appear to be frequently associated with social occasions, fun, and self-gratification.

Treatment   The fundamental treatment for obesity is caloric reduction. The traditional view has been that weight loss depends on reducing the total number, rather than the kind, of calories consumed. While some popular FAD DIETS concentrate on certain types of calorie intake, there is very little evidence of the superiority of such diets to more conventional, calorie-restricted but balanced diets. The degree of caloric restriction required to lose weight depends on the degree of obesity, age, sex, physical activity and general health of the patient. Except for unusually active individuals, it would be difficult to lose weight while consuming more than 1,200 calories per day. Dramatic weight losses commonly result from VERY LOW CALORIE DIETS of fewer than 800 calories; side effects include hypotension, constipation and occasional dizziness. Although initial losses may be impressive, these diets have not effectively encouraged permanent weight loss.

Physical training is widely used for reduction of body fat, although it frequently does not result in a net weight loss because of a parallel increase in muscle mass. With continued training, though, the decrease in body fat generally exceeds the increase in muscle mass so that a net loss in body weight does occur. Studies have shown that at least eight weeks of three-per-week sessions, each lasting a minimum of 30 minutes, is required to reduce fat tissue measurably. Studies have also shown that the initial six to eight months of a training program are characterized by a decline in BODY FAT, after which most individuals reach a plateau in total body weight and in percentage of body fat. One other result of physical training is a general HUNGER-reducing effect of intensive EXERCISE.

For most, exercise is more effective in preventing rather than treating obesity.

In recent years there has been increased interest in BEHAVIOR MODIFICATION for the treatment of obesity. Such techniques as slowing the rate of eating, limiting access to cues that signal eating behavior and keeping records have all resulted in short-term benefits. Unfortunately, these short-term benefits do not seem to be maintained. Newer studies have emphasized spouse training and teaching self-control. Individual therapy rather than group therapy is best used for the person lacking in self-esteem, the immature individual who has had difficulty separating from the mother and the socially isolated person who had little or no contact with his or her mother. GROUP THERAPY is quite effective in treating CHILDHOOD OBESITY, primarily because of the enormous peer pressure among children. It is used with patients who have stronger egos than those who are suitable for individual therapy. Teenage children respond very well to counseling given in groups. They are accustomed to learning in groups, and learning about their diet comes most readily when they are with friends who have similar problems. Most effective with teenagers is a leader who is knowledgeable in the field of nutrition and obesity, who genuinely likes children and wants to help children with this problem. When the cause of childhood obesity is related to family pathology, FAMILY THERAPY is called for. This treatment tends to focus on areas of conflict within the family that foster certain eating habits and patterns.

Research does not support drug therapy as a good primary treatment of obesity. (See PHARMACOTHERAPY.) The use of some drugs, notably AMPHETAMINES, carries a high potential for addiction and abuse, and they are only marginally effective in long-term appetite suppression. At present there are about two dozen APPETITE SUPPRESSANT drugs in use in the United States for which a prescription is not required. The active ingredient in most is phenylpropanolamine. Of the prescription drugs available, amphetamines, methamphetamines and phendimetrazine are the least safe; mazindol, phendimetrazine, chlortermine, benzphetamine and chlorphentermine are safer; FENFLURAMINE, diethylpropion and phentermine are the safest. Antiobesity drugs are not recommended as a sole form of therapy and should be used only with supervision. In treating childhood obesity, appetite suppressants are used primarily in the developmental type of obesity. Stimulants are used to control the impulse disorders of children with minimal brain dysfunction. The use of more potent agents such as the sympathomimetic drugs, which mimic the action of the sympathetic nervous system, amphetamine derivatives and other drugs that act on the nervous system is not advised for children under 12. Such drugs affect the nervous system and the brain differently than in adults and may cause permanent damage. These drugs have also not been proven safe or effective for teenagers. Weintraub and Bray wrote in *Medical Clinics of North America* (January 1989) that anorexiant drugs, the major class of drugs currently available for treating obesity, differ in several important ways, including their effects on noradrenergic and serotonergic systems and in their potential for abuse. New approaches to drug treatment of obesity include thermogenic agents and drugs acting on the digestive system and hormones.

Surgical treatment of obesity has aroused widespread interest and controversy. When used, it is most often as a last resort, after more conventional approaches have failed over a period of at least four years. It is not recommended for patients over the age of 50 and is suggested only for patients who are 125 pounds or more above their desirable body weight. Yet Kral stated in *Medical Clinics of North America* (January 1989) that despite numerous shortcomings and limitations, surgical methods are the only viable alternative for achieving and maintaining substantial weight loss in dangerously obese patients and therefore represent a legitimate, potentially lifesaving intervention. Nevertheless, the magnitude of weight loss varies widely, as does the number of patients who do not return for follow-up treatment or who require multiple operations. The safety of this type of surgery and the recognition and successful treatment of side effects in co-operating patients have improved greatly in recent years. (See BYPASS SURGERY; GASTRIC BUBBLE; GASTRIC PARTITION PROCEDURES; GASTRIC RESTRICTION; GASTROPLASTY; JE-JUNOCOLONIC BYPASS; JEJUNOILEAL BY-PASS.)

A 1988 study conducted by the American Medical Association's Council on Scientific Affairs states that the only effective treatment for obese adults incorporates diet, exercise and behavior modification. The report went on to say that all three practices must also be maintained in order for a person to keep off weight that is lost.

The council also recommended that any obese person considering treatment at a commercial weight loss facility evaluate the program's emphasis on medical supervision by a physician and its exercise curriculum.

David A. Booth of the University of Birmingham, England has performed studies corroborating the council's findings.

> Someone's obesity can be cured only by one or more periods of negative energy balance, with an average null balance at all other times. In practice, this requires permanent changes in the overweight person's own habitual actions of eating, drinking and physical exercise. That is, successful loss of excess weight relies in the end on self-management.

The bottom line, Booth feels, is that unhealthy overweight is not the sort of condition that can be helped by treatment in the usual sense, whether via prescription or behavior modification. He concludes that established treatments for obesity cannot be relied on to effect permanent loss of a clinically significant amount of weight. His research has determined that

> hopes for a future successful treatment are unsound for the same reason. Even if a safe

thermogenesis-inducing drug became available for prescription, any permanent increase in metabolic output is liable to be counteracted by the user allowing an increase in intake within the normal range. The main reason that intestinal bypass, or the likely long-term safer gastric reduction surgery, permanently reduces weight is that it makes restriction of intake much easier; so, even this treatment can be vitiated by continuous eating of readily assimilated foods, if the patient wishes and can afford them.

Booth, D. A. "Holding Weight Down: Physiological and Psychological Considerations." From "A View of Obesity," *Medicographia* 7, No. 3 (1985).

Bray, George A. "Effects of Obesity on Health and Happiness." In *Handbook of Eating Disorders*, edited by Kelly D. Brownell and John Foreyt. New York: Basic Books, 1986.

Brownell, Kelly D., and Wadden, Thomas A. "Behavior Therapy for Obesity: Modern Approaches and Better Results." In *Handbook of Eating Disorders*, edited by Kelly D. Brownell and John P. Foreyt. New York: Basic Books, 1986.

Corcoran, George B.; Salazar, Daniel E.; and Chan, Hannah H. "Obesity as a Risk Factor in Drug-induced Organ Injury." *Toxicology and Applied Pharmacology* 248 (January 1989).

Ernsberger, P. and Haskew, P. "Health Implications of Obesity: An Alternative View." *Journal of Obesity and Weight Regulation* 6 (1987).

"Health Implications of Obesity." *NIH Consensus Development Conference Statement* 5, No. 9.

Jeffrey, D. Balfour; Dawson, Brenda; and Wilson, Gregory L. "Behavioral and Cognitive-Behavioral Assessment." In *Assessment of Addictive Behaviors*, edited by Dennis Donovan and G. Alan Marlatt. New York: Guilford Press, 1988.

Kornhaber, Arthur, and Kornhaber, Elaine. "Psychological Types of Obesity and Their Treatment." In *Childhood Obesity*, edited by Platon J. Collipp. New York: Warner Books, 1986.

Levin, Barry E.; Hogan, Sue; and Sullivan, Ann C. "Initiation and Perpetuation of Obesity and Obesity Resistance in Rats." *American Journal of Physiology* 25 (1989).

Mayer, J. "Genetic Factors in Human Obesity." *Annals of New York Academy of Science* 131 (1965).

Powers, Mary A., and Pappas, Theodore N. "Physiologic Approaches to the Control of Obesity." *Annals of Surgery* 209 (March 1989).

Rodin, Judith; Schank, Diane; and Striegel-Moore, Ruth. "Psychological Features of Obesity." *Medical Clinics of North America* 73 (January 1989).

Stunkard, Albert J. "Obesity: Risk Factors, Consequences and Control." *Medical Journal of Australia* 148 (February 1, 1988).

obesity, attitudes toward   It has been suggested that public derision and condemnation of fat people is one of the few remaining sanctioned social prejudices against any group based solely on appearance. There is evidence that obese people are denied educational opportunities, jobs, promotions and housing because of their weight.

Dennis E. Clayson and Michael L. Klassen stated that "there is considerable evidence to suggest that obese persons are perceived negatively by others. This negative perception seems to be heightened because, unlike many other stereotyped persons, obese persons are seen as personally responsible for their condition." Clayson and Klassen found that obese persons are characterized as lazy, unkempt, lacking self-discipline and self-respect, unhealthy and insecure. (Paradoxically, they are also seen as jolly.) An obese person may be seen as purposely violating a cultural value.

Disdain toward the obese begins before adulthood. Several studies have documented what most people know from experience—that grade school children consistently attribute negative qualities to larger body shapes.

Children appear to develop attitudes about fat at a very early age. They are told repeatedly by parents and physical education teachers that fatness is not only unattractive but leads to sickness, and these attitudes persist throughout their lives. Studies confirm that chubby children are regarded by their peers as ugly, stupid, mean, sloppy, lazy and dishonest and are frequently teased. Samples of adults have rated obese children as less likable than children with a variety of handicaps, disfigurements and deformities.

One study included a preference test to see whether two- to five-year-olds preferred a thin or a fat rag doll. Fifty-three out of 56 children as young as two years of age picked the thin doll. Similar results occurred using drawings of fat and thin children. The team conducting the test had planned to use photographs but were unable to obtain photos of fat children. They visited shopping centers, amusement parks and similar places and asked every parent who passed by to let them photograph their children. No parent of a thin child refused; no parent of a fat child ever consented. Some parents permitted a thin child to be photographed while hiding a fat one behind them. The team ended up with hundreds of photographs of children, and not one of them was fat.

This prejudice is neither natural nor universal. Obesity has been valued highly in many cultures at various periods of history. Some African peoples have been known to lock pubescent females in fattening huts where they are denied exercise and receive extra rations of food for as long as two years. This practice produces an overweight woman who symbolizes the well-to-do status of her family.

Other cultures discriminate in their preference for the location of fat deposits. In our own culture, the attempt to achieve the "right" proportions, those in vogue at given time or in given society, has led women to try a variety of devices, some quite harmful, to alter their natural physique.

Corsets and waist cinches have caused fainting, rib fractures and permanent damage to the respiratory system. Around the turn of the century, some women had ribs removed (a practice not unknown today among fashion models) in order to achieve an hourglass figure. More recently, cosmetic surgery, silicone injections and breast implants have replaced the padded bra and bustle in the relentless pursuit of "beauty."

According to a January 1990 *New York Times* article by Trish Hall, there are some signs that Americans are becoming less critical of overweight people. In a mail survey each year of 2,000 households, the NPD Group, a Chicago research firm, tracks attitudes. In 1984, 55 percent of the respondents agreed with the statement that "people who are *not* overweight are more attractive"; by 1988, that figure had dropped to 42 percent.

See also CULTURAL INFLUENCES ON APPEARANCE.

Clayson, Dennis E., and Klassen, Michael L. "Perception of Attractiveness by Obesity and Hair Color." *Perceptual and Motor Skills* 68 (February 1989).

obesophobic   Having a fear of being fat. A term used by some clinicians to describe people judged underweight by standard measurements but who still think they are too fat and who are preoccupied with their weight.

See also FEAR OF FAT SYNDROME.

Olestra   Trade or proprietary name for a no-calorie fat substitute developed by Procter & Gamble in 1989 after nearly 20 years of research. It is intended for use in shortenings and oils and in the preparation of certain fried snacks, like potato chips. It tastes, feels and, in cooking, functions like fat but is not in any sense a food and is not found naturally in any food.

Also known as sucrose polyester (SPE), it is not absorbed into the bloodstream and therefore, according to Procter & Gamble, should likely produce fewer complications than other food substitutes such as aspartame, a sugar substitute known to cross into the bloodstream. In one study by the company, 10 fat people were fed with up to 60 grams of SPE in their diet for 20 days, so that their caloric intake was reduced by 23

percent and fat intake by 50 percent. On average, the patients lost eight pounds each. Patients on the SPE diet did not crave additional food to make up for their calorie loss. SPE satiates the desire to gorge, as does food made with conventional fats.

Olestra has remained under review by the Food and Drug Administration since 1987. Although Procter & Gamble maintains that Olestra is safe for humans, some scientists have questioned it. Rats in some tests have developed tumors and leukemia, among other diseases, according to the Center for Science in the Public Interest, a consumer advocacy group.

See also FAT SUBSTITUTES.

"Consumers of Fat Substitute Seek Calories Elsewhere." *Atlanta Constitution,* April 24, 1991.
"A Product in Limbo for 20 Years." *New York Times,* September 29, 1991.

Optifast   A commercial PROTEIN-SPARING MODIFIED FAST program, intended for use under medical supervision. This program achieved prominence when television talk-show hostess Oprah Winfrey announced in 1988 that she had lost 67 pounds on the Optifast program. After this announcement, the Optifast company received hundreds of thousands of calls from consumers desperate to lose weight. Sales boomed as people paid $3,000 to $5,000 each to participate in the program. But 18 months later, as reports surfaced about the dangers of VERY LOW CALORIE DIETS, both Oprah and the majority of the Optifast users had regained much of their lost weight (plus added poundage), and the company had cut back on satellite clinics. Today company promotions focus more on the fact that Optifast is a physician-supervised program and less on the weight loss results.

oral expulsion syndrome   Compulsively attempting to lose weight by chewing food and spitting it out instead of swallowing it. People who have experimented with this technique voluntarily have become compulsive about it. They spend hours doing it in secret and in time develop intense anxieties about swallowing. As a consequence, they become isolated, fearful and seriously malnourished.

See also RUMINATION.

oral fixation and obesity Some psychoanalytic theorists relate obesity to a developmental fixation during the earliest, or oral, stage of development. Because the first and most central love attachment to develop is that between mother and infant, and because much of the infant's contact with the mother occurs during feeding, the infant naturally associates eating with maternal care. During normal development, the infant's world expands, and the focus on oral needs becomes integrated with other sensory experiences. If, however, either outside events or internal processes affect development negatively during this oral phase, the child may not easily relinquish the need for oral gratification. And that same child may continue in adult hood to relate to food as the primary symbol of emotional care, turning to it whenever there is a need or desire to recapture the security and comfort experienced in infancy.

According to John S. Daniels, this attempt to link a psychiatric disorder or personality type to obesity has not been successful, even though there is some evidence that this theory of oral fixations holds true for some individuals.

Daniels, John S. "The Pathogenesis and Treatment of Obesity." In *Eating Disorders,* edited by Félix E. F. Larocca. San Francisco: Jossey-Bass, 1986.

oral nutritional supplements Nutrients in liquid form; the least invasive way of supplementing an anorectic patient's food intake during hospitalization.

Because a nutritional supplement is considered a medication, its use is charted in a patient's files and the patient is required to drink it in the presence of a nurse. Not considering it food helps avoid conflicts with the patient over eating or not eating.

oral soft tissues Periodontal tissues, gingival tissues, the lining of the mouth, pharynx and esophagus, the lips and tongue and the salivary glands, are all areas of the oral cavity that can be affected by anorexia nervosa and bulimia. Tissue health is impaired by dry mouth and the resulting reduction of the saliva's membrane-lubricating effects. As a result of dryness and poor oral hygiene, gingivitis, or inflammation of the gums, is quite common in eating-disordered patients. If untreated, this inflammation spreads into the supporting structures of the teeth, causes bone loss and eventually results in loss of the teeth. Vitamin deficiencies from poor diets have very marked effects on soft tissues, including scurvy, inflammation of the tongue and a burning sensation in the tongue. Bulimic patients sometimes evidence abrasions of the lining of the throat due to use of the fingers or foreign objects to induce vomiting. The caustic gastric acid brought up during the purging process inflames esophageal, pharyngeal and salivary gland tissues. Salivary gland enlargement is not an uncommon occurrence in patients with eating disorders.

See also DENTAL CARIES; PERIMYLOLYSIS.

Dalin, Jeffrey B. "Oral Manifestations of Eating Disorders." In *Eating Disorders: Effective Care and Treatment,* edited by Félix E. F. Larocca. St. Louis: Ishiyaku EuroAmerica, 1986.

osteopenia A general term referring to loss of bone, regardless of cause. Bone loss may be due to a number of disorders, the most common of which are osteoporosis, osteomalacia and osteitis fibrosa. There are various causes for these conditions, and treatment and prevention strategies vary accordingly.

Osteoporosis is a condition in which bone mass becomes demineralized, less dense and brittle. It is associated with aging. This is the most common form of osteopenia and has received the most publicity. It accounts for the fragility of the bones in elderly women. A progressive condition, it generally begins at menopause or when there is any loss of hormones. Women are more susceptible to osteoporosis than men for a number of reasons, including their smaller size and lower dietary calcium intake. Other hormones and certain drugs also contribute to the development of osteoporosis.

Osteomalacia is the softening of the bones, characterized by an accumulation of newly created bone mass that has not become mineralized. Hardening of bone mass requires both calcium and phosphorus and will be affected negatively by a deficiency of these minerals or by the presence of certain hormones or drugs. Persons with osteomalacia frequently suffer from generalized bone pain even in the absence of fractures.

Osteitis fibrosa is a condition in which bone degenerates, or is resorbed, very rapidly. It usually results from excessive production of certain substances such as parathyroid hormone or thyroid hormone. In these cases, bone is diminished faster than new bone mass can be formed.

Osteopenia has been recognized as a serious complication of anorexia nervosa within the last 10 years. In 1983, E. R. McAnarney and her colleagues reported a case of pathological rib fracture in a 25-year-old anorectic. Since then there have been at least 10 other reports documenting pathological fractures in anorectics including ribs, vertebrae and hips. In one instance, successful treatment of anorexia nervosa resulted in improvement of the patient's bone density, although she continued to have mild osteopenia.

Reduced bone densities are found in some anorectics, caused by reduced calcium intake and a drop in estrogen levels from self-starvation. Although, in general, a certain level of activity is necessary to promote adequate bone growth, the kind of excessive activity that characterizes some anorectics (such as 1,000 sit-ups a night) may overstress already-weakened bone and lead to fractures.

Rigotti et al. reported in the *New England Journal of Medicine* (December 20, 1984) on a study of the radial bone density of 18 anorectic and 28 normal women, which indicated that the anorectics had a lower bone density. But anorectics having a high level of physical activity had a bone density similar to that of active or inactive nonanorectics, which was greater than that of low-activity anorectics.

Insufficient calcium for bone growth may result from a number of factors besides poor dietary intake. Production of high levels of serum cortisol during FASTING may increase the loss of calcium from the body. PURGING practices such as self-induced VOMITING and LAXATIVE ABUSE can also cause unnecessary elimination by the kidney of essential chemicals required in bone formation. Consequently, eating-disordered patients may have reduced bone mass or may predispose themselves to the future development of osteoporosis through their restrictive dietary practices and purging behaviors.

One study of anorectic women who had been given either calcium or estrogen and who had gained weight showed that bone loss was halted but not reversed. Physical exercise and calcium and estrogen treatments did not affect bone restoration. From this, it was concluded that a period of severe weight loss in young women may be a risk factor for premature osteoporosis.

Brotman, A. W. and Stern, T. A. "Osteoporosis and Pathological Fractures in Anorexia Nervosa." *American Journal of Psychiatry* 142 (1985).

Carmichael, Kim. "How Self-starvation Damages Bone Structure." *BASH Magazine,* January 1990.

Kaplan, F. S; Pertschuk, M.; Fallon, M. D.; and Haddad, J. G. "Osteoporosis and Hip Fracture in a Young Woman with Anorexia Nervosa.'' *Clinical Orthopaedics and Related Research* 212 (1986).

McAnarney, E. R.; Greydanus, D. E.; Campanella, V. A.; and Hoekelman, R. A. ''Rib Fractures and Anorexia Nervosa.'' *Journal of Adolescent Health Care* 4 (1983).

Rigotti, N. A.; Nussbaum, S. R.; Herzog, D. B.; and Neer, R. M. ''Osteoporosis in Women with Anorexia Nervosa.'' *New England Journal of Medicine* 311 (1984).

Overeaters Anonymous (OA)   A nonprofit self-help group formed in 1960 that follows many of the principles of Alcoholics Anonymous; membership is based on free-will donations. OA promotes the belief that ''compulsive eating is a progressive illness that can't be cured but can be arrested.'' Like Alcoholics Anonymous, this group has a 12-step recovery program, based on acceptance of the premise that an overeater is powerless over food and that only a Power greater than oneself can restore one to sanity.

overweight bulimia   Although normal-weight bulimics are the most common, there are substantial numbers of overweight bulimics, who run into difficulties when seeking appropriate treatment. For example, because they binge eat and purge, they are often grouped by providers of therapy with emaciated bulimics or anorectics; or they are classified simply as obese individuals. Overweight bulimics vehemently reject these classifications and the treatment approaches that go with them.

Researchers comparing normal-weight bulimic and obese individuals have found many similaritites between them. Common characteristics include a greater tendency to guilt, alienation, impulsivity, obsessive thinking and preoccupation; there are similarities in eating habits as well. Bulimics, however, display greater distortions in both cognitive and mood disturbances, as evidenced by more pervasive impulsivity as well as BODY IMAGE DISTURBANCE, ANXIETY and DEPRESSION.

The disorders of both groups represent needs from more than one level—physical (the need for weight control) and psychological (the need for increased psychosocial development).

In treating overweight bulimia, clinicians promote the use of SELF-HELP GROUPS in developing self-regulatory abilities. They suggest that it is the development of these abilities that encourages the maintenance of any weight loss that is achieved.

Larocca, Félix, and Goodner, Sherry. ''Self-help as an Adjunct to the Treatment of Overweight Bulimia: An Obesity Variant of Disputed Etiology.'' Paper presented at the satellite conference *Drugs Regulating Food Intake and Energy Balance,* Rome, September 1986.

Williamson, D. A.; Kelley, M. L.; Davis, C. J.; et al. ''Psychopathology of Eating Disorders: A Controlled Comparison of Bulimic, Obese and Normal Subjects.'' *Journal of Consulting and Clinical Psychology* 53 (1985).

Wilson, G. T. ''An Evaluation of Behavioral Therapy in Obesity.'' *International Journal of Obesity* 4 (1980).

P

pagophagia   The craving to eat ice.

pancreatic polypeptide (PP)   A 36–amino acid peptide that is produced by the delta cells of the pancreatic islets and is released in response to feeding. It is thought to be a SATIETY hormone that is deficient in children with hereditary forms of morbid obesity. Whether PP deficiency is the cause of obesity or just a marker is not clear. Administration of pancreatic polypeptide will decrease food intake, although the doses required are believed to be above safe levels.

parental factors in anorexia nervosa

The degree to which parents influence the development of or directly cause anorexia nervosa had not been firmly established, although theories abound. Parents of anorectics have been described in various studies as neurotic, obsessive, rigid or passive. However, the reported incidence of these behaviors in parents of anorectics has varied greatly, ranging from 10 to 40 percent. Controlled research in this area has been sparse, but a few studies of parents have indicated the presence of emotional disturbance. Usually parents do blame themselves for a daughter's anorexia.

HILDE BRUCH suggested that anorexia nervosa develops in a family setting in which the child is not allowed to assume the responsibilities associated with the normal maturational process. She describes these parents as overprotective, overambitious and overconcerned. Consequently, these children often develop unrealistic expectations of themselves. One area of such perfectionism is the body.

See also FAMILY THERAPY.

passive exercise machines   Devices that deliver electrical shocks to muscles, forcing involuntary contractions, which supposedly takes the place of active exercise. A recent fad in weight-reducing gadgetry, these machines are supposed to tone the stimulated muscles, thus firming and trimming objectionable bulges. A forerunner to these latest exercise machines was the Relaxicisor, a device that was banned by a federal court in 1970.

John A. McCurdy wrote that such electrical stimulation is used to maintain muscle tone and flexibility in patients who have suffered localized paralysis from strokes, or who are unable to exercise actively because of coma or other neurological conditions. While properly performed electrical stimulation can enhance muscle tone in healthy people, most researches in this field feel that the machines utilized in "passive exercise"

clinics are not sufficiently sophisticated (and personnel operating these machines not well enough trained) to offer the individual variability necessary to deliver the proper frequency, magnitude and duration of electrical stimulation required for efficient muscle toning. And unfortunately, muscle toning has no effect on overlying fat deposits that usually contribute the bulk of the objectionable figure deformity.

See also FRAUDULENT PRODUCTS.

McCurdy, John A., Jr. *Sculpturing Your Body: Diet, Exercise and Lipo (Fat) Suction.* Hollywood, Fla.: Frederick Fell Publishers, 1987.

pathophysiology   The study of abnormal function as related to body structure.

The late physiologist William Sheldon speculated that a genetic trait common to the overweight is a long intestinal tract. He estimated that in long, thin body types, ECTOMORPHS, the length is about 20 feet; thus food reaches the colon in a matter of hours, before many calories can be absorbed. Heavy ENDOMORPHS, however, might have up to 40 feet of intestine, which gives them additional absorptive surface and more time to absorb and store every bit of fat and sugar. Sheldon believed that MESOMORPHS have about 30 feet of bowel and tend to be neither fat nor thin. Sheldon's theories are not considered valid, although the terms associated with them frequently appear in books and articles.

perfectionism   Extreme or obsessive striving for perfection; a trait often exhibited by young people with eating disorders. One definition of perfectionistic thinking is that it involves the setting of unrealistic standards, rigid and indiscriminate adherence to these standards and the equating of self-worth and performance. Others go a step further and argue for a distinction between "normal" perfectionism, a useful characteristic, and neurotic perfectionism, a dysfunctional or self-defeating one. The latter is

characteristic of those who are predisposed toward developing an eating disorder, according to Peter Slade, reader in clinical psychology at the New Medical School, University of Liverpool, England.

For perfectionists, eating disorders are another side of the "all-or-nothing" mind set. The more they focus on being perfect, the more aware they become of their faults. Feelings of worthlessness set in. Especially if they think they are being dominated in other areas of their life—family, school, work—they may decide to take charge of at least one area: eating. Controlling and monitoring their food intake is something within their power. Other areas of perfectionistic tendencies have also been documented. In one study of 20 anorectics, school achievement was found to be significantly greater than would be predicted by standard tests. Many women with eating disorders also admit to feeling pressured to be "the perfect person." Often they share low SELF-ESTEEM and a deep fear of making mistakes.

See also DICHOTOMOUS REASONING.

Slade, Peter D. "The Misery That Neurotic Perfectionism Can Create." *BASH Magazine*, July 1989.

perimylolysis   A loss of enamel and dentin from the surfaces of the teeth as a result of repeated contact with regurgitated gastric acids, rubbed in by movements of the tongue. Destruction can range from slight (smooth and polished surface of the teeth) to extremely severe (the complete dissolution of tooth structure through to the nerve). In more severe cases, all surfaces of the teeth are affected by acid erosion. This decay can be caused by a number of factors, but once other problems are ruled out, the patient can be assumed to have an eating disorder.

Perimylolysis is generally seen in the bulimic or bulimic/anorectic patient and not in the patient exhibiting restrictive anorexia alone, since the latter does not usually vomit to purge. The chronic vomiting characteristic of bulimics (sometimes five to 10 or more times daily) brings gastric acids into the oral cavity; these acids dissolve tooth structure. Enamel will not usually erode until repeated regurgitation has occurred for two years. The surfaces most commonly affected are the lingual, or tongue-side parts of the upper teeth. The other teeth are protected by the position of the tongue, lips and cheeks. It has been suggested that acidic gastric juices accumulate among the papillae of the tongue and that tongue movement continually deposits the acid on the lingual surfaces of the teeth.

See also DENTAL CARIES; ORAL SOFT TISSUES.

Dalin, Jeffrey B. "Oral Manifestations of Eating Disorders." In *Eating Disorders: Effective Care and Treatment,* edited by Félix E. F. Lacorra. St. Louis: Ishiyaku EuroAmerica, 1986.

personalities of eating disorder victims   Bulimics and anorectics seem to differ in personality. People who succumb to bulimia are more impulsive and more likely to abuse alcohol and drugs than anorectics. Anorectics tend to be "too good to be true." They rarely disobey, keep their feelings to themselves and tend to be perfectionists, good students and good athletes.

Bulimics and anorectics, however, do share feelings of helplessness, a lack of SELF-ESTEEM and fear of fat (see FEAR OF FAT SYNDROME). In both disorders, eating behaviors seem to develop as a way of handling stress and anxieties. The bulimic person consumes huge amounts of food, often junk food, in search of comfort and to ease stress. This BINGE EATING, however, brings guilt and depression. Relief comes only with PURGING. The anorectic restricts food, particularly carbohydrates, to gain a sense of control in her life. Having followed the wishes of others, for the most part, she has not learned to cope with the problems of adolescence and growing up.

In a University of Georgia study, 15 bulimics and five anorectics were tested with the California Psycholgical Inventory, the EATING DISORDERS INVENTORY, the Revised Children's Manifest Anxiety Scale and the House-Tree-Person Projective Test to determine if there were any personality differences between the two groups of women diagnosed with these two types of eating disorders. The bulimics scored significantly higher on extroversive personality characteristics and the anorectics high on introversive.

A connection was made between eating disorders and addiction to drugs or alcohol, with alcoholism present in the families of three of the women interviewed. The parents were described as perfectionistic and critical with regard to appearance, especially weight. The results of this study support the distinction of bulimia from anorexia nervosa as a separate disorder.

See also ANXIETY; MULTICOMPULSIVE; PARENTAL FACTORS IN ANOREXIA NERVOSA; PERFECTIONISM.

Allinder, Rose. "The Personality Differences between Women Diagnosed with Anorexia Nervosa versus Bulimia." Ph.D. diss., University of Georgia, 1987.

Aronson, H.; Fredman, Marla; and Gabriel, Marsha. "Personality Correlates of Eating Attitudes in a Nonclinical Sample." *International Journal of Eating Disorders* 9, no. 1, 1990.

personality disorder   A condition, as defined by the *American Medical Association Encyclopedia of Medicine,* "characterized by a general failure to learn from experience or adapt appropriately to change, resulting in personal distress and impairment of social functioning." The *Comprehensive Psychiatric Nursing* definition is "a mental disorder that originates within the character structure of a person."

Recent research has found personality disorder to be a possible risk factor for bulimia. JOEL YAGER et al. administered the Personality Diagnostic Questionnaire (PDQ) to 628 eating-disordered women: 300 with normal-weight bulimia, 15 with anorexia nervosa with bulimic features and 313 with subdi-

agnostic eating disorders. Three-quarters (75 percent) of subjects with normal-weight bulimia had personality disorder diagnoses, compared with 50 percent of those with subdiagnostic eating disorders. The most common PDQ diagnoses were schizotypal, histrionic and borderline disorders, but avoidant and dependent personality features also occurred.

In another study, Yates et al., of the University of Iowa College of Medicine, compared 30 bulimic patients with 30 age- and sex-matched controls (see CONTROL GROUP) on DSM-III personality measures. The bulimic patients were more likely to display cluster B (histrionic, narcissistic, antisocial and borderline) personality abnormalities and cluster C (avoidant, dependent, compulsive and passive-aggressive) personality abnormalities than were the controls.

Yager, Joel; Landsverk, John; Edelstein, Carole K.; and Hyler, Steven E. "Screening for Axis II Personality Disorders in Women with Bulimic Eating Disorders." *Psychosomatics* 30(3) (Summer 1989).

Yates, William R.; Sieleni, Bruce; Reich, James; and Brass, Clint. "Comorbidity of Bulimia Nervosa and Personality Disorder." *Journal of Clinical Psychiatry* 50 (February 1989).

pharmacotherapy   The use of drugs in the treatment of psychological disorders. An outgrowth of research in the neurobiological sciences, pharmacotherapy has made great inroads in the treatment of psychological disorders and psychiatric illness.

By studying medications used in the treatment of depression, researchers have found clues to the potential role of drugs in the treatment of eating disorders. Although drug treatments do currently have a place in the management of some patients with eating disorders, they have not yet proven sufficiently effective to be employed on other than an experimental basis.

Unfortunately, not much data have been collected in studies of medications in the treatment of anorexia nervosa. According to

B. Timothy Walsh, author of "Pharmaco-therapy of Eating Disorders," a chapter in *Modern Concepts of the Eating Disorders,* edited by B. J. Blinder et al., only three drugs have been tested for their effects on anorexia nervosa, and these have shown only marginal effects.

More studies have been done on medication treatments for bulimics; ANTIDEPRESSANTS, anticonvulsants (see ANTICONVULSANT TREATMENT) and others have been tested. Studies have shown that antidepressants do cause short-term improvements of bulimic behaviors. Even bulimic patients without symptoms of depression show improvement on antidepressants.

In a trial conducted of 50 women by Walsh et al. at the New York State Psychiatric Institute, phenelzine (an MAO inhibitor–type antidepressant) was significantly superior to PLACEBO in the reduction of binge frequency (64 percent versus 5 percent). However, there was a problem with side effects, so researchers determined the usefulness of phenelzine to be limited among bulimics.

Drug studies lasting more than 16 weeks have revealed a difficulty in getting patients with bulimia to continue taking their medication even when it has been effective.

Pharmacotherapy can interfere with necessary behavioral change if it removes the cue that triggers binge eating, without which behavior to counteract it cannot be adopted. Moreover, when medication ceases, the cue may reappear, setting off binge eating again.

W. A. Price wrote that

pharmacologic management in anorexia nervosa and in bulimia nervosa is especially helpful when it is part of a multimodal treatment approach that includes individual, family and behavioral therapy. Care must be taken to guard against side effects, abuse and noncompliance in a group of patients that tends to be prone to all three.

Garfinkel, Paul E., and Garner, David M., eds. *The Role of Drug Treatments for Eating Disorders.* New York: Brunner/Mazel, 1987.

Price, W. A. "Pharmacologic Management of Eating Disorders." *American Family Physician* 37 (May 1988).

Rockwell, W. J. Kenneth. "Pharmacological Approaches to the Treatment of Eating Disorders." In *Eating Disorders,* edited by Félix E. F. Larocca. San Francisco: Jossey-Bass, 1986.

Tolstoi, Linda G. "The Role of Pharmacotherapy in Anorexia and Bulimia." *Journal of the American Dietetic Association* 89 (November 1989).

Tupoin, J. P., and Shader, R. I. *Handbook of Clinical Psychopharmacology.* Northvale, N.J.: Jason Aronson, 1988.

Wilson, G. Terence. "Cognitive-Behavioral and Pharmacological Therapies for Bulimia." In *Handbook of Eating Disorders,* edited by Kelly B. Brownwell and John P. Foreyt. New York: Basic Books, 1986.

phenylpropanolamine (PPA)   An AMPHETAMINE-like agent available without prescription and approved for sale as an APPETITE SUPPRESSANT. It is used in over-the-counter diet products like Dietac and Dexatrim. PPA is also the decongestant in such cold remedies as Contac, Robitussin CF and Vicks Formula 44D. It is potentially harmful for those with high blood pressure.

physiological   arousal   Physical response to stimuli; for instance, the development of a feeling of hunger in response to the sight of food.

Although several studies have suggested that physiological arousal is an important factor in overeating by obese persons, a 1988 study by Rick M. Gardner et al. of the University of Southern Colorado found no differences in arousal between weight groups. They examined differences in arousal between obese and normal-weight persons while exposed to food stimuli, during eating and during exposure to visual imagery of both food and nonfood stimuli.

The only sex differences in arousal occurred during the auditory presentation of food imagery; men displayed higher arousal than women. Significant sex differences were not present during any of the other intervals.

The study concluded that there is no support for the notion that obese subjects are differentially aroused by food-related stimuli. Although the presentation and eating of pizza did produce significant changes in arousal, there was no differential arousal between the obese and normal-weight persons. Both food and nonfood imagery tasks proved ineffective in increasing arousal in both obese and normal-weight persons.

Gardner, Rick M.; Espinoza, Tracy, Martinez, Renee. "Physiological Responses of Obese Subjects to External Stimuli" *Perceptual Motor Skills* 66 (1) (February 1988).

pica   An appetite disorder; the craving for and ingestion of strange or repulsive substances not normally considered suitable for food. The phenomenon occurs throughout the world and has been recorded for centuries. The most common explanation is that those who evidence pica are seeking trace minerals or inorganic minerals missing from their diet and desperately needed by their bodies. Seen most often in malnourished people, it also occurs in some severe psychiatric disorders.

Horner, Ronnie D.; Lackey, Carolyn J.; et al. "Pica Practices of Pregnant Women." *Journal of the American Dietetic Association* 91 (January 1991).

pimozide   An antipsychotic medication.

In a Dutch study, anorexia nervosa patients treated with pimozide gained weight faster than another group administered PLACEBO, but overall the difference from placebo was not statistically significant. There was also no significant difference in the pimozide patients' attitudes.

pituitary obesity   The pituitary gland influences most body functions and is particularly important in growth, sexual maturity and reproduction. It does this through the release of hormones (thyroid, adrenals and gonads). Pituitary obesity may result from a

disorder of the pituitary, including the loss of more than one of these pituitary hormones.

The major cause of pituitary obesity is CUSHING'S DISEASE, caused by an excess of ACTH (which stimulates the adrenal glands to secrete hormones, with multiple effects on metabolism); it is also associated with hypothyroidism. Pituitary obesity is slow to develop, is of a generalized type and can be diagnosed by a dryness of the skin, shortened growth of the eyebrows and diminished function of the reflexes. Other characteristics that suggest a pituitary disorder include pallor, a generalized obesity and, in both sexes, lack of fully developed sexual characteristics. In men with this disorder there is a tendency for the adipose tissue to concentrate in the pelvic region. Secretion of the growth hormone becomes sluggish in the obese, compared with people of normal weight. Yet it returns to normal with weight reduction, indicating that this is the result rather than the cause of the obesity. When pituitary obesity is treated by correcting the basic disorder, it is possible for the patient to lose weight by restricting calories.

Frawley, Thomas F., "Obesity and the Endocrine System." In *The Psychiatric Clinics of North America, vol. 7, no. 2: Symposium on Eating Disorders,* edited by Félix Larocca. Philadelphia: W. B. Saunders, 1984.

placebo   A harmless inactive substance (or ineffective procedure) given to a CONTROL GROUP in a study as if it were an effective treatment, used as a comparison for the substance or procedure being tested. A placebo substance is made to look and taste identical to the active preparation; subjects are not told which they are taking.

pleasure foods   A term used for typical "craving" foods, those containing sugar, starch and fat, which are part of the "addiction" dilemma. Because they are a common part of the everyday diet, a person with an addictive type of eating disorder may not be aware of the consequences of consuming them. Those around such a person are generally aware of the problem long before he or she senses that something is wrong.

See also FOOD ADDICTION.

polyphagia Excessive craving for all types of food; very great HUNGER.

ponderosity Body weight relative to height. Individual differences in ponderosity are important determinants of health status. In a family study by Trudy L. Burns, P. P. Moll and R. M. Lauer reported in *American Journal of Epidemiology* (May 1989), the researchers determined that if the specific environmental exposure associated with differences in ponderosity could be identified, strategies could be devised to prevent the development of excess ponderosity in high-risk children and to reduce the risk of development of chronic diseases associated with obesity in adulthood.

post-traumatic effect A specific form of ANXIETY that appears following a stressful or frightening event. There have been numerous cases recorded of anorexia nervosa and bulimia apparently precipitated by physical trauma such as surgery or an automobile accident. Trauma resulting in either temporary or permanent body disfigurement may in turn bring on or make worse DEPRESSION, BODY IMAGE DISTURBANCE, family or social stresses and may possibly affect hypothalamic function, thereby contributing to the onset of eating disorders.

See also STRESS AND EATING DISORDERS.

Prader-Willi syndrome A birth defect whose victims are always hungry and do not know how to stop gorging. About one child in 10,000 to 15,000 is born with this incurable syndrome, identified in 1956 by Swiss doctors. Characteristics include short stature, unusually small hands and feet, hyperphasia (excessive talkativeness), hypo-

gonadism (retarded sexual development) and some degree of learning disability or mental retardation. Unless people with this syndrome are strictly supervised, their compulsion to gorge (hyperphagia) can cause them to swell two or three times their ideal weight. That can lead to heart or respiratory problems and early death. At the First International Scientific Conference on Prader-Willi Syndrome and Other Chromosome 15 Deletion Disorders (The Netherlands, 1991), specialists noted that hyperphagia is first manifested between ages one and six, and that while victims do reach SATIETY, it is only after consuming three times more calories than controls. Their hunger also returns more quickly. Many patients develop diabetes during adult life.

pregnancy and obesity In her studies, HILDE BRUCH found that obesity that develops during or after pregnancy often develops in response to stress (see REACTIVE OBESITY). Some women gain weight after each pregnancy, some only after one. Bruch's studies determined that the most frequent causes of stress underlying obesity following pregnancy are disappointment with the marriage, unfulfilled, unrealistic expectations about what the child might do for the mother or frank envy of the care the child receives and resentment about the demands it makes.

Though noting that "much has been written about obesity indicating a desire for pregnancy," Bruch argued against this theory. While agreeing that some fat women have pregnancy fantasies, she cautioned that those who are not fat do also.

"Occasionally," Bruch added,

a father may become fat after the birth of a child; this occurs in extremely dependent men who, even before the baby is born, feel that they never received quite enough [attention]. They will resort to overeating to combat their anger and jealousy and to compensate themselves for what they feel they are missing.

Physical Effects Bray wrote that body weight before pregnancy and weight gain during it both affect pregnancy. He cited a study of 3,939 women who delivered babies between 1963 and 1965, in which the "heavy" women (averaging 169 pounds) had significantly higher frequency of toxemia and hypertension, and longer duration of labor, than "light" women. Because cesarean section was performed on 5.5 percent of the heavy patients but only on 0.7 percent of the light, more obstetrical complications occurred in the heavy group.

Diets to control weight during pregnancy must account for the increased need for protein, iron, folic acid and most other minerals and vitamins. For this reason, during pregnancy weight is best controlled through small decreases in calorie intake, with increased energy expenditure through exercise. VERY LOW CALORIE DIETS are to be avoided during pregnancy unless specifically prescribed by a physician.

Bray, George A. "Effects of Obesity on Health and Happiness." In *Handbook of Eating Disorders*, edited by Kelly D. Brownell and John P. Foreyt. New York: Basic Books, 1986.
Bruch, Hilde. *Eating Disorders: Obesity, Anorexia Nervosa, and the Person Within*. New York: Basic Books, 1973.

preloading   During experimentation and research testing, the eating of individuals on restricted diets of some food or quantity of food normally forbidden them, before regular meals. In tests, subjects ate more after they had "preloaded" with more food (e.g., two milk shakes) than those who had preloaded with less (e.g., one milk shake). Once their normal restraints on eating were overcome, they ate as if their controls were no longer functioning. Research concluded that people who are on diets, regardless of how much they weigh, are inclined to overeat once they have eaten something they believe contains a large number of calories. Their belief that control has been lost appears to be the decisive factor in this situation, rather than the actual number of calories consumed.

protein-sparing modified fast (PSMF)
A diet regimen designed to be safer than formula diets and to produce loss primarily of fat tissue rather than lean body tissue by adding PROTEINS and electrolytes to the FASTING regimen. It was developed by pioneers such as Bistrian and Blackburn, who defined the conceptual framework and nutritional profile of a diet that produces rapid and significant fat loss while minimizing or eliminating many of the adverse health consequences of the earlier LIQUID FORMULAS.

The PSMF is recommended for the moderately obese (see OBESITY) when undertaken under close medical supervision. It is not recommended for the mildly obese because the risk from the treatment outweighs the risk from mild obesity; nor for the morbidly obese, because they are more safely and effectively treated with GASTRIC PARTITION PROCEDURES; nor for children and adolescents, because there is some loss of lean body mass, which may interfere with growth.

Bistrian, B. R. "Clinical Use of a Protein-Sparing Modified Fast." *Journal of the American Medical Association* 240 (1978).
Lindner, P. G., and Blackburn, G. L. "Multidisciplinary Approach to Obesity Utilizing Fasting Modified by Protein Sparing Therapy." *Obesity/Bariatric Medicine* 5 (1976).
Powers, Pauline S., and Rosemurgy, Alexander. "Current Treatment of Obesity." In *Eating Disorders: Effective Care and Treatment*, edited by Félix E. F. Larocca. St. Louis: Ishiyaku EuroAmerica, 1986.

proteins   One of the three major types of nutrients (see CARBOHYDRATES and FATS) found in food. Proteins constitute about 20 percent of the body's cell mass. They are necessary for the building and repair of all kinds of body tissues, especially of muscles and organs such as the heart, liver and kidneys. Skin, hair, ligaments, tendons, muscle and nails are composed of protein. Major sources of protein are animal products such as meat, eggs, fish and milk.

Digestion breaks down protein into its component elements, amino acids, which pass into the blood, some to be used as structural proteins for the building of body tissues, others to be used as enzymes and the rest to be carried to various parts of the body as a reserve. Because they are drawn on directly as a source of energy, there is no noticeable weight gain when high-protein foods are eaten in reasonable amounts. Proteins provide about four CALORIES per gram.

Protein deficiency manifests itself in weakness, poor resistance to disease and swelling of body tissues due to accumulation of fluid in the tissue spaces. When eaten in large amounts, protein-rich foods can cause constipation, kidney dysfunction and heart failure.

Prozac Proprietary name for fluoxetine, a long-lasting ANTIDEPRESSANT drug that acts by selectively and effectively blocking the reuptake (reabsorption) of the neurotransmitter SEROTONIN into nerve terminals in the brain. It was introduced in the United States early in 1988 and within a year became one of the most widely prescribed antidepressants in the country.

Experiments on more than 1,000 patients showed that fluoxetine works at least as quickly and effectively as IMIPRAMINE and other tricyclic antidepressants. The main side effects, according to researchers, are nausea and vomiting, insomnia and nervousness. It is less likely than other antidepressants to cause constipation, dry mouth, drowsiness, sexual difficulties or urinary problems. Obese patients given fluoxetine at fairly high doses lost eight to 10 pounds in two months without dieting, even when the drug caused no nausea or upset stomach.

There is hope that fluoxetine and other serotonin regulators (still in the approval state) will help bulimics. Early research shows that bulimics suffer from diminished serotonin activity. In a University of Illinois at Chicago study of 15 patients suffering from DEPRESSION accompanied by BULIMIA, binge/

purge episodes dropped dramatically (93 percent) within the first four weeks on Prozac, compared with a 42 percent drop in a CONTROL GROUP on a placebo. After four weeks of treatment, the fluoxetine group lost an average of four pounds, while the placebo group lost between one and one and a half pounds. Patients reported that CARBOHYDRATE craving diminished considerably. Those who lost the most weight were overweight bulimics. The one subject who was at normal weight lost very little. It appears that fluoxetine helps considerably in controlling bulimic behavior, affecting carbohydrate METABOLISM, decreasing APPETITE and reducing weight. Further study with a larger group, however, still needs to be done.

Clifton, P. G.; Barnfield, A. M. C.; and Philcox, L. "A Behavioral Profile of Fluoxetine-induced Anorexia." *Psychopharmacology* 97 (1090).

Cowley, Geoffrey, with Karen Springen, Elizabeth Ann Leonard, Kate Robins, and Jeanne Gordon. "The Promise of Prozac." *Newsweek*, March 26, 1990.

Gomez, Evaristo. "Promising Results of Fluoxetine When Tried on Depressed Bulimics." *BASH Magazine*, June 1989.

Schatzberg, Alan F. "Forum." *Harvard Medical School Mental Health Letter*, March 1989.

psychodrama A form of GROUP THERAPY in which patients act out their responses to difficult or conflicted situations from their daily lives. Psychodrama was developed by a psychiatrist, J. L. Moreno (1890–1974) during the 1930s to liberate the "spontaneous" self from the constrictions of Victorian social morality. Today, psychodrama offers adolescents and adults whose "real self" is hiding from hurtful or shameful traumas of the past to reenact these scenes that have led to the disordered behavior of the present. It's a nonconfrontational format intended to make it possible for patients to gain insight into their own conflicted or self-defeating behavior. Psychodrama has been used as treatment for eating disorders.

Veronica O. Bowlan, psychodrama consultant at the Renfrew Center in Philadelphia explains that psychodrama is not merely role-playing and not acting class.

> In psychodrama, a patient gets a chance to deal with people and events in her past, present, or future. She gets a chance to begin to resolve unsettled or hidden feelings and often learns new ways of handling conflicts in real situations.
>
> Psychodrama . . . [uses] action rather than talking to help patients deal with difficult feelings. The patient creates and actually steps into a situation to confront the problem and her feelings about it. It is difficult, but it is also very real and powerful . . . [she] demonstrates to each player how the character should behave. She does this throughout the whole drama. This is called role reversal. Reversing roles gives her a chance to see the situation from other perspectives and discover new solutions or ways of interacting.

Baaklini, George. "Psychodrama: A Timely Therapeutic Procedure." *Renfrew Perspective,* Fall 1992.

Bowlan, Veroncia O. "Psychodrama: Taking Action to Discover Feelings." *Renfrew Perspective.*

Hudgins, Kate. "Using Psychodrama as a Therapeutic Tool." *Addiction Letter,* October 1990.

psychodynamic approach to obesity An understanding of obesity on the belief that overweight people eat in response to stress-engendered emotional states, especially ANXIETY and DEPRESSION, rather than simply to internal HUNGER cues. The stress is due to conditions such as marital or work problems, mother-daughter conflict and PERSONALITY DISORDERS.

The eating response recurs because it works: it relieves emotional distress. Psychodynamic theorists discuss overeating as a means of diminishing anxiety, achieving pleasure, relieving frustration and emotional deprivation, expressing hostility (conscious or unconscious) and so forth (see ORAL FIXATION AND OBESITY).

Opponents of this theory believe that these stress factors are consequences rather than causes of obesity, due largely to diminished SELF-ESTEEM from the discrimination obese people experience today.

psychogenic malnutrition Weight loss from psychological causes; the noneating associated with it is incidental. The term covers a wide range of psychiatric disorders including chronic schizophrenia, acute catatonic schizophrenia, mental retardation and schizophrenic disorganization and forms of DEPRESSION. Cases of this type have sometimes been included in anorexia nervosa literature but do not qualify as a true anorexia eating disorder.

psychosomatic medicine A field of medicine begun in the 1930s; Joan Brumberg describes it as "the scientific study of emotion and the bodily changes that accompany different emotional states." She continues,

> Psychosomatic medicine involved practitioners from many different specialty areas, not just psychiatry. Followers of the psychosomatic movement shared a common interest in a more integrated approach to etiology and therapy. Body (soma) and mind (psyche) were considered as one.

Brumberg added that anorexia nervosa was particularly suited to psychosomatic research because of "the manner in which bodily changes accompanied neurotic mechanisms," but the attempt to explain it with a simple, single formula was ultimately doomed because of the complexity of the disorder. After World War II, HILDE BRUCH led the way to a broader and more complex view of the significance of food behavior and its relation to individuals' lives.

Brumberg, Joan Jacobs. *Fasting Girls.* Cambridge: Harvard University Press, 1988.

psychotherapy Treatment of mental and emotional disorders by any of various means involving communication between trained therapists and patients, including counseling, psychoanalysis and other types of therapy. Through psychotherapy, patients are helped to understand why they have followed certain behavior patterns and to change those patterns. Psychotherapy aims to help individual suffering from eating disorders achieve a more competent, less painful way of handling their problems. It may involve patients singly or in COUPLES THERAPY, FAMILY THERAPY or GROUP THERAPY.

Individual psychotherapy is generally recommended for all eating-disorder patients and usually forms the foundation for all other treatment. Initially, individuals begin to accept their eating disorders as attempts to solve psychological dilemmas, and they explore attitudes about weight, food and body image. As a feeling of trust is established through the therapists' acknowledgement of the patients' pain, the patients begin to recognize the multiple origins and influences of disorder (social, psychopathologic, genetic, biological, behavioral and familial). Through psychotherapy, individuals can explore concerns, test new behaviors and receive constructive and nonjudgmental commentary. It provides an opportunity for them to develop self-confidence, self-esteem and feelings of power and control. Therapy also helps conquer DEPRESSION, guilt, ANXIETY and STRESS, alleviating the need to turn to, or away from, food to deal with problems. Effective psychotherapy avoids simplistic explanations and solutions. Some anorectics and bulimics will terminate psychotherapy prematurely, unable to relinquish their own control or to see it as a problem.

After HILDE BRUCH and ARTHUR H. CRISP, among others, concluded that traditional insight-directed psychotherapeutic approaches aimed at personality reorganization had failed to deliver a permanent resolution of the eating-disorders dilemma, GARNER AND GARFINKEL advocated a cognitive-behavioral approach, in which misstatements and mis-

conceptions are challenged in a systematic way. This technique is useful, though it has not proven the most effective approach.

According to the results of a five-year experiment conducted by the National Institute of Mental Health and reported in the November 1989 issue of *Archives of General Psychiatry,* weekly sessions with a psychologist or psychiatrist have a measurable effect on mental distress. The experiment measured the effects of short-term psychotherapy on patients suffering mild to severe depression. The experiment was an attempt to see if the effects of psychotherapy could be measured in the same way as the effects of drugs and surgical operations—that is, with controlled clinical trials. If so, the agency believed, the experiment could be a model for testing psychotherapeutic effects in other areas of mental and emotional distress besides depression.

In the experiment, the CONTROL GROUP consisted of patients given the antidepressant drug IMIPRAMINE, which has proven over the years to be effective for straightforward depression. The control patients also saw a doctor weekly who offered support and encouragement but didn't attempt any formal psychotherapy. To make sure the effects of imipramine were being gauged correctly, a second control group of patients received a PLACEBO in addition to the weekly support sessions. The treatment groups consisted of depressed patients, half of whom received cognitive behavior therapy and half of whom received interpersonal psychotherapy.

Patients in all four groups showed an improvement—that is, their scores on the tests for depression dropped. But the patients undergoing drug treatment and those receiving psychotherapy showed greater improvement than the patients receiving the placebo.

Generally, the researcher concluded that there is no evidence that psychotherapies are less effective than antidepressant drugs but that there is evidence that psychotherapies are better than a placebo. There were indications that interpersonal therapy might be better than COGNITIVE THERAPY in certain specific areas, particularly for severely depressed patients, but generally one form of psychotherapy does not appear superior to the other.

Researchers at the University Department of Psychiatry at Royal Edinburgh Hospital reported on a randomized controlled trial of different types of psychotherapy for bulimia. Thirty-two women were assigned to receive cognitive-behavior therapy, 30 received behavior therapy, 30 received group therapy, all for 15 weeks, and a further 20 (controls) were assigned to remain on a waiting list for 15 weeks. At the end of the trial, the control group had significantly higher scores than the treated groups on all measures of bulimic behavior. In terms of behavioral change, all three treatments were effective, 71 (77 percent) of 92 women having stopped BINGE EATING. In addition, scores on eating and depression questionnaires were lowered, and SELF-ESTEEM improved. Of 24 women available at one-year follow-up, 21 were not binge eating and had maintained their improved scores on psychometric scales. The researchers concluded that bulimia nervosa is amenable to treatment by once-weekly structured psychotherapy in either individual or group form.

Anderson, Arnold E. "Inpatient and Outpatient Treatment of Anorexia Nervosa." In *Handbook of Eating Disorders*, edited by Kelly D. Brownell and John P. Foreyt. New York: Basic Books, 1986.

Freeman, Barry, and Dunkeld-Turnbull, Henderson. "Controlled Trial of Psychotherapy for Bulimia Nervosa." *British Medical Journal* 20 (February 1988).

Muslin, H. D., and Val, E. R. *The Psychotherapy of the Self*. New York: Brunner/Mazel, 1987.

Siegel, Michele; Brisman, Judith; and Weinshel, Margot. *Surviving an Eating Disorder*. New York: Harper & Row, 1988.

psychotropic drugs   Drugs that affect psychic (mind) functioning and/or experi-

ence, sometimes used in the treatment of bulimics. These include the phenothiazine-derivative tranquilizers (Compazine, Phenergan, Stelazine, Temeral, Thorazine), tricyclic ANTIDEPRESSANTS (Elavil, Nardil, Tofranil, Triavil) and other hallucinogenic, sedative, tranquilizing and antipsychotic drugs.

The use of psychotropic medication is not the primary approach for treating eating disorders. This is because such medication usually accounts for only a temporary reduction in symptoms and thus is generally considered an addition to intensive psychotherapy.

One exception is the case of women who have, one way or another, dealt with issues likely to have been among the most significant causes of their eating disorders but who are unable to control their symptoms. With a medication-related decrease in symptoms, they may be able to gain more from PSYCHOTHERAPY and eventually be able to control the symptoms without medication.

Occasionally, overwhelming reactions to thoughts, feelings or memories long suppressed and replaced in consciousness by symptoms of an eating disorder require the short-term use of medication. Psychotropic medications are also indicated when patients are sufficiently depressed, anxious or thought-disordered that they cannot respond to other treatment techniques, or when their eating-disorder symptoms remain completely out of control.

Garfinkel, Paul, and Garner, David, eds. *The Role of Drug Treatments for Eating Disorders*. New York: Brunner/Mazel, 1987.

Rockwell, W. J. Kenneth. "Pharmacological Approaches to the Treatment of Eating Disorders." In *Eating Disorders*, edited by Félix E. F. Larocca. San Francisco: Jossey-Bass, 1986.

Wilson, G. Terence. "Cognitive-Behavioral and Pharmacological Therapies for Bulimia." In *Handbook of Eating Disorders*, edited by Kelly D. Brownell and John P. Foreyt. New York: Basic Books, 1986.

puberty The stage of physical development when secondary sex characteristics develop and sexual reproduction becomes possible. It usually occurs between the ages of 10 and 12 in girls and between 12 and 14 in boys. However, the onset of puberty has been shown to be more closely related to weight and percentage of BODY FAT than to chronological age. In the United States, the mean weight of girls at menarche (first menstrual cycle) is 105 pounds (and about 22 percent *body fat*), according to studies. Delayed menarche often occurs with dieting, exercise and extreme thinness and can be as late as age 19 or 20 for athletes and ballet dancers.

"High Body Fat Brings Early Puberty." *Obesity and Health*, October 1990.

purging A term used to cover the forced expulsion of ingested foods by bulimics. Purging has been called a purification rite for bulimics, a means of overcoming self-loathing by gaining self-control. Having regained their self-discipline, they once again feel like "good" persons who are fresh and clean.

Forced VOMITING is the most common method of purging. Other methods of purging unwanted calories are LAXATIVE ABUSE, DIURETIC ABUSE, emetic abuse, FASTING, enemas and excessive exercising (see EXERCISE).

R

reactive obesity An increase in body weight resulting from overeating as a response to stressful life events. It is widely accepted that all aspects of human growth, development and disease are conditioned by social and interpersonal environment, and case reports and surveys suggest that obesity is no exception. Obesity has been found to follow stressful experiences such as financial reverses, hospitalization, instances of social or intellectual failure, marriage, failure of marriage, childbirth, illness or death of parents or close relatives.

There are numerous references in the medical literature to obesity as a possible symptom of nervous disturbance since the 19th century. These include women who, grieving over the loss of their loved ones during World War I, were observed to put on weight that could not be accounted for otherwise. Similarly, during World War II there were many instances of severe obesity in young women who had been exposed to bombing or other hardships. HILDE BRUCH observed frequent cases of newly developed obesity following the deaths of family members, separations from home, breakups of love affairs or other situations involving fear and loneliness.

Bruch observed that reactive obesity occurred more commonly in adults and infrequently in children.

See also COMPULSIVE EATING; NIGHT EATING SYNDROME; PREGNANCY AND OBESITY.

Bruch, Hilde. *Eating Disorders: Obesity, Anorexia Nervosa, and the Person Within.* New York: Basic Books, 1973.

religion and eating disorders Because there had been no consensus among researchers on the etiology of the anorexia syndrome, a 1987 Loyola University of Chicago study attempted to examine critically the background from which anorexia develops. Because medical literature places great emphasis on family environmental factors in the development of anorexia, a primary focus of this study was on rituals in the family, particularly of a religious nature.

Conclusions reached were that religion functioned as a reinforcer in developing a personality profile that reflected poor SELF-ESTEEM and that religion was found to be associated with the instillation of guilt feelings. Fear of offending God inhibited the subjects from doing things in their own best interest. It was also found that even though all respondents had left their childhood religions, those who adopted new religions committed themselves to more formalized, structured and controlling belief systems. Consistently, God was portrayed as a controller, a protector and a judge.

Lavallee, Patricia Anne. "Religiosity, Rituals and Patterns in Anorexic and Bulimic Families." Ph. D. diss., Loyola University of Chicago, 1987.

Renfrew Centers   The country's first residential facility exclusively devoted to the treatment of women with eating disorders. It was founded by Samuel E. Menaged, an attorney, and Allen R. Davis, administrator of a private psychiatric clinic. They bought the Renfrew farm in 1984 and secured a license making it a Community Residential Rehabilitation Service. The center received $2.9 million in funding from banking and private sources. In 1985, when the Philadelphia program opened, its philosophy of respect for and empowerment of women and its location in a serene 27-acre environment contrasted sharply with hospital-based, coercive programs offered in psychiatric units or drug and alcohol facilities. International in its scope, the Renfrew Center now has a second facility near Fort Lauderdale, Florida and has treated more than 2,500 women from the United States, Canada, Europe and South America. Follow-up studies conducted by the Renfrew Foundation indicated that 88 percent of their residents have never been rehospitalized.

Restraint Scale   A test administered by clinicians in the form of a questionnaire, the results of which are used to measure "restrained eating" or chronic dieting. It was composed originally in 1980 by Janet Polivy and Peter Herman in the attempt to assess the tendency toward COMPULSIVE EATING in chronically dieting college coeds. However, the scope of the testing soon expanded beyond eating behavior itself to encompass attitudes and other indices of chronic dieting. By analyzing results, clinicians are able to assess attitudes and evaluate the resulting behaviors and the fluctuations in weight accompanying them.

Restrained eaters have been shown to differ from unrestrained eaters in a number of respects, displaying greater emotionality, distractibility and salivary responsiveness as well as different eating patterns. In addition, restrained eaters seem to be more likely to be or become bulimic, and patients with anorexia nervosa score significantly above average on the Restraint Scale, particularly if they are also bulimic. A high score on the Restraint Scale may thus indicate a susceptibility or tendency to bulimia, although it is by no means a certain indicator.

Stunkard, A. J., and Messick, S. "The Three-Factor Eating Questionnaire to Measure Dietary Restraint and Hunger." *Journal of Psychosomatic Research* 29 (1985).

restrictor anorectics   So-called pure anorectics who restrict their intake of food rather than binge eat or purge. (See ANOREXIA NERVOSA.)

rumination   The voluntary regurgitation of partially digested food into the mouth, where it is subsequently rechewed and reswallowed. The human syndrome is named after a normal digestive process carried out by ruminant animals, such as cattle, sheep and goats, which results in improved digestibility of ingested material. One of the less commonly recognized of the eating disorders, it occurs much more frequently in young infants and mentally retarded children and adults than it does in adults of normal intelligence. However, rumination does plague a number of bulimics. It is often unrecognized by victims or professionals and is often diagnosed as a "digestive problem," secondary to bulimic behaviors.

Rumination in infants typically develops between three and six months of age, although cases developing as late as 12 months have been reported. It is believed to be a psychosomatic illness resulting from a poor mother-infant relationship. Mothers of ruminating infants are often characterized as having difficulty in enjoying their babies and in sensing what gives the baby satisfaction, resulting in the infant's turning to self-stimulating behavior. The appearance of infants during rumination has been described as "withdrawn and self-absorbed," as though they were deriving gratification from the process.

Because rumination can lead to growth failure, weight loss to the point of emaciation, electrolyte imbalances and dehydration, it is considered a serious medical condition. Because of the electrolyte imbalance, ruminating children can die early in life from cardiac and other complications. The condition is often overlooked initially as the primary cause of weight loss, because rumination usually occurs when infants are left alone and the behavior is not observed. Once established, it is difficult to interrupt. Treatments attempted with minor success have included behavioral, medical and surgical. The most effective treatment has been shown to be increased social stimulation and reestablishment of a positive interaction between the mother and infant.

Rumination in mentally normal adults is increasingly being recognized as a distinct clinical syndrome. There appear to be two types of adults ruminators: those in whom the behavior develops during childhood and apparently persists without severe negative consequences, and those in whom rumination is associated with bulimia nervosa.

In one study of patients with bulimia nervosa, a small but significant proportion were found to ruminate. Because this behavior is often performed in secret, diagnosis, especially in bulimics, can be very difficult and is frequently missed.

Comparisons of ruminating bulimics with nonruminating bulimics have found a higher incidence of history of anorexia nervosa and previous psychiatric treatment for an eating disorder among the ruminators. Most of the patients have reported the activity as being "soothing," regardless of whether they felt the practice was shameful or innocuous.

Bulimic ruminators display a greater tendency to spit out, rather than reswallow, the regurgitated food in an attempt to reduce the amount of food absorbed. The medical consequences of rumination in bulimics can be very similar to those in bulimics who induce VOMITING, which adds to the difficulty of making a correct diagnosis. The most serious consequence is probably electrolyte depletion. The presence of digestive acids, mixed with undigested food, in the mouth can also affect the mucosal membranes and the teeth. A ruminator can also develop esophageal ulcers as a result of the passage up and down of hydrochloric acid. In the chronic ruminator, the salivary glands become quite enlarged. There is a tendency in adult rumination for weight loss because food is not properly digested and the nutrient value is reduced.

Rumination occurs throughout the day, not specifically after meals. Patients have reported ruminating from five or six times a day to as many as 30 times a day. One who ruminated all the time consumed dozens of mints and used toothpaste to hide the smell. The process is not unconscious at all; ruminators can bring the undigested food into the mouth at will.

Treatment of rumination in adults can be very difficult, owing to the apparent pleasure derived from it. Patients have described a sense of relief during the reswallowing. For those with bulimia nervosa, treatment resulting in reestablishment of control over eating has led to cessation of rumination. In nonbulimics, behavioral treatment directed at training them to relax before and after meals has largely proven unsatisfactory, mostly because there is less incentive than for bulimics to stop the behavior. In two reported cases of pharmacologic treatment, administration of paregoric prior to eating completely inhibited after-meal rumination; and premeal administration of dopamine-blocking agents reduced after-meal rumination. In other cases, paregoric at first had a PLACEBO effect, with patients feeling a beneficial impact, but it soon wore off. More successful has been a combination of COGNITIVE THERAPY and ANTIDEPRESSANTS.

Fairburn, C. G., and Cooper, P. G. "Rumination in Bulimia Nervosa." *British Medical Journal* 288 (1984).

Larocca, Félix E. F., and Della-Fera, Mary Anne. "Rumination: Its Significance in Adults with Bulimia Nervosa." *Psychosomatics* 27 (March 1986).

Russell, Gerald F.M. Professor of psychiatry and consultant psychiatrist at the Institute of Psychiatry and the Maudsley Hospital, London. Dr. Russell in 1979 published the first extensive description of an "ominous new variant of anorexia nervosa," which he named BULIMIA NERVOSA. At the time, Dr. Russell was a professor in the Academic Department of Psychiatry at Royal Free Hospital in London.

Russell's principal works include "Anorexia Nervosa: Its Identity as an Illness and Its Treatment," in *Modern Trends in Psychological Medicine*, edited by John Harding Price (London: Butterworths, 1970); "Anorexia Nervosa and Bulimia Nervosa," in *Handbook of Psychiatry*, vol. 4, *The Neuroses and Personality Disorders*, edited by G. F. M. Russell and L. A. Hersov (Cambridge: Cambridge University Press, 1983); and "Bulimia Nervosa: An Ominous Variant of Anorexia Nervosa," *Psychological Medicine* 9 (1979).

S

satiety A state of fullness and satisfaction (see APPETITE). Factors that affect how much a person eats include palatability of food, emotional state (stress turns off hunger in animals, but humans may eat more or less; see STRESS AND EATING DISORDERS), hormones and general state of health.

After eating, digestion breaks down food for immediate energy needs (carbohydrate), tissue repair (protein) and energy reserve (fat). Digestion is controlled by the hypothalamus, which determines how we utilize food and energy. The hypothalamus controls the pituitary gland, which regulates feeding behavior. The venteromedial hypothalamus is said to be the locus of the feeling of satiety—if it is injured, a person becomes hyperphagic (eats excessively) and obese. If the lateral hypothalamus is destroyed, a person becomes aphagic (noneating) and eventually starves to death. (See HYPOTHALAMIC DISEASE.)

On a reducing diet, hunger stress might be alleviated by the use of certain menus and even occasionally an APPETITE SUPPRESSANT drug to increase the satiating effect of the food that has been eaten. This would help reduce the desire to snack between meals or take second helpings.

A number of digestive hormones have been thought to be satiety hormones, and the best known of these is CHOLECYSTOKININ (CCK), though, according to Herzog and Copeland, its locus of action remains controversial. Receptors in the vagus nerve or in the central nervous system may be involved. Cholecystokinin inhibitors increase food intake, suggesting that cholecystokinin has a role in inducing satiety.

Herzog, David B., and Copeland, Paul M. "Bulimia Nervosa—Psyche and Satiety." *New England Journal of Medicine* 319 (September 15, 1988).

Woods, Stephen C., and Brief, Deborah J. "Physiological Factors." In *Assessment of Ad-*

dictive Behavior, edited by Dennis M. Donovan and G. Alan Marlatt. New York: Guilford Press, 1988.

secondary amenorrhea Cessation of menstruation after menarche (the first menstrual period of a girl in PUBERTY), a condition most common in anorectics but not uncommon among bulimics, particularly those who rely heavily on FASTING and/or extreme DIETING as means of PURGING. In many instances it is attributed to undernourishment. In addition, the menstrual cycle can be interrupted by environmental stress, a primary factor in bulimia.

See also AMENORRHEA.

self-control therapy A psychological treatment method in which clinicians help patients control their own behavior without the aid of drugs or other outside controls. Self-control treatment techniques for obesity attempt to help dieters achieve increased control over their eating to enable them to reduce their food intake. The self-control approach has been very widely adopted; nearly 80 percent of published studies of behavior therapy are of the self-regulation approach. As D. A. Booth of the University of Birmingham, England wrote in *Medicographia,* curing obesity "requires permanent changes in the overweight person's own habitual actions of eating, drinking, and physical exercise." He goes on to say that this self-management must be achieved if weight loss is to be permanent.

The core components of the self-control approach to treating obesity are changing mealtime eating behavior, rearranging eating cues, self-monitoring and "deprogramming" inappropriate behaviors. (See BEHAVIOR MODIFICATION.)

self-esteem Belief in one's own value; self-respect. Low self-esteem is often a symptom of eating disorders. People with eating disorders feel inadequate, and this adversely affects their recovery.

A 1987 study conducted by Debra Lorraine Mandel of the California School of Professional Psychology in Los Angeles compared two groups of bulimic women— those who compensate for binges by means of laxatives/diuretics, vomiting and/or spitting out food (B-L) and bulimics who compensate by fasting (B-F)—with each other and with a third group of nonbulimic women (NB) on self-esteem and self-role concept. All women were of normal weight and were selected from a nonclinical population of undergraduate college students.

Self-esteem was assessed using the Coopersmith Self Esteem Inventory. Three components of sex-role concept, real self (RS), ideal self (IS) and imagined male ideal (IMI), were assessed using the Sex Role Attribute Inventory. It was hypothesized that the three groups would differ on self-esteem with the B-L group measuring lowest; that the groups would differ on each component of sex role with B-L measuring lowest on RS femininity and highest on IS and IMI femininity; and that low self-esteem in bulimics would correlate with discrepancies between components of sex role. Contrary to expectations, however, although the bulimic groups combined averaged lower self-esteem measurements than the NB group, only the B-F group had lower self-esteem than the NB group. In addition, while results indicated that low self-esteem is related to an RS sex-role concept (incorporating both masculine and feminine characteristics) for B-F and NB, no relationship was found between RS sex-role concept and self-esteem measurements for B-L.

Self-esteem is also considered a factor in adolescent obesity. In a 1988 University of Arkansas study, the Rosenberg Self-esteem Scale was administered to 550 14- to 16-year-old girls. Self-esteem scores were categorized by weight and by height. Results indicated that self-esteem of adolescent girls is related to their weight. As obesity increased, self-esteem decreased. These results tend to confirm the observation that

adolescent girls do internalize social attitudes about body size, which result in continued low self-esteem in overweight girls.

Martin, Sue, et al. "Self-esteem of Adolescent
Girls as Related to Weight." *Perceptual and
Motor Skills* 67 (1988).

self-help groups   Therapy groups that rely
on their members to supply one another with
support, assistance and positive influence,
so that individual members do not have to
try to help themselves in isolation.

Eating-disorders self-help organizations are
a recent addition to the treatment of anorexia
nervosa, originating only within the past 15
to 20 years. With more than 100 groups
developing independently in different parts
of the country, their structures, formats and
goals are quite varied. Standardized group
procedures are still to be developed.

The "ideal" self-help (or mutual-aid) group
does not involve professionals. In practice,
however, the most stable groups do involve
them. Although an association with professionals appears to infringe on the self-help
premise of "equal-status" relationships, when
groups are formed without such assistance,
they tend eventually to deteriorate into un-
productive complaint sessions, which may
erode the members' motivation. Some authors also suggest that the poor interpersonal
and leadership skills of many anorectics and
bulimics prevent long-term commitment to
such groups. Professional therapists can assist by acting as organizers, teachers of social skills, role models and consultants and
can provide a structure for meetings without
infringing on the primary purpose of groups,
mutual support. Groups that maintain
connections with professionals have the potential to train group leaders capable of fa-
cilitating constructive group interaction. These
"lay" leaders may be parents of anorectics
or bulimics who are motivated to help other
parents, or individuals who have themselves
recovered, or who are recovering, from eating disorders.

Various attempts have been made to study
the effectiveness of self-help groups, since
such groups may divert people from seeking
professional help. A 1976 study demonstrated that the degree of distress felt by a
person is inversely related to the number of
people in his or her social network who
provide frequent emotional support. Self-
help groups extend members' social networks. They may thus discourage them from
seeking professional help, but they may also
refer them to it.

A 1979 study examined help-seeking behavior in members of self-help groups and
in individuals who enter PSYCHOTHERAPY. It
concluded that social networks and self-help
groups share the following features: they
buffer the experience of stress; they obviate
the need for professional assistance through
provision of instrumental and affective support; they act as screening and referral agencies for professional services; and they
transmit attitudes about values and norms of
help-seeking.

In the literal sense, self-help means helping oneself without the assistance of others.
In the context of multidimensional treatments of eating disorders, the term is really
misleading. Members of a "true" self-help
group become interdependent for support,
understanding and acceptance as they gradually grow to trust one another and share
feelings and experiences.

Families of members also benefit from
these groups. The setting reduces social isolation and provides a noncritical environment for issue exploration. Through shared
experiences, parents can learn how to cope
with their children's problems and their own
feelings. In groups that mix parents and
children of different families, the greater
emotional distance can sometimes enable the
older generation to hear and appreciate better
what the younger generation has to say. For
previously unresponsive therapy patients, the
contact with people who have "been there"
and found themselves capable of changing
has proven particularly beneficial.

Self-help groups are not a substitute for other forms of treatment. They differ significantly from individual or group therapy, whose purpose is to free patients from disabling forms of psychological disorder by developing insight into and understanding of underlying causes, eventually enabling changes in dysfunctional behavior. But one valuable function groups often perform is to refer individuals to qualified professional treatment. Some groups are parts of multimodal treatment programs. Self-help groups sometimes are also the preferred resource of anorectics and their families for financial reasons or by personal choice, especially if they fear professionals or have had previous unsuccessful encounters with them.

Because self-help groups for eating disorders have originated so recently, no standardized nationwide procedures have been developed. Effective guidelines based on the successful experience of existing groups, however, are beginning to emerge. According to recent social science literature on self-help, the ideal mutual-aid group provides members with information (factual knowledge and referrals to appropriate professionals); opportunity to share and learn from one another's experience; mutual support; positive association (members can identify with group goals); collective willpower; and benefit from the exchange itself.

A Model Program In general, self-help groups intended to provide peer support for overweight bulimics and the obese focus on weight reduction. Activities are aimed at promoting this goal for each individual and for the group. These methods do not provide the resources to engage individuals in a meaningful effort to deal with other complicating factors in their lives.

While running a successful eating-disorders program (see BASH), the psychiatrist Félix E. F. Larocca became aware that many patients and their families felt that something was lacking. Issues other than eating disorders, such as DEPRESSION, suicide, aggression and sexual behavior, were not being

addressed. Larocca designed a self-help care unit that combined treatment for both eating disorders and related disorders. As the program developed, its design changed; today, meetings are held exclusively for those suffering from mood disorders; meetings are held for those with eating disorders; meetings are held for both categories of patients.

Dr. Larocca's BASH program proposes that self-help must get past the focus on concerns of weight alone. The major goal of group interactions is not only to promote education but also to encourage support and communication between group members as well as encouraging self-awareness and individual insight. Group members have an opportunity to express feelings in an atmosphere that guarantees unconditional acceptance. Such changes are known to enhance self-esteem; motivation for weight loss soon follows.

See also ANOREXIA NERVOSA; BULIMIA NERVOSA; OBESITY; GROUP THERAPY; PSYCHOTHERAPY.

Larocca, Félix E. F., with Nancy J. Kolodny. *Facilitator's Training Manual*. St. Louis: Midwest Medical Publications, 1983.
Rubel, Jean A. "The Function of Self-help Groups in Recovery from Anorexia Nervosa and Bulimia." *Psychiatric Clinics of North America* 7, #2 (June 1984).

self-monitoring The process of keeping a careful record of one's own body weight, food intake and its caloric value, physical activity and, in some cases, the circumstances (time, place, occasion, company) of eating. Self-monitoring is a key element in almost all BEHAVIOR MODIFICATION programs and typically the first behavior change requirement. In obesity treatment, it is frequently prescribed before any attempts to diet or increase exercise are made. Originally intended strictly as an information-gathering tool, it has proven to have other value.

Monitoring eating habits affects eating behavior in a number of ways. First, the very act of recording can force awareness of previously unconscious patterns of behavior. For example, because snacking usually becomes a routine, automatic behavior, most people express surprise at the amount of food—and calories—they discover they eat in a day. This awareness can be a first and necessary step in their efforts to control how much they eat. It can also reveal behaviors likely to have defeated previous attempts to lose weight or keep it off. Second, self-monitoring provides specific information that allows eating-disordered persons to evaluate their progress and then reward or punish accordingly. Third, records of eating behavior can provide information useful to therapists in assisting the obese to make behavior changes.

Therapists suggest that self-monitoring is most effective and successful when patients have convenient forms for recording the information, when behavior is recorded soon, or immediately, after it occurs and when feelings, degree of HUNGER and concurrent problems are also noted.

self-mutilation   The act of deliberately injuring oneself. Mutilation of one's own or another's body has always been a part of human existence and continues to be a normal part of some cultures even today. Many cultures have long used mutilation of the body in religious or other social rituals, such as circumcision (of both sexes), tattooing or scarring the skin during rites of passage into adulthood or the binding of feet to make women more attractive. These forms of mutilation or self-mutilation are not meant to be harmful; on the contrary, they often signify strength or rebirth.

In our culture, self-mutilation generally is not an attempt to commit SUICIDE but a way of dealing with anxieties and stress. Many self-mutilators find bleeding to be comforting and scarring a welcome sign of healing.

The mentally retarded may do things that result in injury to themselves, and psychotics sometimes perform drastic acts such as poking out their eyes or cutting off extremities. The most common cases of mutilation are more subtle in nature. Typically they involve cutting or burning parts of the body or interfering with the healing of wounds.

The literature suggests that self-mutilators have a high incidence of eating disorders. Out of four studies mentioned by Armando R. Favazza, associate chairman of the Department of Psychiatry at the School of Medicine, University of Missouri–Columbia, the percentages of self-mutilators who also had a history of an eating disorder (anorexia nervosa, bulimia or overweight) ranged from 57 to 93 percent. In a study by Paul Garfinkel (see GARFINKEL AND GARNER) in 1989, only 9.2 percent of the bulimics in the study practiced self-mutilation; however, in another study, 38 percent of the female eating-disorder patients also practiced self-mutilation. In a third study, reported in the September 1990 *American Journal of Psychiatry*, female eating-disorder patients demonstrated significantly higher levels of dissociative psychopathology than non–eating-disordered subjects. This appeared to be specifically related to a propensity for self-mutilation and suicidal behavior.

Favazza reported on some of his own cases of self-mutilators who also suffered from eating disorders. One patient developed a fear of becoming overweight after being treated on an outpatient basis for self-mutilation at age 16. After this treatment her mutilating behaviors decreased; however, at 19, when she was hospitalized for her eating disorder, the self-mutilating behaviors intensified. After one year in treatment, both behaviors stopped; but when events in her life became stressful, she relapsed once again into the eating disorder. For another of his patients with a history of alcohol abuse, eating disorder and self-mutilation, the three behaviors were "interchangeable ways of hurting myself."

According to Favazza, an impulse-control problem seems to be the basis for self-mutilation, eating disorders and substance abuse;

he feels that a good number of those with one of these problems may also be affected by another.

Although psychotherapeutic treatment is currently available for self-mutilators, researchers are now speculating that a deficiency of SEROTONIN, a neurotransmitter that influences HUNGER, SATIETY, sexual drive and pain response, among other feelings, may be a biological contributor to self-mutilation.

Jewell, Regina. "Self-mutilation and Its Kinship to Eating Disorders." *BASH Magazine*, November 1989.

serotonin   One of a family of NEUROTRANSMITTERS that mediate the passing of impulses through the nervous system. The chemical is produced in the brain when an impulse passes between two nerve endings. Most is then reabsorbed by the nerves; that which remains improves mood and turns off APPETITE once HUNGER is satisfied.

A link between eating disorders and serotonin is assumed, since eating CARBOHYDRATES stimulates the production of serotonin in the brain. It paves the way for other neurotransmitters that stimulate an appetite for protein and fat. It is thought that bulimics, who suffer from diminished serotonin activity, become depressed as their serotonin level drops. As a result they develop a CRAVING for foods that trigger production of the substance, as if they were using pasta and sugar as a "natural" antidepressant (see ANTIDEPRESSANTS). This theory is controversial.

Fairburn, Christopher; Cooper, Zafra; and Cooper, Peter. "The Clinical Features and Maintenance of Bulimia Nervosa." In *Handbook of Eating Disorders*, edited by Kelly D. Brownell and John P. Foreyt. New York: Basic Books, 1986.
Goodwin, G. M., et al. "Plasma Concentrations of Tryptophan and Dieting." *British Medical Journal* 300 (June 9, 1990).

set-point theory   There is persuasive evidence that animals and humans naturally maintain, and thus will always return to, a constant weight range, just as the body naturally returns to its own temperature level following illness or external influence. This weight level is referred to as the body's set point. In support of this theory, studies have shown that once "starved" volunteers are given free access to food, they eat ravenously until their weight returns to its normal level, when appetite and caloric intake level off at prediet amounts. Similarly, after experimental forced feeding to increase weight as much as 25 percent, weight rapidly returns to normal levels when volunteers are once again allowed to eat whatever they want, with no attempt to control weight in either direction.

It is this set point, proponents say, that explains why dieters invariably return to their prediet weight once they cease to restrict food intake. An individual's set point can vary as much as 10 to 20 pounds over time. It is believed that a combination of factors, including METABOLISM and number of FAT CELLS, work together to "set" a level of fat (weight) that's "normal" for that person. If weight drops below the set point, HUNGER increases and the body burns fewer CALORIES until weight once again stabilizes.

It is believed, but not proven, that the set point can sometimes be changed by EXERCISE, certain drugs such as nicotine, hormonal changes and aging.

Bennett, William I. "Dieting." *Psychiatric Clinics of North America* Vol. 7, no. 2 (June 1984).
Daniels, John S. "The Pathogenesis and Treatment of Obesity." In *Eating Disorders*, edited by Félix E. F. Larocca. San Francisco: Jossey-Bass, 1986.
Keesey, Richard E. "A Set-Point Analysis of the Regulation of Body Weight." In *Obesity*, edited by A. J. Stunkard. Philadelphia: W. B. Saunders, 1980.
———. "A Set-Point Theory of Obesity." In *Handbook of Eating Disorders*, edited by Kelly D. Brownell and John P. Foreyt. New York: Basic Books, 1986.

McCurdy, John A., Jr. *Sculpturing Your Body: Diet, Exercise and Lipo (Fat) Suction.* Hollywood, Fla.: Frederick Fell Publishers, 1987.

sexual abuse and eating disorders

There is an increasing awareness that many survivors of sexual abuse develop eating disorders. Root and Fallon report in *Bulimia: A Systems Approach to Treatment* that 60 percent of 172 bulimics studied had been sexually and/or otherwise physically victimized, and other authors have indicated an even higher rate. Current studies at the RENFREW CENTER also reveal the high correlation between sexual abuse and eating disorders—61 of a sample of 100 women had been sexually abused before the age of 18. Of these, 24 were victims of incest, 47 were molested by acquaintances and 18 by strangers. Realizing that this population had a need for specific treatment, the Renfrew Center of Florida, in June 1992, opened a program for survivors of abuse.

Jane Shure, a consulting therapist at Renfrew, writes that

> the development of an eating disorder such as bulimia or anorexia is a logical response to the emotional experiences and messages received throughout the abused child's formative years. As the young child moves into adolescence and young adulthood, she turns to food as a means of comfort and a tool for avoiding feelings. Fasting, or bingeing and then purging, both help create an illusion of being in control—while also reinforcing her shame and feeding the desperate need to isolate [herself].

(See BINGE EATING; FASTING; PURGING.)

Recent findings at the Johns Hopkins Eating and Weight Disorders Clinic show that 50 percent or more of bulimic and anorectic women have histories of sexual abuse, including rape and incest.

However, not all researchers support the connection between sexual abuse and eating disorders. Pope and Hudson, for example, reviewed the scientific literature on childhood sexual abuse as a risk factor for the development of bulimia nervosa. They concluded that

> controlled studies generally did not find that bulimic patients show a significantly higher prevalence of childhood sexual abuse than control groups. Furthermore, neither controlled nor uncontrolled studies of bulimia nervosa found higher rates of childhood sexual abuse than were found in studies of the general population that used comparable methods. Therefore, current evidence does not support the hypothesis that childhood sexual abuse is a risk factor for bulimia nervosa.

Waller found that bulimics were substantially more likely to report a history of unwanted sexual experience than anorectics. He suggested that sexual abuse may not cause eating disorders but may determine the nature of those disorders when they have been prompted by other factors.

Bulik, Cynthia M.; Sullivan, Patrick F.; and Rorty, Marcia. "Childhood Sexual Abuse in Women with Bulimia." *Journal of Clinical Psychiatry* 50 (December 1989).

Palmer, R. L., et al. "Childhood Sexual Experiences with Adults Reported by Women with Eating Disorders: An Extended Series." *British Journal of Psychiatry* 156 (May 1990).

Pope, Harrison G., Jr., and Hudson, James I. "Is Childhood Sexual Abuse a Risk Factor for Bulimia Nervosa?" *American Journal of Psychiatry* 149 (April 1992).

Waller, Glenn. "Sexual Abuse as a Factor in Eating Disorders." *British Journal of Psychiatry* 159 (November 1991).

sexuality and eating disorders

Restricting anorectics demonstrate significant immaturity and inhibition in sexual and social experience; however, in their attempt to meet all social expectations, they sometimes present a facade of good social adjustment.

Bulimic women, on the other hand, although less sexually and socially mature than borderline women, are more so than anorectic women. But bulimia usually results in a sharp decrease in sexual desire, attributed to both psychological and physiological causes.

Bulimic patients often have irregular menstrual cycles, pointing to disruption of the pattern of sex-hormone secretion. Their obsession with food leaves them little time to think about other aspects of life, and they characteristically feel worthless and flawed. They also often fear that if anyone becomes closely involved with them, they will learn their secret. Likewise, psychiatrists contend that many people overeat to cover up feelings of sexual inadequacy. If they do not seem attractive to the opposite sex, they will avoid occasions of stress and humiliation.

However, it is not unusual for those bulimics who lack control over their impulses to participate in sexual promiscuity and extramarital affairs.

Andersen, Arnold E. *Practical Comprehensive Treatment of Anorexia Nervosa and Bulimia.* Baltimore: Johns Hopkins University Press, 1985.

Garfinkel, P. E.; Moldofsky, H.; and Garner, D. M. "The Heterogeneity of Anorexia Nervosa: Bulimia as a Distinct Subgroup." *Archives of General Psychiatry* 37 (1980).

Strober, M.; Salkin, B.; Burroughs, J.; and Morrell, W. "Validity of the Bulimia-Restrictor Distinction in Anorexia Nervosa." *Journal of Nervous and Mental Disease* 170 (1982).

sialodenosis   Swelling of the salivary glands, most evident in the parotid glands; frequently seen in bulimics. "Puffy cheeks" may be an indication of this problem.

simple overeating   The most common form of eating disorder; what results when people do not reduce their food intake in response to the natural lowering of energy output that accompanies aging. (See ENERGY INTAKE/EXPENDITURE IN OBESITY.)

For overeaters, the desire to eat almost always exceeds their need for food, and when they allow their APPETITE free rein, they become fat. Overeaters who attempt to deal with their problem resist focusing their attention on their appetite. They worry instead about their bodies, which they see as disfigured with excess fat. They are often dieting or looking for a simple and easy cure that will cause the fat to melt away.

Simplesse   A FAT SUBSTITUTE developed by NutraSweet. It can replace fat, and thus reduce calories, in such foods as frozen desserts, mayonnaise, salad dressing and margarine. One of dozens of fat substitutes being developed by food manufacturers, Simplesse is composed of proteins from milk and egg whites, which are heated and whipped to create tiny spheres one-tenth the size of a grain of powdered sugar. On the tongue, Simplesse particles taste and feel like cream. The first product made with Simplesse to be marketed to the American public was Simple Pleasures, an ice "cream" with half the calories of the real thing and virtually no fat.

sitomania (sitophobia)   Interchangeable terms included as diagnostic categories in American medical dictionaries during the mid-1850s to describe a "phase of insanity" characterized by "intense dread of food." Sitophobics were not classified among the FASTING GIRLS of that period. They claimed no special powers, and no public pronouncements were made about the duration of the fasting or the patients' miraculous inspiration. Sitophobic girls came from middle-class families, well educated and well situated. No organic explanation could be found for their not eating. In *Fasting Girls*, Joan Jacobs Brumberg refers to sitomania as a "prehistory of anorexia nervosa."

size discrimination   Systematic restrictions in employment, housing, child adoption and other areas based on weight rather than ability, training or other qualifications.

In 1989, University of Vermont researchers reported the results of a survey they conducted on employment, medical and housing discrimination against fat people. The survey included 367 women and 78 men. It found that more than 40 percent of fat men and 60 percent of fat women claimed to have been refused a job because of their weight. In contrast, almost none of the non-fat respondents indicated that this had ever occurred. More than 30 percent of fat men and women indicated that they had been denied promotions or raises, and over 25 percent that they had been denied benefits (such as health and life insurance), because of their weight. Nearly 70 percent of fat men and women had been questioned about their weight on the job or urged to lose weight; and this was also true of about 30 percent of moderately fat people and 10 percent of nonfat people. In general, fat people were employed in jobs that had lower prestige.

Some employment discrimination cases have been won by fat plaintiffs using state disability laws, defining their obesity as a perceived disability. The Trump Shuttle airline reportedly scrapped size requirements for its flight attendants after considering the costly legal battles waged by other airlines. Pan Am, for instance, settled a suit by 116 female flight attendants by paying $2.35 million.

"Results of the NAAFA Survey on Employment Discrimination." *NAAFA Newsletter*, April 1989.

skin fold measurement   The thickness of a fold of skin at a selected body site, usually the upper arm or triceps, the subscapular region or the upper abdomen. The measurements are used to calculate body fat, in order to evaluate nutritional status.

In the National Health Survey, 1960–62, the average right arm skin fold measured over the middle of the triceps muscle was 11 mm for male subjects 18 to 24 years and 14 mm for males 25 to 34 years. In the same study, the average triceps skin fold for women was 22 mm. Between 18 and 24 years, the average skin fold measurement was 18 mm, 21 mm between 25 and 34, and increased to 25 mm between 55 and 64, after which there was a slight drop to 24 mm between 65 and

74 years. There are no statistical differences between triceps skin folds measured on either arm.

Triceps skin fold measurements are based on the assumption that 50 percent of the fat is subcutaneous. The midpoint between the shoulder and elbow process is located, with the arm folded. The person making the measurement pinches up a full fold of skin and subcutaneous tissue with the thumb and forefinger of the left hand at a distance 1 cm above the site at which the measurement is to be taken. The fold is pulled away from the underlying muscle. The pressure on the fold is exerted by the calipers and not the fingers. The dial of the calipers is read to the nearest 0.5 mm, after releasing the handle and applying pressure to the skin fold. Skin fold measurements are then translated into percentage of body fat by means of standard equations.

When carefully used, skin fold measurements provide a good indication of body fatness. (See BODY FAT.) They are most accurate when applied to healthy subjects who are not either grossly obese or severely underweight. Measurements are more accurate when extremes in temperature are avoided. Extreme heat can cause skin fold swelling. Edema, which in severe cases can cause a great increase in body weight, can cause errors in skin fold measurements. Recent weight loss may also have an effect on tissue tension or the pattern of subcutaneous fat thickness.

Gray, David S.; Bray, George A.; et al. "Skin-fold Thickness Measurements in Obese Subjects." *American Journal of Clinical Nutrition* Vol. 51, No. 4 (April 1990).

Must, Aviva; Dallal, Gerard E.; and Dietz, William H. "Reference Data for Obesity: 85th and 95th Percentiles of Body Mass Index and Triceps Skinfold Thickness." *American Journal of Clinical Nutrition* 53 (4) (April 1991).

social factors in obesity   In industrialized societies obesity is more prevalent in lower social classes, whereas the reverse pattern has been observed elsewhere, as in rural India. Stunkard wrote that social mobility has also accompanied changes in the incidence of obesity; in America, upward mobility has been associated with decreasing obesity, and downward mobility is associated with increasing obesity. In New York City, incidence of obesity has been found to be seven times higher in the lowest than in the highest social class. There also is a tendency for slim women to move up the social scale and overweight women to move down.

The proliferation of cars and labor-saving devices is blamed for much of today's rise in obesity. A sedentary life-style means that APPETITE is not a trustworthy guide to energy needs.

See also OBESITY.

Goldblatt, P. B.; Moore, M. E.; and Stunkard, A. J. "Social Factors in Obesity." JAMA: Journal of the American Medical Association 192 (1965).
Stunkard, Albert J. "The Control of Obesity: Social and Community Perspectives." In Handbook of Eating Disorders, edited by Kelly D. Brownell and John P. Foreyt. New York: Basic Books, 1986.

sodium pump   A metabolic process that maintains balance in the concentrations of sodium and potassium ions inside and outside cell walls. It has been shown that obese people have lower pressure differentials across cell membranes than do normal weight subjects. This means that the sodium pump consumes less ENERGY in obese people, who therefore survive on fewer CALORIES.

spot reducing   Exercising a particular group of muscles such as those of the stomach or upper arms in order to lose weight, tone muscles or reduce fat in that area.

Exercising specific muscles does tighten and increase the tone of these muscles but does not preferentially mobilize fat from storage cells overlying these muscles. AEROBIC EXERCISE is required for mobilization of fat; the sequence of mobilization from various areas of the body varies from person to person.

McCurdy, John A., Jr. "Spot Reducing: Myth or Reality?" In Sculpturing Your Body: Diet, Exercise and Lipo (Fat) Suction. Hollywood, Fla.: Frederick Fell Publishers, 1987.

starch blockers   Substances derived from concentrated protein from certain beans that inhibit digestion of starch by preventing complete METABOLISM of CARBOHYDRATES. They are marketed as aids in weight reduction.

Any weight loss that starch blockers may effect is due to the malnutrition this process causes, along with flatulence and gastric upset. In 1984, starch blockers were taken off the market pending Food and Drug Administration approval. Those currently available are effective only in preventing breakdown of complex carbohydrates and have no effect on the digestion of the simple sugars abundant in the American diet.

"Automatic Weight Loss with Cal-Ban? Send for Your Refund Now!" Consumer Reports Health Letter, June 1990.

starvation   syndrome   Studies   have shown that starvation influences behavior and reasoning, from preoccupation with food to mood swings to social isolation. Garfinkel and Kaplan wrote that all the symptoms described in studies of starving people are also prominent in anorexia nervosa. "That they result from starvation per se and not from a pathophysiological process unique to anorexia nervosa has allowed greater diagnostic specificity and more emphasis on weight gain as a critical aspect of treatment."

Garfinkel, Paul E., and Kaplan, Allan S. "Anorexia Nervosa: Diagnostic Conceptualizations." In Handbook of Eating Disorders, edited by Kelly D. Brownell and John P. Foreyt. New York: Basic Books, 1986.

steatopygia   Having abnormal fatness of the buttocks; it is seen to an extreme in certain parts of Africa. Location of this excess fat accumulation in the buttocks apparently represents an evolutionary adaptation to a very hot climate. If this fat were spread throughout the subcutaneous tissue, normal cooling of the skin would be severely limited.

Stein-Leventhal syndrome   A disorder in women characterized by irregular menses, mild obesity and hirsutism, usually beginning during the years of puberty and worsening with time. Chronic anovulation, and therefore infertility, is present as a result of inappropriate feedback signals to the hypothalamic-pituitary unit. Also known as polycystic ovary syndrome or PCO, this disorder is benign (not life threatening), and there is no ideal therapy for it. Treatment to induce ovulation is administered when pregnancy is desired.

Cheung, A. P., et al. "Polycystic Ovary Syndrome." *Clinical Obstetrics and Gynecology* Vol. 33, No. 3 (September 1990).

Franks, S., et al. "Obesity and Polycystic Ovary Syndrome." *Annals of New York Academy of Science* 626 (1991).

stimulus control   A BEHAVIOR MODIFICATION technique, also called cue elimination, stimulus control attempts to alter the circumstances that may trigger the impulse to eat, while also including measures used in traditional weight reduction programs. Every effort, for instance, is made to limit the amount of high-calorie food kept in the house and to limit accessibility to the food that is kept. Foods that require preparation replace those that require none. Spare change is kept to a minimum to decrease the likelihood of impulse buying of candy or snacks. Eating is confined to scheduled mealtimes and places. (See EATING HABITS MONITORING.)

At the same time, new stimuli for eating are established. For example, the obese adult might restrict all eating to special table settings or unusually colored place mats and napkins—anything to make the eating process special and intentional (as distinct from habitual, almost subconscious snacking). Emphasis is put on the eating process rather than the amount of food eaten.

Brownell, Kelly D., and Wadden, Thomas A. "Behavior Therapy for Obesity: Modern Approaches and Better Results." In *Handbook of Eating Disorders*, edited by Kelly D. Brownell and John P. Foreyt. New York: Basic Books, 1986.

Fairburn, C. G. "Cognitive-Behavioral Treatment for Bulimia." In *Handbook of Psychotherapy for Anorexia Nervosa and Bulimia*, edited by D. M. Garner and P. E. Garfinkel. New York: Guilford Press, 1985.

Wheeler, M. E., and Hess, K. W. "Treatment of Juvenile Obesity by Successive Approximation Control of Eating." *Journal of Behavior Therapy and Experimental Psychiatry* 7 (1976).

stomach stapling   A general term used for about 20 surgical operations that create artificially smaller stomachs out of portions of the original stomachs. Usually the stomach is closed off with a staple gun, although other means are sometimes used, such as the insertion of plastic mesh. Some involve gastric bypass, in which the intestine is severed and reattached to a hole punched in the stomach pouch. These operations cause weight loss by limiting food intake; as soon as a few mouthfuls are eaten, the person feels nauseated and must stop eating to avoid vomiting.

When these procedures were first developed, the stomach was reduced from its original capacity of more than a quart to five ounces. Currently, a two-ounce capacity is most common; one-half ounce is not uncommon.

See also BYPASS SURGERY; GASTRIC PARTITION PROCEDURES; GASTRIC RESTRICTION PROCEDURES.

Ernsberger, Paul. *Report on Weight-Loss Surgery*. Bellerose, NY: National Association to Advance Fat Acceptance (NAAFA), 1986.

stress and eating disorders   Some eating-disorder patients, particularly those who ruminate, use their eating-disordered behaviors as a way to improve stress or anxiety. It is thought that infants may use RUMINATION to decrease the stress of poor maternal bonding.

The precise role stress plays in the development of eating disorders remains unclear, however. One theory is that biological changes within the body that occur during times of stress may promote the development of eating disorders. Another is that psychological changes accompanying life stresses may affect the response to such stresses.

Stress may influence the development of eating disorders because of the effect it can have on various biochemical systems within the body, especially those that govern APPETITE. Changes may occur within the hypothalamic-pituitary-adrenal axis, within the endorphin system. Because the body is a complex system of biochemical processes, there may be changes in one or all of these systems as a result of stress. Therefore, the exact relationship between stress and eating disorders remains unknown. It is evident, however, that stress requires a response of some type from the organism. As Thomas P. Donohoe, of the University of Nottingham, England concludes in his paper, "Stress-induced Anorexia" (1984), "Psychosocial stress may combine with dieting behavior to produce changes in hypothalamic function or other systems to generate or shape the symptoms of anorexia nervosa."

In 1986, Michael Rutter (professor of child and adolescent psychiatry, University of London, England) examined the work of Adolf Meyer (1866–1950; professor of psychiatry at the Johns Hopkins University; introduced the concept of psychobiology) to understand the role of life experiences as stressors and the effect they have on personality development. Although he acknowledged that certain negative life experiences could have such "an impact on psychological function . . . that in some circumstances they play a part in the genesis of psychiatric disorder," he also acknowledged that perspective was an essential factor. Individuals respond in a variety of ways to life experiences, depending on their point of view and previous history. A particular life experience may be viewed as negative by one individual and positive by another.

Some researchers suspect that it is this perspective on the life experience that actually determines the degree of stress involved. Physiologically, physical illness is more stressful for some individuals than for others and can play a role in the development of an eating disorder. For example, because of the many physical changes accompanying the aging process, older adults more often succumb to physical illness and may experience more stress from them than they would if they were younger. And following the Gulf War, the Washington, D.C. health commissioner announced that war-related anxiety had caused an increase in eating disorders, as well as drug and alcohol abuse.

The stress of fear is also being studied for its effect on eating disorders. Research suggests that film-induced negative affect (exposure to a frightening film) may prompt overeating in persons who are attempting to restrict their caloric intake.

Although the precise role of stress and DIETING in the development of eating disorders remains unknown, that they can be precipitating factors is not in doubt. Concerns about body image or physical changes affecting peer group approval can often be sources of stress. Social emphasis on thinness may also be accentuated in peer groups, regardless of age, encouraging further self-consciousness and dieting behaviors. Issues of social or financial independence may become chronic strains for older persons. Such stresses may promote dieting to regain a sense of control but may lead to the development of an eating disorder.

Donohoe, T. P. "Stress-induced Anorexia: Implications for Anorexia Nervosa." *Life Sciences* 34 (1984).

Fischman, Ben. "Unsweetened Stress." *Psychology Today*, March 1989.

Rutter, M. "Meyerian Psychobiology, Personality Development, and the Role of Life Experiences." *American Journal of Psychiatry* 143, no. 9 (1986).

Schotte, David; Cools, Joseph; and McNally, Richard. "Film-induced Negative Affect Triggers Overeating in Restrained Eaters." *Journal of Abnormal Psychology* 99 (3) (August 1990).

Strober, Michael Associated with the Neuropsychiatric Institute at UCLA, he and his colleagues have carried out extensive studies of the families of patients with eating disorders. He is executive editor of the *International Journal of Eating Disorders*.

Strober's principal works include "Disorders of the Self in Anorexia Nervosa: An Organismic-Development Paradigm," in *Psychodynamic Treatment of Anorexia Nervosa and Bulimia*, edited by C. L. Johnson (New York: Guilford Press, 1991); and "Family-Genetic Studies of Eating Disorders," *Journal of Clinical Psychiatry* Vol. 52, No. 10 (October 1991).

sucrose polyester (SPE) See OLESTRA.

sugar A sweet-tasting simple CARBOHYDRATE containing carbon and hydrogen usually in the ratio of 1:2. The food we call sugar is refined from sugarcane, but sugars are found universally in plants and animal tissues. Americans consume about 133 pounds of sugar a year from all sources; that accounts for 20 to 25 percent of all calories, about 500 to 600 calories per day per person. Glucose, the main sugar in the blood and a basic fuel for the body, is essential to the functioning of all cells, particularly brain cells.

Sugar is not the leading cause of obesity. Eating more calories than one uses is the basic problem, and for most people most excess calories come from FAT, not sugar.

So concluded two studies in the *American Journal of Clinical Nutrition*, which found that lean people tend to eat more sugar and less fat than obese people. Not only does fat have more calories than sugar (about 36 versus 16 calories per teaspoon), but studies have also suggested that dietary fat may be more efficiently converted to body fat than carbohydrates (sugars) are.

People often blame sugary foods for weight gain, forgetting that the cakes, ice cream, chocolate and cookies they're eating derive most of their calories from fat, not sugar. Many a "sweet tooth" may actually be a "fat tooth."

Studies have failed to show that artificial sweeteners keep people from gaining weight, much less help them lose significant amounts. One problem is that instead of eating artificially sweetened foods *in place of* high-calorie ones, many people simply add them to their diet. Moreover, artificial sweeteners do not suppress appetite—they may even increase it.

Sugar can lead to tooth decay; however, so can all forms of carbohydrates if decay-producing bacteria are also present. Between-meal sugary snacks play a bigger role in dental caries than sugar eaten during a meal, according to studies.

Sugar is *not* a cause of diabetes. It—along with other simple carbohydrates, total caloric intake or stress—can contribute to a rise in blood glucose levels in persons who already have diabetes.

"The Healthy Eater's Guide to Sugar." *University of California, Berkeley Wellness Letter*, December 1989.

Krause, Marie, and Mahan, L. Kathleen. *Food, Nutrition, and Dirt Therapy*. Philadelphia: W. B. Saunders, 1984.

Williams, Sue Rodwell. *Nutrition and Diet Therapy*. St. Louis: Times Mirror/Mosby College Publishing, 1989.

suicide Suicidal behavior (attempts and threats) is common with bulimia; several researchers report that approximately one-third of their samples have attempted suicide. Others report lower but still significant rates. In one study of 142 bulimic women, researchers found that 49 percent of their sample had suicidal thoughts and 20 percent had attempted suicide. According to Fairburn, Cooper and Cooper, "few are a true suicide risk."

Root, Fallon and Friedrich write in *Bulimia: A Systems Approach to Treatment* that

it is surprising that suicidal behavior in the bulimic population has not been studied more extensively. Irritability, depression, mood swings, and anxiety are commonly observed and reported in the bulimic. While these affective states do not necessarily predict suicidal behavior, they have been correlated with increased suicidal ideation and threats.

(See ANXIETY, BULIMIA NERVOSA AND DEPRESSION.)

Fairburn, Christopher G.; Cooper, Zafra; and Cooper, Peter J. "The Clinical Features and Maintenance of Bulimia Nervosa," In *Handbook of Eating Disorders*, edited by Kelly D. Brownell and John P. Foreyt. New York: Basic Books, 1986.

Reto, C.; Root, M. P. P.; and Fallon, P. "Incidence of Suicide in a Bulimic Population." Paper presented to the Washington State Psychological Association, Vancouver, B.C., 1985.

Root, Maria P. P.; Fallon, Patricia; and Friedrich, William N. *Bulimia: A Systems Approach to Treatment*. New York: W. W. Norton, 1986.

sulpiride   An antipsychotic medication experimented with in treating anorexia. In a 1984 study, there was a slight trend favoring the drug compared with a PLACEBO, but no statistically significant effect was demonstrated either on weight gain or on patient attitudes or behavior.

See also ANTIDEPRESSANT.

Vandereycken, W. "Neuroleptics in the Short-Term Treatment of Anorexia Nervosa: A Double-Blind Placebo-Controlled Study with Sulpiride." *British Journal of Psychiatry* 144 (1984).

superobesity   Extreme morbid OBESITY. It affects less than one-half of 1 percent of the population. Superobesity appears to shorten life expectancy by nearly five years. The superobese often find themselves the objects of unwanted public attention.

Superobese people have received more clinical attention in recent years, since reducing by starvation or LIQUID FORMULAS has become popular. Though they are capable of losing enormous amounts, they are likely to regain their weight, bringing their hypercellular ADIPOSE TISSUES back into metabolic balance (see SET-POINT THEORY). HILDE BRUCH noted that "some of these superobese people accept themselves with more equanimity than the many people who struggle with minor weight deviations." (See HUDSON, WALTER.)

superstitious (or magical) thinking Thinking based on a belief that there is a cause-and-effect relationship between unrelated events, a belief common among anorectic patients, according to GARFINKEL AND GARNER. They found that anorectics often assume that every last calisthenic in their exercise regimen must be completed or they will gain weight: "One patient developed an elaborate set of exercise rituals in which various situations required her to perform specific rigorous exercise routines. Passing post boxes or street lamps had to be followed by jogging for one block."

As with superstitious behavior in general, the rituals are designed to avoid or mitigate either specific or, more often, obscure but ominous consequences. This behavior is so powerfully controlled by the belief in bizarre internal relationships and contingencies that it is hardly affected even by extremely punishing external consequences. Like other avoidance behavior, superstitious rituals are resistant to critical examination because the beliefs governing them insulate the believer from acknowledging contradictory information and experience. (See ANOREXIA NERVOSA.)

Garner, David M., and Garfinkel, Paul E. *Handbook of Psychotherapy for Anorexia Nervosa and Bulimia*. New York: Guilford Press, 1985.

support groups A term sometimes used interchangeably with SELF-HELP GROUPS. Generally, support groups are free of charge and members may enter or leave at any time. Support groups are considered an adjunct to therapy, not a substitute for professional treatment. They are useful because they provide a social network, emotional support, self-help techniques and information.

T

---

taste The bodily sense that distinguishes flavors; it is dependent on sense organs located on the surface of the tongue. These organs, called taste buds, when appropriately stimulated, produce one or a combination of the four fundamental taste sensations: sweet, bitter, sour and salty.

Both anorectic and bulimic women tested for perception of taste quality and intensity exhibited impaired sensitivity in estimating the magnitude of higher concentrations of all four different taste qualities, with bitter and sour tastes most severely affected. Bulimics' cravings for sweets have been hypothesized as the outcome of an impaired sense of taste. One mechanism for this change in gustatory sensitivity may be the saliva, because saliva is important for taste perception and because endocrinological changes occurring in eating disorders influence the composition of saliva. No data, however, support this hypothesis.

Results of testing by a Yale University research team headed by Judith Rodin provided evidence of a taste disturbance in bulimia nervosa, most likely caused by the acid in vomit damaging palate receptors. Rodin suggested that, because of this taste disturbance, bulimics may be less responsive to the taste of vomit as the disorder progresses, which could prolong its existence. Rodin stressed that this research does not reveal whether bulimics' taste disturbances are consequences of, or predisposing factors to, bulimia nervosa, but she suspects they are the result of bulimia nervosa.

Jirik-Babb, P., and Katz, J. L. "Impairment of Taste Perception in Anorexia Nervosa and Bulimia." *International Journal of Eating Disorders* 7 (1988).

Rodin, Judith, et al. "Bulimia and Taste: Possible Interactions." *Journal of Abnormal Psychology* 99, no. 1 (February 1990).

Rosenbaum, Joshua. "Taster's Choice." *Avenue*, March 1990. Reprinted in *Review* (in-flight magazine of Eastern Airlines), September 1990.

television and obesity With television watching the nation's most time-consuming activity after sleeping and working, the role it plays in the development of health-related attitudes and behaviors is of growing interest. Studies of this powerful medium suggest that many health messages are conveyed to viewers but that the information is sometimes unrealistic, distorted and misleading, particularly regarding food, nutrition and obesity.

William Feldman, medical professor at the University of Ottawa and author of a report in *Pediatrics* on children's attitudes toward weight, blames television for most girls' belief that they are fatter than they really are. On television shows during the prime evening viewing hours, he said, women in prestigious positions are typically thin. Ubiquitous television imagery delivers the message that thinness equates with beauty and the good life.

Although many of these "lessons" to which Americans are regularly exposed promote misconceptions that may lead to unhealthy eating habits, television's primary offense may be simply its very existence, which has profoundly altered American leisure. When the TV is on, activity ceases; time spent exercising is reduced significantly. The heart and other muscles are not strengthened, and CALORIES are not expended beyond the resting METABOLISM level during television viewing.

When Larry A. Tucker (then of Auburn University in Alabama) examined the relation between television viewing and physical fitness, he found that, among 379 high school males, as TV watching increased, multiple measures of physical fitness decreased markedly and systematically. Similarly, other researchers have shown that as TV viewing increases among children, obesity increases substantially.

Tucker and Glenn M. Friedman measured the extent of the association between TV viewing and obesity among adult males. Study subjects were 6,138 adult male employees of more than 50 different companies. Those who viewed TV more than three hours a day were twice as likely to be obese as those who viewed less than one hour per day.

Tucker and Friedman caution that with the growth of cable television, home video recording and video games, television viewing is likely to increase in the coming years. The findings of their study and other recent research show that the impact of television on fitness and health (especially obesity) cannot be ignored.

Tucker, Larry A., and Friedman, Glenn M. "Television Viewing and Obesity in Adult Males." *American Journal of Public Health* 79 (April 1989).

"Girls, at 7, Think Thin, Study Finds." *New York Times*, February 11, 1988.

therapy   Any treatment designed to mitigate or eliminate disease or disorder, physical or psychological. Among the therapies often used in treating eating-disordered persons are individual PSYCHOTHERAPY, FAMILY THERAPY, GROUP THERAPY and various physical treatments. Which type of therapy or combination of therapies to use depends upon the age, needs and living situation of the person seeking treatment.

In individual psychotherapy, patients meet with therapists alone, usually at least once a week for 45 minutes to an hour at a time. Patients in therapy work to understand the role that eating or PURGING has served in their lives and to find replacements for destructive behaviors while developing healthier coping mechanisms.

In family therapy, sessions include not just eating-disordered persons but members of their families. These may include parents and siblings, spouses and even grandparents or other relatives. In family therapy, the eating disorder is seen as a "red flag," signaling that whole families are troubled, not just the persons with the eating disorders.

A therapy group usually consists of five to 12 people who meet with a therapist weekly. The group therapy approach is particularly helpful in countering feelings of isolation, of being all alone with the problem. Groups can provide feedback and support for those attempting to change their eating patterns. They are also safe places for members to learn new ways of relating, to express feelings and to develop trusting relationships of the kind whose absence led in the first place to their self-destructive relationship to food.

thermodynamic approach to obesity
From this perspective, obesity is understood in terms of energy balance. Since the law of conservation of energy must be preserved, obesity is the outcome of energy (food) intake in excess of energy (heat) output. HILDE BRUCH described this as a limited approach because it does not consider the underlying reasons for this disturbed energy balance, such as possible endocrine and biochemical factors. The reasons for variations in energy needs, and the underlying mechanisms, remain a matter of controversy.

Bennett, Gerald A. "Behavior Therapy in the Treatment of Obesity." In *Eating Habits*, edited by Robert A. Boakes, David A. Popplewell and Michael J. Burton. New York: John Wiley & Sons, 1987.

Bruch, Hilde. *Eating Disorders: Obesity, Anorexia Nervosa, and the Person Within*. New York: Basic Books, 1973.

thermogenic drugs   Drugs that increase resting metabolic activity. In a study reported in the *International Journal of Obesity* (April 1988), it was suggested that the main effect of one of these drugs, BRL 26830A, is in maintaining the rate of weight loss in subjects in a state of negative energy balance (expending more energy than they take in) by preventing the metabolic reduction in energy expenditure that normally occurs following dieting (see OBESITY).

thin fat people   A term used by HILDE BRUCH to describe obese people who succeed in becoming and staying thin but whose problems are far from solved by having lost weight. On the contrary, their difficulties now have a chance to flourish, since obesity no longer prevents them from putting their unrealistic dreams to the test. She was referring to those people who blame all their difficulties on being fat and who hope that their lives will change when they get thin. Such people, though no longer obese, are far from transformed.

The term was originated by Heckel, who stated in 1911 that a fat person cannot be considered cured even though he has lost weight, unless all other symptoms of dysfunction have also disappeared.

Heckel, F. *Les grandes et petites obésités*. Paris: Mason et Cie, 1911.

thymoleptic medications   Medications effective in the treatment of major DEPRESSION or bipolar disorder; ANTIDEPRESSANTS. These have been used in treating bulimia on the theory that it may be closely related to MAJOR AFFECTIVE DISORDER—the family of psychiatric illnesses that includes depression and manic-depressive illness.

thyroid disease (hypothyroidism)   A deficiency of thyroid gland activity, resulting in underproduction of the hormone thyroxine. Among its consequences are a lowered BASAL METABOLIC RATE and weight gain.

Probably nothing has been blamed more often as the cause of obesity than hypothyroidism, but studies show that thyroid function in obese people is usually within normal limits. Thyroid disease is not diagnosed unless there is strong laboratory evidence of reduced thyroid function accompanied by findings of classic physical symptoms and a medical history that includes a long-standing goiter, thyroiditis or thyroid surgery. Weight gain develops insidiously rather than suddenly. Associated features include some coarsening of scalp hair, dryness of skin, yellowing of palms, generalized obesity, some thinning of the eyebrows and sluggish and delayed reflexes. Hypothyroid patients frequently complain of constipation. Menstrual periods are usually characterized by excessive bleeding; a history of dysfunctional bleeding may be the earliest clue to thyroid disease. In cases in which thyroid disease is the true cause of obesity, weight control is achieved in over 90 percent of these cases through treatment with thyroxine (see THYROID HORMONE).

Frawley, Thomas F. "Obesity and the Endocrine System." *Psychiatric Clinics of North America*. Vol. 7, no. 2 (June 1984).

thyroid hormone (thyroxine)   Prescribed for patients suffering from hypothyroidism (see THYROID DISEASE), whose thyroid glands produce it in insufficient amounts; it raises the basal metabolic rate (see METABOLISM), causing more calories to be burned.

It is also the metabolic medication most commonly prescribed and marketed as a weight reduction agent, even to people whose thyroid glands are in good working order. But for overweight people without thyroid disease, thyroxine is of no value. Thyroid hormones are especially dangerous for people with heart disease.

According to some authors, use of this hormone increases breakdown of muscle protein rather than fat. In addition, the body quickly adapts to the administration of extra thyroid hormone by reducing its natural production of this hormone, thus returning metabolism to its normal rate. Excess thyroid hormone causes anxiety, irritability, sweating, rapid heartbeat and other possible side effects.

TOPS (Take Off Pounds Sensibly)   A nonprofit support organization for overweight people founded in 1948 that incorporates some of the principles of behavior therapy into its program. There are about 12,000 chapters throughout the United States, Canada and 20 other countries. It is patterned after Alcoholics Anonymous and employs group dynamics, competition and recognition (for those who have achieved greatest weight loss) to aid the overweight. There are weekly meetings with weigh-ins; programs vary, but all in some way provide members with motivation and reinforcement. TOPS is medically oriented and asks members to obtain their individual weight goals and dietary regimens from their personal physicians. The organization has had an active research program for several years, headquartered at the Medical College of Wisconsin in Milwaukee. Areas of study have included the relative importance of heredity and environment in the development of obesity, psychosocial differences between those successful and those unsuccessful in losing weight, the effect of obesity on pregnancy and the relationship of overweight to infertility and various diseases.

total parenteral nutrition (TPN)   See HYPERALIMENTATION.

Traffic Light Diet   A simplified diet developed for children. It divides food into three colors, the same as the ones in traffic lights, green, yellow and red. Green foods contain fewer than 20 calories per serving. Yellow foods have 20 calories per average serving. Red foods are those whose caloric value exceeds those of yellow foods and thus have lower nutrient density.

See also CHILDHOOD OBESITY.

Epstein, Leonard H. "Treatment of Childhood Obesity." In *Handbook of Eating Disorders*, edited by Kelly D. Brownell and John P. Foreyt. Basic Books, 1986.
Epstein, Leonard H., and Squires, Sally. *The Stoplight Diet for Children: An Eight-Week Program for Parents and Children*. Boston: Little, Brown, 1988.

trichophagia   The (compulsive) habit of eating hair, considered to be a variant of an atypical eating and/or mood disorder. It also could be considered a perilous disorder, as trichobezoars (hairballs) can form and obstruction of the bowel may occur, requiring surgical intervention.

trichotillomania (trichologia)   A compulsion or irresistible urge to pull out one's hair. Considered to be a variant of an atypical eating and/or mood disorder, trichotillomania has been described only scantily in the psychiatric literature. Recent reviews agree that the degree of incidence of the disorder has not been established and that most of the medical and psychological literature consists primarily of single-case reports.

"Chemistry of Compulsive Hair Pulling." *Science News*, September 9, 1989.
Christenson, Gary, et al. "Characteristics of Sixty Adult Chronic Hair Pullers." *American Journal of Psychiatry*, 148, no. 11, 1991.
Goldberg, Nancy. "Trichotillomania: Compulsive Hair Pulling." *Ms.*, January 1992.

tube feeding   Forced feeding through a nasogastric tube is a method sometimes used to supplement nutrition and replace body fluids in anorectic patients. GARFINKEL AND GARNER find several disadvantages to this method: it represents a direct intrusion into the gastrointestinal tract of someone who is already preoccupied with (and misguided about) bodily functions; it may be perceived as an assault or act of hostility that will only serve to confirm the patient's sense of her own worthlessness; it is done with minimal patient cooperation and may lead to increased mistrust; and the physiological side effects are not insignificant. According to Garfinkel and Garner, it is almost always unnecessary.

Usually tube feeding is only recommended in life-threatening situations, although Larocca and the BASH Unit staff have used tube feeding for a greater number of patients than Garfinkel and Garner had prior to their findings, and their work supports the thesis that tube feeding is beneficial when properly done.

Larocca, Félix E. F., and Goodner, Sherry A. "Tube Feeding: Is It Ever Necessary?" In *Eating Disorders*, edited by Félix E. F. Larocca. San Francisco: Jossey-Bass, 1986.

tummy tuck   The commonly used name for an ABDOMINOPLASTY.

Turner's syndrome   A syndrome resulting from defective gonad development, characterized by retarded growth, sterility, heart defects, webbing of the neck, low posterior hairline and other deformities. It is associated with absence or structural abnormality of the X chromosome.

The association of Turner's syndrome and anorexia nervosa was first described by Pitts and Guze in 1963. Since then the coexistence of these two conditions has been the subject of speculation and various interpretations. Because of the mention of low mood in at least three of the 13 cases reported involving both syndromes, the association of Turner's syndrome and a major mood disorder with secondary anorexia nervosa has been considered. It has been suggested that in these cases, the anorexia nervosa may not result from social influences during puberty but from the genetic influence of Turner's syndrome, which may also predispose the patient to DEPRESSION. Some support for

this possibility comes from suggestions that affective disorders and eating disorders may be related. (See MAJOR AFFECTIVE DISORDER.)

Fieldsend, B. "Anorexia Nervosa and Turner's Syndrome." *British Journal of Psychiatry* 152 (February 1988).
Larocca, Félix E. F., "Concurrence of Turner's Syndrome, Anorexia, and Mood Disorders: Case Report." *Journal of Clinical Psychiatry* 46 (July 1985).
Pitts, F. N., and Guze, S. B. "Anorexia Nervosa and Gonadal Dysgenesis (Turner's Syndrome)." *American Journal of Psychiatry* 119 (1963).

V

very low calorie (VLC) diets   Programs for achieving rapid weight loss through eating as few as 400 calories per day. These diets can result in serious side effects, the most common of which are inability to tolerate cold, dizziness, diarrhea, constipation, dry skin, hair loss and gout. Mood changes ranging from elation to DEPRESSION may occur, and acute psychosis has been reported.

Most VLC diets are not tailored for individual needs. Fatter people, for instance, can tolerate more drastic cuts in calorie consumption than less obese individuals. The best VLC diets are closely supervised and monitored by physicians, behavioral psychologists and dietitians. VLCs have been recommended as viable treatment for people whose obesity puts them at risk for such problems as diabetes, hypertension and heart disease.

VLC diets are accomplished by consuming powdered protein mixes available by prescription only. According to the University of California, Berkeley Wellness Letter, they contain 33 to 75 grams of egg- or milk-derived protein, varying amounts of carbohydrate and RDA (recommended daily allowance) levels of most other nutrients. The formulas, mixed with liquid, are taken three to five times a day at meal and snack times. Usually nothing else other than water is allowed; a few programs do allow raw vegetables. In addition to the formula, patients receive regular electrocardiograms and blood and urine tests and regularly visit their doctors. This regimen is augmented by required exercise, nutrition education and participation in support groups.

These programs can cost as much as $2,000 including weigh-ins and clinic visits and usually last three months, followed by a gradual "refeeding" phase. Some include a maintenance phase of up to 18 months devoted to educating patients in long-term weight-management techniques. For persons with medically significant obesity, a very low calorie diet yields an average weight loss of greater than 44 pounds and a significant reduction in health risks in 12 weeks.

One argument against the formula VLC diet is that it teaches reliance on patented products, not on sound, lifelong eating habits. The permanency of the results of VLC diets is not dissimilar to that of other types of diet.

A San Diego State University study found that while people who actually completed a VLC program (45 percent of those enrolled) lost an average of 84 percent of their excess weight, they regained 59 to 82 percent of it within 30 months. Although intensive BEHAVIOR THERAPY MODIFICATION can help reduce the dropout rate to one-third, three-year follow-up checks show that by then 40 percent of patients have regained all their excess weight. Those who do not return for retreatment gain back, on average, all but 10 pounds of the weight they've lost.

A three-year study reported in 1986 compared long-term results after a very low calorie diet, a conventional 1,200-calorie diet plus behavior modification and a very low calorie diet plus behavior modification. In the initial therapeutic phase, patients lost an average of 31.1, 31.5 and 42.6 pounds respectively. Three years later, average weight had returned to within 8.4, 10.6 and 14.3 pounds of prediet weights.

Assessing VLC Diet Programs   According to the American College of Healthcare Executives, an adequate obesity treatment program that uses a very low calorie diet must include:

- Mandatory medical supervision provided by a multidisciplinary team of well-trained health care professionals (physicians, dietitians, nurses, behaviorists and exercise physiologists). Training of professional staff is critical to the success of an obesity treatment program.
- A high-quality nutritional beverage with adequate protein and calories and with an appropriate nutrient composition. The dietary beverage should have a high nutritional profile, meeting the protein recommendation of 1.5 grams of protein per kilogram (2.2046 pounds) of ideal body weight. Studies show that at this protein level, lean body mass is preserved and subjects quickly attain nitrogen balance. Lower protein levels are not adequate for the calorie deficit of the modified fasting state, and the addition of CARBOHYDRATE is not an equivalent protein-sparing replacement for protein. Some products are nutritionally incomplete, requiring vitamin and mineral supplementation in addition to the beverage. This can place patients who neglect to take their supplements at nutritional risk.
- A comprehensive educational program that emphasizes behavior change and long-term weight maintenance. Without doubt, it is the comprehensive educational program, in conjunction with the diet, that determines long-term weight maintenance. The components of a comprehensive program include nutrition education, behavior mod-

ification (e.g., planned behavior change and cognitive restructuring) and EXERCISE.

See also LIQUID FORMULAS; PROTEIN-SPARING MODIFIED FAST; BEHAVIOR MODIFICATION; DIETING.

Atkinson, R. L. "Low and Very Low Calorie Diets." *Medical Clinics of North America* 73 (January 1989).
Healthcare Executive Briefings, July/August 1989.
Paulsen, Barbara K. "Position of the American Dietetic Association: Very-Low-Calorie Weight Loss Diets." *Journal of the American Dietetic Association* 90 (May 1990).
Segal, Marian. "A Sometime Solution to a Weighty Problem." *FDA Consumer*, April 1990.
Wadden, Thomas A.; Van Itallie, Theodore B.; and Blackburn, George L. "Responsible and Irresponsible Use of Very-Low-Calorie Diets in the Treatment of Obesity." *JAMA: Journal of the American Medical Association* (January 5, 1990).

vibrator belts　Gadgets sold as a means of eliminating localized fat deposits, based on the premise that localized stimulation breaks down fat cells, releasing fat stores into the bloodstream so that they can be effectively eliminated from the body. The localized vibration also stimulates blood circulation in the treated area, thus purportedly enhancing the transport of released fat. There is no scientific evidence to support this concept.

See also FRAUDULENT PRODUCTS; NOVELTIES.

McCurdy, John A., Jr. *Sculpturing Your Body: Diet, Exercise and Lipo (Fat) Suction*. Hollywood, Fla.: Frederick Fell Publishers, 1987.

vitamin deficiency　An insufficiency of vitamins in the diet, a form of malnutrition that can result from malabsorption of fat by the intestines of bulimics (caused by abuse of laxatives) or from self-starvation by anorectics. Vitamin deficiency can also result from taking drugs that have side effects of reducing absorption of vitamins in the intestines. When physicians prescribe these drugs, they will frequently also prescribe vitamin supplements to correct the situation.

vocational bulimics　Some of the best-known bulimics are those who started PURGING because thinness is important to them vocationally. In this category are models, actresses, athletes and dancers who use VOMITING or laxatives (see LAXATIVE ABUSE) as a means of weight control and become dependent on it. Vocational bulimics present a special obstacle to treatment, because it would be unreasonable to try to convince a dancer, for instance, that she doesn't have to weigh 90 pounds when that is the current standard for dancers.

See also ATHLETES; BALLET DANCERS.

vomiting　Forcible ejection of contents of the stomach through the mouth. Self-induced vomiting is the most dramatic, quickest and most common method employed by bulimics and anorectics to eliminate unwanted CALORIES. They can do so before the calories "take effect," and it provides instant relief for the painfully overstuffed stomachs of bulimics. Vomiting can also be "justified" as a means of getting rid of what is regarded as protrusion of the stomach.

To induce vomiting, many patients use "starters" such as Q-tips; they are effective and have been described as less "disgusting" than fingers. Drinking large amounts of liquids makes the vomiting easier. Eventually, most patients can vomit at will.

Patients have reported self-induced vomiting as frequently as 18 times a day or more. Vomiting has led to severe tearing and bleeding in and around the esophagus, hiatal hernias and severely infected salivary glands, not to mention serious electrolyte disturbances.

According to Neuman and Halvorson in *Anorexia Nervosa and Bulimia*, there is a subgroup of anorectics consisting of individuals who resort to vomiting regardless of whether they also restrict their food intake or binge. Other authors have theorized that vomiting may be the driving force in bulimia nervosa rather than BINGE EATING. They feel that binge eating might not occur if the person could not vomit afterward, citing cases in which once bulimic individuals begin to vomit, they binge eat more frequently. These patients also discover that it is easier to vomit after eating a lot and therefore prolong their binges. Some patients report that the only reason they binge eat is to make it physically easier to vomit.

Casper, R.; Eckert, E.; Halmi, K.; Goldberg, S.; and Davis, J. "Bulimia: Its Incidence and Clinical Importance in Patients with Anorexia Nervosa." *Archives of General Psychiatry* Vol. 37, no. 9 (September 1980).
Neuman, Patricia A., and Halvorson, Patricia A. *Anorexia Nervosa and Bulimia.* New York: Van Nostrand Reinhold, 1983.

W

weight phobia   Fear of gaining weight. A term coined by ARTHUR H. CRISP to describe the anorectic's attitude toward being of a normal body weight.

Crisp, Arthur H. "Diagnosis and Outcome of Anorexia Nervosa: The St. George's View." *Proceedings of the Royal Society of Medicine* 70 (1977).

Weight Watchers   A commercial corporation that markets a line of packaged, reduced-calorie "diet" foods, meant to be used according to a company-sponsored diet and BEHAVIOR MODIFICATION plan. Weight Watchers also sponsors fee-collecting support groups. The company was purchased in 1978 by H. J. Heinz, which took control of both the diet program and a prepackaged food line.

Y

Yager, Joel   Medical director of the UCLA Eating Disorders Clinic, started in November 1980 to help anorectic patients. The clinic program was soon expanded to accommodate bulimics as well.

Yager's principal works include "Bulimia Nervosa," *Western Journal of Medicine* 155 (November 1991); Yager, Joel, et al., "Attitudes toward Mental Illness Prevention in Routine Pediatric Practice," *American Journal of Diseases of Children* 143 (September 1989); and Kurtzman, Felice D.; Yager, Joel; Landsverk, John; Wiesmeier, Edward; and Bodurka, Diane C., "Eating Disorders among Selected Female Student Populations At UCLA," *Journal of the American Dietetic Association* 89 (January 1989).

yo-yo dieting   A habitual cycle of weight loss by dieting followed by weight regain; an inability to maintain weight loss. Studies have shown that yo-yo dieting increases body fatness and may ultimately result in an inability to lose weight even on a very low caloric intake.

People who get caught up in the yo-yo cycle take progressively longer each time to shed pounds and gain them back progressively faster. Kelly Brownell, a psychologist then at the University of Pennsylvania, found in 1986–87 that yo-yo dieting increased the activity of lipoprotein lipase, an enzyme that promotes the storage of body fat. And because fat tissue is metabolically less active than muscle, with each diet cycle the daily caloric needs dropped and weight was gained on fewer calories. Dr. Brownell concluded that yo-yo dieting increases the body's efficiency in using food for fuel and may ultimately make weight loss impossible.

In agreement with this is David A. Booth, a psychologist at the University of Birmingham, England, who says that yo-yo dieting "may have physiological and psychological consequences which would make weight loss more difficult when it became medically more important.'' A constantly repeated yo-yo dieting cycle has been shown to be more of a health risk than remaining at a stable weight, even if high, particularly for those who are genetically predisposed toward obesity.

In a 1989 report in the *American Journal of Clinical Nutrition,* Djoeke van Dale and Wim H. M. Saris of the University of Limburg, The Netherlands compared body composition (fat to lean ratio), resting metabolism rate and conversion of fats into fatty acids among those with a history of yo-yo dieting with those of dieters without such a history. After 14 weeks, significant differences in weight loss and fat loss were revealed between dieting-only and diet-and-exercise groups, but not between yo-yo and non—yo-yo dieters. Resting metabolic rate decreased in all groups, but there was a significantly smaller decline after 14 weeks for the diet-exercise groups. No effects of frequent dieting or exercise on basal and fat-burning activity were observed.

Evidence continues to mount that yo-yo dieting makes subsequent weight loss more difficult. In the Van Dale and Saris study, researchers examined the weight loss patterns of obese patients participating in a university weight loss program for the second time. The dieters had all lost weight on the program but had regained at least 20 percent—more typically 120 percent—of their lost weight in the intervening years. Though they were placed on the same weight loss regimen, and compliance was monitored by a battery of laboratory tests, the dieters lost significantly less weight the second time. The researchers speculate that chronic dieting leads to a slowdown in METABOLISM, which sets the stage for weight gain and makes future attempts at weight loss more difficult.

Most recently, Dr. Brownell, now at Yale University, led a research team that studied and analyzed data collected from 3,200 participants in the Framingham (Mass.) Heart Study over a period of 32 years. The much-heralded results of the study were reported in the June 27, 1991 *New England Journal of Medicine.* Among the conclusions: ''Persons whose body weight fluctuates often or greatly have a higher risk of coronary heart disease and death than do persons with relatively stable body weights.'' Controversy remained because the study did not address the issue to whether weight fluctuations are more dangerous than obesity.

Z

zinc deficiency   Zinc is necessary in the body in small amounts. A shortage of zinc, the result of malnutrition or starvation, can greatly alter taste perception and may play a role in the bizarre food combinations eaten by starving anorectics. It also leads to hair loss, brittle nails and anemia.

APPENDICES

APPENDIX I
CHRONOLOGY*

1873

The term *anorexia nervosa* is first used in England by physician Sir William Gull, who described the symptoms in several young upper-middle class English girls. In a speech in 1868 he described the symptoms of a "peculiar form of disease," which he then called "apepsia hysterica," later deciding "anorexia" was a more appropriate term.

Charles Lasègue, a French neurologist, publishes a paper, "On Hysterical Anorexia," which details the symptoms of anorexia nervosa, which he refers to as a form of hysteria.

1900

C. Von Noorden classifies obesity into two types: exogenous, due to overeating and under-exercising; and endogenous, due to metabolism.

1920s

Behavioral science pioneers Ivan Pavlov, Edward Thorndike and B. F. Skinner each begin important behavioral studies relating to eating responses.

1921

Skinfold test to measure obesity is introduced, in which the thickness of a "pinched" fold of skin indicates the ratio of body fat to muscle tissue.

1929

Invention of constant-tension calipers by R. Frazen improves accuracy of skinfold obesity test.

1933

Reducing drug called dinitro-ortho-creso is introduced by Drs. E. C. Dobbs and J. D. Robertson.

*Adapted from *Library in a Book: Eating Disorders*, by John R. Matthews. Copyright 1991 by Facts On File.

1935

Surgeons in Budapest, Hungary remove 93 pounds of fat from 379-pound poultry dealer by making many small surgical incisions on his body.

1936

Hormone Lipocaic, which controls utilization of fat, is discovered by Drs. L. R. Dragstedt, J. van Prohaska and H. P. Harms.

1947

Dr. H. E. Richardson advocates treating non-glandular obesity in women as neurosis.

1948

Scientists at Brown University link obesity to heredity.

1950

Dr. H. Millman reports on emotional factors in obesity.

E. H. Rynearson reports on "emotional factors in overeating" and recommends formation of an organization to be called "Calories Anonymous."

1951

Metropolitan Life Insurance Company starts drive to curb obesity and promote sound nutrition.

1953

Dorset Foods begins marketing canned foods with calorie information printed on label.

Knickerbocker Hospital in New York establishes obesity treatment center.

1954

Dr. W. S. Kroger patents weight reducing belt that checks hunger pangs by pressing against upper part of stomach.

Pituitary hormone adipoteinin is studied for its fat burning properties.

J. Wolpe, in describing "avoidance conditioning" attempts to treat overeating with classical aversion methods using electric shock.

1957

Hilde Bruch postulates that obesity is consequence of personality defects in which body size becomes expressive of underlying psychological conflicts.

U.S. House subcommittee holds hearings on misleading remedies for weight loss. Better Business Bureau says Americans spent $100 million in 1956 on worthless remedies. The drug Phenyl propanolamine in reducing pills is declared harmful.

1959

J. M. Strang reclassifies Von Noorden's metabolic obesity type, endogenous, to include breakdowns in the physiological or psychological regulation of food intake, and a type related to various endocrinological dysfunctions.

First Metropolitan Life Insurance Company height and weight tables are published.

In a criminal case in New York, the District Attorney calls Regimen brand reducing tablets fraudulent, raids office and seizes ads and television commercials. Later in a criminal trial in 1965, the drug company, its ad agency and their executives are found guilty and fined: the ad agency is fined $50,000; the drug company president is given an 18-month prison sentence and fined $50,000; and the drug company is fined $53,000.

Dr. Albert Stunkard and Mavis McLaren-Hume complete watershed analysis of obesity research, setting forth criteria for evaluating obesity research and reducing to eight the vast number of research studies that met criteria.

1960

The Federal Trade Commission (FTC) charges Stauffer Labs with false claims of weight loss from "magic couch."

Milk companies begin to market skim milk as diet food.

Federal Drug Administration (FDA) seizes falsely labeled diet mixes.

1961

Yale doctors find link between tendency to gain weight and heart problems.

1962

Major study is published by U.S. Public Health Service (PHS) of weight, height and body dimensions of adults throughout the U.S.

"Midtown Manhattan Study" directed by Dr. Lee Srole, establishes relation of obesity to social status, showing greater obesity in the lower socio-economic classes.

W. L. Laurence reports new synthetic ACTH (pituitary hormone) compound that breaks down fat tissue into liquids.

Reducing drug phenmetrazine (Preludin) causes deformities in newborns in Germany.

1964

French women discover "cellulite" and rush to spas and salons for treatment.

1965

First intestinal bypass operation for weight loss is reported by American College of Surgeons.

1966

M. Mendelson, in a pioneer study, delineates a continuum of the range of psychological disturbance in obesity causes.

New York State appellate court upsets Regents Board's 1964 censure of Dr. Walter Sherman for negligence in treating obesity patients. Dr. Sherman, who specialized in treatment of obesity, overlooked conditions such as diabetes and prescribed amphetamine sulphate, desiccated whole thyroid and phenobarbital.

The U.S. Public Health Service (PHS) reports on obesity as a major health problem and finds diets are of limited value and urges exercise. The report rejects height and weight charts for tests for obesity and recommends skinfold pinch test instead.

PHS publishes nationwide study of adult heights and weights and finds males are seven pounds and females 11 pounds heavier than found in the 1959 Metropolitan Life charts.

New York state superior court awards Mrs. Elizabeth Ostopowitz $1,205,000 for injuries caused by taking anti-cholesterol drug Mer-29 to lose weight. The drug was withdrawn from the market in 1962 by its maker, the Richardson-Merrell Corporation, after its toxic effects were discovered. Mrs. Ostopowitz, who had Cushing's disease, suffered from cataracts, baldness and scaling skin, caused by the drug.

Harvard University Public Health School study finds that colleges discriminate against obese in admissions.

NAAFA (National Association to Aid Fat Americans) is founded.

1967

Dr. Herman Taller, author of *Calories Don't Count,* is charged in federal court in Brooklyn with mail fraud and making false claims in promoting his book along with safflower oil diet pills marketed by Cove Vitamins and Pharmaceuticals. Taller is convicted and fined $7,000; charges against the book's publisher, Simon & Schuster, and its ad agency are dropped.

Professor A. Feinstein, on American Physicians College panel, asserts that being mildly obese poses no health risks.

Scientists at Iowa University Medical College report that people who become obese, especially early in life, activate internal biological mechanisms that tend to keep them obese. The report hypothesizes an alternative pathway for disposing of excess glucose intake. Studies of obese children found that they produced low levels of the hormone dehydroepiandrosterone (DHA), which regulates the process of disposing of the excess glucose.

Senator Philip A. Hart's (D., Michigan) subcommittee begins probe into diet pill industry, charging that manufacturers recruit doctors to promote drugs and also charges that obesity specialists use mass production procedures in treating patients.

Dr. Alvan Feinstein at a meeting of the American College of Physicians proposes that otherwise healthy, slightly obese persons not diet and cites harm of fad dieting. Dr. Jules Hirsch of Rockefeller University reiterates his contention on lack of scientific knowledge about obesity.

Dr. Jean Mayer of Harvard reports on research to locate the seat of hunger and satiation signals in the brain. He describes the hypothalamus, a tiny region at the base of the brain. Studies show animals with an injured hypothalamus display confusion about hunger and satiation signals and consequently overeat.

1968

Senator Philip A. Hart's (D., Michigan) subcommittee hearings produce evidence of indiscriminate dispensing of dangerous diet drugs containing thyroid extract, digitalis, amphetamines, barbiturates and prednisone at about 1,000 clinics across the U.S. Two companies, Western Research Labs and Lanpar Company, are charged. Companies are ordered to cease marketing pills containing amphetamines and digitalis. In a related investigation, Illinois Narcotics Control Division probes death of nurse who died from amphetamine accumulation in her body after taking reducing pills.

Dr. J. Hirsch of Rockefeller University claims that some persons with chronic obesity continue to "remember" and think of themselves as fat even after reducing.

Hypnosis cure for obesity becomes briefly popular.

J. Knittle, et al., conduct a series of studies showing that adipose cells remain constant throughout life and that by adulthood increases in body size are caused by increase in cell size, not cell number.

1969

Drs. I. B. Perlstein, B. N. Premachandra and H. T. Blumenthal report to the American Therapeutic Society on study showing that some obese people produce antibodies against their own thyroid hormone, and gain weight because of the resulting metabolic imbalance.

A study by R. Half Personnel Agency finds that higher-paid executives are thinner than lower-echelon employees.

In a study on metabolism at Lankenau Hospital in Philadelphia it was found that the metabolic rate in a well-fed obese person and a starving lean person are similar because they both burn relatively more fat and less blood sugar than normal persons, and it is thought that this is a vestige of early human behavior similar to some wild animals.

1970

February 8: Two slightly overweight mothers, aged 24 and 27, in Monroe County, New York, are reported to have died after taking diet pills containing thyroid hormones, digitalis and amphetamines.

July 30: National Research Council criticizes practice of limiting weight gain by pregnant women and recommends weight gains of 20–25 pounds during pregnancy, plus diet supplements.

August 6: FDA proposes limiting the manufacture of amphetamines, an important ingredient in diet pills.

September 13: Research report indicates overfeeding children produces excess of fat cells, which remain for life, hampering future weight loss.

November 17: Drug industry promotions to doctors of reducing drugs is linked by the Narcotics and Dangerous Drugs Bureau of the U.S. Justice Department to increasing drug abuse.

1970

January 20: Weight Watchers International, Inc. launches Operation HOPE in New York City to help people unable to leave home or function normally because of extreme obesity.

September 7: Dr. J. L. Knittle, National Institutes of Health researcher, finds that adult obesity can be predicted by age two because number of fat cells in body can be closely determined by that age.

September 12: Weight loss fad Hot Pants, product name for inflatable shorts that allegedly reduces weight by increasing expenditure of energy, is investigated by the U.S. Postal Service. Test shows no weight loss by using the product.

1972

Joseph Cautela introduces "covert conditioning" in treatment of obesity, which is based on "escape-avoidance" paradigm that punishes particular eating responses and reinforces responses antagonistic to eating.

September 28: The Better Business Bureau of Metropolitan New York mounts campaign against medical quackery relating to obesity control. It claims that Americans spend between $2 billion and $10 billion annually on useless gadgets and pills.

October 11: FDA reports on study it undertook to test claims of diet pills; study reveals that diet pills are no aid in weight reduction. It recommends imposing manufacturing quotas on amphetamines.

November 14: British study reports that babies born underweight suffer from educational and behavioral problems by the time they reach school age. Dr. N. Butler, director of the study, says effects were found in all social classes but most pronounced in lower socioeconomic levels.

December 14: FDA moves to restrict harmful diet pills. FDA director E. Simmons mails bulletins to 600,000 health professionals warning of hazards of diet pills. In defending FDA's original action in permitting prescribing of diet pills for weight loss, Mr. Simmons said that a small number of people are able to lose weight taking the pills, and because the treatment of obesity is so difficult and includes high rates of failure, they believe that physicians should have use of all therapeutic aids.

December 14: In testimony before Senator Gaylord Nelson's (D., Wisconsin) subcommittee Drs. Jean Mayer, J. Tepperman and T. E. Prout accuse the medical profession and drug companies of pandering to public misbeliefs about obesity and weight loss. Dr. Mayer cites diets such as "Drinking Man's Diet," rice diet, Mayo and Atkins diets as extreme and dangerous.

December 26: The $220-million salon and health spa industry is said to be permeated with fraud. Consumer agency investigators focus on deceptive ads, high pressure sales pitches and long-term contracts to attract customers. Health clubs run by Jack LaLanne and Nu-Dimensions are target of probe. Complaints include misleading ads, promise of improbable weight loss, dirty and overcrowded facilities and untrained instructors.

1973

February 7: A federal grand jury in Newark, New Jersey, indicts G. Maisonet, E. Axel, D. Bradwell and V. Lynch for selling $1.1 million in phony diet pills by mail.

February 8: The Federal Office on Consumer Affairs warns against inflated claims and high pressure sales tactics used by spas and salons. The Federal Trade Commission (FTC) investigates sales tactics and claims of health clubs and spas; recommends limiting contracts to $500 rather than $1,000 and forbidding sellers to assign contracts to banks or others, and recommends triple damages to buyers who bring successful deceptive-practices suits.

March 9: AMA in warning against the book, *Dr. Atkins' Diet Revolution,* says the diets are unscientific and potentially dangerous; book recommends diet that activates fat-mobilizing hormone, converting stored fat to carbohydrates; advocates unlimited intake of fats and cholesterol rich foods.

March 14: New York County Medical Society calls Atkins' diet unscientific, unbalanced and potentially dangerous to persons prone to kidney or heart disease and gout; it is called especially dangerous to pregnant women and unborn children. Dr. Atkins claims diets are based on clinical observation of 10,000 obese subjects over nine years.

March 21: U.S. District Judge F. B. Lacey asks postal service to begin probe of mail order sales of diet pills and upheld postal service's right to withhold mail delivery to Baslee Products Corporation of Bayonne, New Jersey which had been found guilty in nine counts of false advertising relating to sales of the diet pill Marvex.

March 22: Dr. Atkins, author of *Dr. Atkins' Diet Revolution,* is sued for $7.5 million in suit claiming his diet is responsible for heart attack as result of negligence and malpractice. Superior Court names Atkins, his associate I. Mason and publisher David McKay Company as co-defendants.

March 31: O. N. Miller, associate director of biological research for Hoffman-La Roche, granted patent for obesity control product using nicotinic acid to inhibit growth of fatty substances known as lipids. Hoffman-La Roche is testing product on animals.

April 2: FDA and Bureau of Narcotics and Dangerous Drugs recall diet drugs containing amphetamines. Action includes injectable amphetamines and closely related chemicals and all combination diet pills that contain amphetamines and other ingredients such as sedatives or vitamins.

April 9: New York City Consumer Affairs Department passes regulation prohibiting noncancellable contracts for "future service" aimed especially at reducing salons and spas.

June 7: American Chemical Society in a study conducted at Loyola University's Stritch School of Medicine in Maywood, Illinois reports on fat-reducing agent FMS (fat-mobilizing substance) found in urine of those who are fasting. It is thought to play a role in rapid breakdown of fat during starvation. FMS appears to stimulate the release of a form of adenosine monophosphate known as cyclic-AMP, which promotes the enzyme lipase that breaks down fats. The chemical structure of FMS is unknown, but it is thought to be a protein.

June 14: Bureau of Narcotics of the Justice Department places restrictions of prescription nonamphetamine diet pills which include ingredients such as benzphetamine, fenfluramine and phendimetrazine, and are sold under many trade names as appetite suppressants. Illicit drug world begins underground sales in an effort to replace lost sales because of unavailability of amphetamines.

August 7: E. Axel pleads guilty of conspiring to commit mail fraud in the sales of $1.1 million in diet pills advertised as Slim-Tabs 33 slenderizing tablets and admits to being principal of Stanford Research Corp., arranging "fronts" as corporate officers.

August 21: Cassette tape recording designed to help in weight loss is marketed by Accomplishment Dynamics Company and narrated by Dr. R. E. Parrish, who says tape uses technique similar to hypnosis.

September 22: D. R. Salata receives patent for Rollslim, massaging device consisting of two rollers, for overweight women.

October 19: Liberty Life Insurance Company announces hospitalization program with premium rates based on insured's weight; overweight persons will pay higher premiums.

October 21: A Brooklyn College study involving mice finds that over-weight mice live only half as long as normal-weight mice, and many of the overweight develop diabetes, become sluggish, inactive and almost sterile, and have low sex drive; process is reversed by reducing mice's weight. Professor G. H. Fired says experiment corroborates accepted theories about proper exercise and nutrition. Study is based on more than 1,000 mice over 10-year period.

November 11: National nutritional study of more than 20,000 Canadians finds more than half the population are overweight and attributes cause to sedentary lifestyle rather than overeating.

November 26: Drug Guild Distributors, manufacturer of X-11 Reducing Plan Tablets, agrees to discontinue misleading and harmful advertising. Tablets are considered by medical authorities as potentially harmful to those suffering from heart disease, high blood pressure, diabetes or thyroid disease, despite ad statement that they are safe for everyone.

December 27: Dr. J. Hirsch and J. Knittle and colleagues report on people who have been fat since childhood and have larger than normal number of fat cells and claim that earlier in life obesity begins, the larger the number of fat cells.

December 27: Dr. Jean Mayer says persons of particular body type—slender ectomorphs with long, narrow hands and feet—are unlikely to become fat; other researchers note that infant feeding practices lead to overfeeding, which in turn creates a greater number of fat cells. Researchers found that mothers of fat children tend to respond to their infants' distress by feeding; later these children react to emotional stress or frustration by eating.

1974

January 23: Operator of weight reducing products company, Raymond Carapella, pleads guilty to mail fraud in multi-million dollar per year sales of diet pills and bust-developing products.

May 6: FTC begins New York regional investigation of sales of future service contracts by reducing salons.

June 15: Brewster Produce, a mail order house, admits in federal court in Newark, New Jersey, that it sold almost $2 million worth of phony diet pills.

August 31: Patent is issued for mirror device that shows how obese person will look after considerable weight loss.

September 15: Woman on fast weight loss diet dies of heart attack after fasting for four days.

September 16: Several weight loss clinics are the subject of federal investigation into fraudulent practices for falsely advertising medical supervision and using unapproved drugs. Chain-operated clinics charge fees of $175 to $500 for 21- to 40-day treatment consisting of low calorie diet and daily injections of hormone HCG (human chorionic gonadotropin) obtained from urine of pregnant women, which clinics admit may be worthless.

November 10: Citing studies showing anorexia nervosa as having a fatality rate higher than any other psychiatric disorder, the Philadelphia Child Guidance Clinic claims 100% cure rate for children who remain in treatment.

December 12: U.S. postal service bars mailing of fraudulent products Slimmer Shake and Joe Weider's Weight Loss Formula XR-7 made by Weider Distributors Inc. of Norwood, New Jersey.

December 15: FDA announces that drugs containing hormone HCG must be labeled as worthless for weight loss.

1975
March 27: Jack Fried, operator of Phase Method, is indicted in Newark, New Jersey on mail fraud charges for selling weight reduction plans based on clients' handwriting samples. Fried is latter convicted and sentenced to three years in prison.

April 4: Pillsbury Company announces it will acquire Weight Watchers International Inc. for $43 million.

May 14: Slim-Tabs Slenderizing Tablets producer Arnold Mandell pleads guilty to mail fraud, admitting pills are worthless.

December 15: Federal Trade Commission (FTC) prohibits Stuart Frost Inc. from advertising body wrapping devices called Slim-Quick or services used for weight reducing.

1976
March 3: Americans for Democratic Action issue a report attacking the weight reducing industry, citing $90 million annually wasted by consumers.

March 26: A study is published showing that early puberty and menstruation of girls is associated with stoutness and late menstruation with thinness.

June 9: FTC Judge Daniel H. Hanscom rules that Porter & Dietsch Inc., makers of X-11 Diet Tablets, and its ad agency, Kelly Ketting Furth, falsely advertised that users could lose weight while eating as much as they wanted.

December 4: Two government employees patent a method of controlling obesity with purified "miracle fruit" grown in West Africa.

1977
March 12: Because of saccharin's role in causing cancer, FDA announces plans to classify saccharin as a drug instead of a food additive.

April 11: Dr. John E. Farley, Jr., Head of the Rhode Island Medical Society drug abuse commission, announces his organization's opposition to the use of amphetamines in treating obesity; Utah Medical Association also opposes amphetamine use.

June 21: In the first major malpractice suit under a new Pennsylvania law, Marlene Baumiller, who underwent intestinal bypass operation for weight loss, is awarded $100,000 from Dr. Robert Cassella, who accidentally punctured her spleen and had to remove it; $25,000 from Pittsburgh Podiatry Hospital; and $225,000 from Medical Professional Liability Catastrophe Loss Fund.

July 21: FDA opposes strict rules for labeling foods as low calorie.

August 29: At annual American Psychological Association meeting Dr. Judith Rodin says overweight people secrete more insulin when stimulated by food sights and smells. Increased insulin secretion increases hunger, leading to overeating.

September 20: In Porter County (Indiana) superior court Cora Staniger is awarded $50,000 in damages from doctors who put her on a protein deficient diet during her pregnancy, causing mental retardation of her daughter.

November 3: FDA and Center for Disease Control (CDC) begin inquiry into 12 deaths suspected to be caused by liquid protein diet formula, which supplies 300 calories per day in a liquid made of fibrous protein collagen from animal tissue. Investigators suspect it may deprive users of potassium. FDA names a panel to investigate.

November 24: Federal Disease Control Center reports 10 more deaths suspected tied to crash dieting with predigested liquid proteins. FDA Commissioner Donald Kennedy requests 35 manufacturers of product to label compounds as hazardous under some conditions. Senator Charles Percy urges FDA to reclassify these diet products as prescription drugs.

December 1: At an American Heart Association meeting, California heart specialists claim that liquid protein diets can result in death even if used under strict medical supervision.

December 21: Figures from National Health Statistics Center show that American adults weigh an average of about four pounds more than in the previous decade.

December 29: At a House Subcommittee on Health and Environment hearing about liquid protein diets Dr. Robert Linn, author of *The Last Chance Diet,* questions the accuracy of the government report linking the diet to deaths.

1978

January 27: FDA asks 800,000 professional health workers to report cases of liquid protein-caused health problems; 46 deaths and 200 injuries from product are to be investigated. Sales of the product plummet.

February 12: Luciano Pavarotti, having lost 90 pounds on diet, disproves myth that obesity helps opera singers project strong voices.

March 12: Fat Liberation Front announces drive to free fat people from stigma and claims that no health problems result from obesity. Dr. Robert Sherwin of Yale comments that organizations such as the Fat Liberation Front help the obese psychologically but warns that obesity still needs to be treated.

April 22: Dr. Feridun Gundy of Queens, New York is convicted in federal court of illegally dispensing $2.5 million worth of amphetamines to obese patients.

May 16: Dr. George Blackburn, whose research was partially the basis for liquid protein diets, warns that the diets dangerously deplete essential nutrients.

May 16: H. J. Heinz Company announces that it will acquire Weight Watchers International Inc. for over $71 million.

September 22: Drs. Arthur Hartz and Alfred Timm, and mathematician Eldred Geifer announces that research at the Medical College of Wisconsin shows that environment is more important than heredity in determining tendency to obesity, disputing previous studies showing heredity as more important. Study observed behavior among natural and adopted siblings with overweight mothers, who were selected from weight reduction organization TOPS (Take Off Pounds Sensibly).

October 15: Substantial decline in sales of liquid protein diets is reported; decline is attributed to FDA findings of deaths by users of products. All deaths reported were of women who all died of myocarditis, inflammation of heart tissue.

December 17: Survey by British shirt manufacturer shows that fewer than 20% of women are attracted to skinny men, while 34% prefer men to have "slight suggestion of a paunch and 31 percent like a bit more of a paunch."

December 30: FDA revises order for warning labels on liquid protein diets and now requires warning on all protein products that provide more than 50% of a person's calories and are promoted for weight loss or as a food supplement.

1979

February 20: New research study challenges heredity-caused theories on obesity; the new study shows overeating as primary cause.

May 13: FDA panel headed by Dr. John W. Norcross reports that phenylpropanolamine and benzocaine, found in several nonprescription diet aids, may help some dieters; calls for further study on other ingredients; and reports that dozens of others are worthless.

July 1: FDA requirements for strict labeling of diet foods goes into effect. Foods labeled "low calorie" are required to contain no more than 40 calories per serving and must be lower in calories than food normally found in grocery stores. Foods labeled "reduced calorie" must contain at least one-third fewer calories than similar products for which it is substituted. Comparisons must be shown on label.

July 17: FDA proposes crackdown on illegal amphetamine use by banning their use in weight reduction. FDA says ban would reduce pill production by 80 to 90%. Three and one-third million prescriptions for amphetamines were written in 1978.

December 15: A study is reported in medical journal *Lancet* claiming that bypass surgery is safe and quick way to loose weight. *Lancet* editorial questions validity of study, criticizing research design and calling project ethically unsound.

1980

February 10: Essex County, New Jersey chapter of NOW (National Organization for Women) sponsors program called Food, Fat and Feminism, which explores reactions to fat and fat people, and food and diet.

May 1: Five drug companies agree to FDA request to stop shipments of new nonprescription diet products containing twice the current legal limits of phenylpropanolamine hydrochloride (PPA), an appetite suppressant drug. FDA determines that recalls are not necessary because pills are not considered a health risk.

May 4: A study is reported that finds that although death rates are higher for people who are above average weight, death rates are higher still for those weighing less than average.

May 29: A report by the Food and Nutrition Board of the National Academy of Sciences says healthy Americans need not worry about fat and cholesterol and admits its stand dissents from other major organizations that urge curbs on fat and cholesterol. Government experts criticize the report, saying board members ignored important scientific data.

July 5: Diet preparation that suppresses appetite for calories but not proteins is patented by Richard J. Wurtman, Judith J. Wurtman and John D. Fernstrom and licensed for production by Massachusetts Institute of Technology.

September 28: Research linking stress to obesity is reported. Rats reportedly overate when their tails were pinched, but their appetites abated when given naloxone, an opiate antagonist. This research has implications for understanding stress-related overeating.

October 30: A study is reported showing evidence that obese people have a biochemical defect involving enzyme adenosine triphosphatase (ATPase), which helps pump sodium and potassium across the membranes of the body cells. ATPase may be responsible for 10 to 50% of the body's heat energy production. The amount of ATPase in the red cells on the obese group was 22% lower than in the nonobese in the study.

December 12: A study by Drs. Eugene Lowenkopf and L. M. Vincent finds that 15% of students in professional ballet schools suffer from anorexia nervosa and many others are borderline. The study attributes dancer's obsession with body weight to the ballet profession's emphasis on thinness.

1981

August 4: New York State passes law making amphetamine prescription for sole purpose of weight loss illegal.

August 11: Study by Drs. Linda Craighead, Albert Stunkard and Richard M. O'Brien finds that appetite suppressant drugs may be counterproductive to long-term weight loss.

October 31: Psychotherapists report that bulimia nearly always begins with stringent weight loss diet.

November 16: An *AMA Journal* report criticizes the book, *The Beverly Hills Diet,* saying it is filled with medical inaccuracies.

1982

February 13: A report is published saying 10,000 poisoning cases per year result from taking PPA (phenylpropanolamine).

March 9: Study by Richard Weindruch and Roy L. Walford finds that undernutrition begun in middle age can lead to longer and healthier life for mice.

July 2: FDA announces that starch blockers, sold as diet aids, are possibly dangerous drugs and must be removed from market. Bio-Tech Laboratories, manufacturer of the pills, sues FDA to prevent defining starch blockers as drug.

August 22: Federal judge in Chicago denies request by FDA for ban on starch blockers despite a report of 75 illnesses related to the pills.

October 10: Federal court classifies starch blocker diet aids as drugs and ends all sales until determination of their safety can be made.

October 24: Gastroplasty, new operation that seals off most of stomach, is reported.

November 22: Suction lipectomy, new surgery that removes body fat by suction, is reported.

1983

March 2: Metropolitan Life Insurance Company publishes new height and weight tables showing ideal weights have increased for men by two to 13 pounds and three to 8 pounds for women.

April 28: Dr. Edward R. Woodward warns of life-threatening side effects resulting from jejunoileal bypass, a surgical procedure to lose weight by bypassing small intestine.

July 5: Cornell University study finds exercise after eating is the best way to get rid of extra calories and finds exercise crucial in maintaining stable weight when daily caloric intake fluctuates.

July 23: Dr. Thomas R. Knapp of the University of Rochester recommends people abandon concept of "ideal weight" because it is based on inconsistent data.

1984

December 16: A new eating disorders program is reported at Phelps Memorial Hospital in North Tarrytown, New York that treats anorexic and bulimic patients who require extensive care.

December 16: Pump therapy for anorexic patients is reported to pump up to 2,000 calories a day into severely underweight patients.

December 21: A study at Massachusetts General Hospital by Dr. Nancy A. Rigotti finds that women with anorexia nervosa often have weak bones, but can be treated with exercise.

1985

February 14: A National Institutes of Health panel defines obesity as a disease and says it should receive the same medical attention as high blood pressure, smoking and other factors that cause serious illness and premature death, and that overweight should be treated when it reaches 20% above "desirable" weight.

March 19: A study reported in *Journal of Abnormal Psychology* finds that women have negatively distorted view of their bodies; men also have distorted image of their bodies, but it is more positive.

March 22: Physicians and psychotherapists specializing in anorexia nervosa and bulimia treatment ask FDA to ban over-the-counter sales of syrup of ipecac, a drug used to induce vomiting, because of its potential use by bulimics.

May 6: A study of Dr. William Dietz, of the New England Medical Center, and Dr. Steven Gortmaker, of the Harvard School of Public Health, finds that children who watch lots of television exercise less, eat more and become obese.

August 6: Dr. Reubin Andres challenges Metropolitan Life height and weight tables, saying weight ranges given in tables do not reflect ideal weights.

September 2: First free-standing residential facility in U.S. devoted exclusively to treatment of anorexia nervosa and bulimia, Renfrew Center in Philadelphia, is reported.

1986
May 22: Scientists report that anorexia nervosa sufferers have high levels of cortisone, hormone excreted by adrenals in response to fear.

1987
March 24: Dr. George Blackburn, obesity specialist at Harvard Medical School, comments on study on causes of obesity and finds that dieting is ineffective for many people because when they reduce food intake, their metabolic rate drops to protect them from starvation.

1988
February 11: A study by Dr. William Feldman of Ottawa University reports that girls come to believe thin is beautiful as early as age seven and links that attitude to rising incidence of eating disorders in young girls.

February 25: Two studies are published showing evidence of genetic causes of obesity: one study was of Pima Indians in Arizona, the other of infants in Britain. These studies confirm theories of Dr. Jules Hirsch of Rockefeller University, who has promoted the idea for over two decades.

March 22: Doctors specializing in bulimia report that use of antidepressant drugs can help some patients reduce binge eating and purging, but warn that they cannot replace psychotherapy needed to get to the root problems.

April 17: Wilkins Center for Eating Disorders in Greenwich, Connecticut survey says among anorectics and bulimics, number of those who are 12 years old or younger has doubled in the last two years from 3 to 7% and says rise indicates increasing social pressure for thinness.

1989
January 3: Researchers at Rockefeller University announce discovery that abnormally low levels of protein adispin, which is secreted directly into the bloodstream by fat cells, may be linked to tendency to gain weight when not enough adispin is secreted. It may be a factor in genetic tendency to obesity.

February 23: A University of Michigan study is released that finds American women aged 18 to 34 have been getting fatter over past several decades; black and poor women and women with low education levels show the greatest weight gains.

March 18: Ronald T. Stunko patents chemical method of preventing fat formation in humans.

July 1: Pharmacologist Mark Hohenwarter patents biamine, chemical for treating addictions such as food or cocaine. Biamine works by replenishing certain neurotransmitters in the brain.

September 16: Cardiologists Jackie R. See and William E. Shell patent ''Fat Magnets'' diet pills, made from bovine bile, that prevents the body from absorbing some fat and cholesterol in food.

October 3: Merck Sharp & Dohme announce discovery of manner in which hormone cholecytokinin triggers brain to tell body when to stop eating. They also discovered two chemicals that block hormone's action.

1990

January 3: Nationwide survey by Calorie Control Council finds that pounds almost always return after dieting and that only fundamental changes in eating behavior will keep them off. Survey also found a 26% drop in the number of people on diets.

March 20: Research team led by David Williamson of the Federal Centers for Disease Control announces findings that people are most likely to gain weight as young adults and that black women are especially vulnerable; women of all races are twice as likely as men to gain large amounts of weight; and women form 25 to 44 who were overweight at the beginning of the study gained the most weight of all subjects.

March 28: Representative Ron Wyden (D., Ore.) chairman of the House Regulation, Business Opportunities and Energy subcommittee opened hearings into questionable practices of the weight-loss industry amid charges that health risks, false advertising and profiteering are "bedrock" in the industry.

April 1: Five-year study by Dr. Thomas Wadden shows that 98 percent of all dieters regain their weight within five years.

April 1: New York Times story says recent studies suggest that formula diets can lead to psychological and physiological burdens that limit diets' long-term effectiveness; some people develop fear of food and become dependent on formula diets, while others binge and suffer humiliating weight gains, while few maintain their lower weights.

APPENDIX II

TABLES

Table 1 Physical Manifestations of Anorexia Nervosa and Bulimia

Manifestation	Anorexia Nervosa	Bulimia

Endocrine/metabolic	Amenorrhea
	Osteoporosis
	Euthyroid sick syndrome
	Decreased norepinephrine
	  secretion
	Decreased somatomedin C
	Elevated growth hormone
	Decreased or erratic
	  vasopressin secretion
	Abnormal temperature
	  regulation
	Hypercarotenemia
		Menstrual
		  irregularities

Cardiovascular	Bradycardia Hypotension Arrhythmias	Ipecac poisoning

Renal	Increased blood urea
	  nitrogen
	Renal calculi
	Edema
		Hypokalemia (diuretic
		  induced)

Gastrointestinal	Decreased gastric emptying
	Constipation
	Elevated hepatic enzymes
		Acute gastric dilation,
		  rupture
		Parotid enlargement
		Dental-enamel erosion
		Esophagitis
		Mallory-Weiss tears,
		  esophageal rupture
		Hypokalemia (laxative
		  induced)

Hematologic	Anemia Leukopenia Thrombocytopenia	
Pulmonary		Aspiration pneumonia

SOURCE: David B. Herzog and Paul M. Copeland, "Eating Disorders," *New England Journal of Medicine* 313, no. 5 (August 1, 1985), p. 297.

Table 2   DSM-III Criteria for Diagnosing Anorexia Nervosa and Bulimia

Anorexia Nervosa
1. Refusal to maintain normal body weight
2. Loss of more than 25 percent of original body weight
3. Disturbance of body image
4. Intense fear of becoming fat
5. No known medical illness leading to weight loss

Bulimia
1. Recurrent episodes of binge eating
2. At least three of the following:
   a. Consumption of high-calorie, easily ingested foods during a binge
   b. Termination of binge by abdominal pain, sleep, social interruption or self-induced vomiting
   c. Inconspicuous eating during a binge
   d. Repeated attempts to lose weight by severely restrictive diets, self-induced vomiting or use of cathartics or diuretics
   e. Frequent weight fluctuations greater than 10 pounds due to alternating binges and fasts
3. Awareness of abnormal eating pattern and fear of not being able to stop voluntarily
4. Depressed mood and self-deprecating thoughts after binge
5. Bulimic episodes not due to anorexia nervosa or any known physical disorder

SOURCE: David B. Herzog and Paul M. Copeland, "Eating Disorders," *New England Journal of Medicine* 313, no. 5 (August 1, 1985), p. 300.

Table 3   Possible Medical Complications of Commonly Used Weight Regulation/ Weight Loss Methods

Vomiting
Parotid gland enlargement (neck area)
Erosion of tooth enamel and increased cavities
Tears in esophagus
Chronic esophagitis
Chronic sore throats
Difficulty swallowing
Stomach cramps
Digestive problems
Anemia
Electrolyte imbalance

Diuretic Abuse
Hypokalemia (low potassium): fatigue; diminished reflexes; if severe, possible cardiac arrhythmia; if chronic, serious kidney damage
Fluid loss: dehydration, lightheadedness, thirst

Laxative Abuse
Nonspecific abdominal complaints, cramping, constipation
Sluggish bowel functioning ("cathartic colon")
Malabsorption of fat, protein and calcium

(Combinations of these methods can dangerously affect potassium regulation and fluid balance.)

SOURCE: *An Overview of Eating Disorders* by the National Anorexic Aid Society Inc., copyright © 1991 by NAAS, Ohio.

Table 4 Danger Signals

Eating disorders may be prevented or more readily treated if they are detected early. A person who has several of the following signs may be developing or has already developed an eating disorder.

Anorexia
The individual:
- has lost a great deal of weight in a relatively short period.
- continues to diet although bone-thin.
- reaches diet goal and immediately sets another goal for further weight loss.
- remains dissatisfied with appearance, claiming to feel fat, even after reaching weight loss goal.
- prefers dieting in isolation to joining a diet group.
- loses monthly menstrual periods.
- develops unusual interest in food.
- develops strange eating rituals and eats small amounts of food, e.g., cuts food into tiny pieces or measures everything before eating extremely small amounts.
- becomes a secret eater.
- becomes obsessive about exercising.
- appears depressed much of the time.
- begins to binge and purge (see below).

Bulimia
The individual:
- binges regularly (eats large amounts of food over a short period of time), and
- purges regularly (forces vomiting and/or uses drugs to stimulate vomiting, bowel movements and urination).
- diets and exercises often but maintains or regains weight.
- becomes a secret eater.
- eats enormous amounts of food at one sitting but does not gain weight.
- disappears into the bathroom for long periods of time to induce vomiting.
- abuses drugs or alcohol or steals regularly.
- appears depressed much of the time.
- has swollen neck glands.
- has scars on the back of hands from forced vomiting.

SOURCE: National Institute of Mental Health.

Table 5   How to Handle the Anorexic/Bulimic Child in the Family

DON'T

1. Do not urge your child to eat, or watch her eat, or discuss food intake or weight with her. Leave the room if necessary. Your involvement with her eating is her tool for manipulating parents. Take this tool out of her hands.

2. Do not allow yourself to feel guilty. Most parents ask: "What have I done wrong?" There are no perfect parents. You have done the best you could. Once you have checked out her physical condition with a physician and made it possible for her to begin counseling, getting well is her responsibility. It is her problem, not yours.

3. Do not neglect your marriage partner or other children. Focussing on the sick child can perpetuate her illness and destroy the family. The anorexic must be made aware by your actions and attitudes that she is important to you, but no more important than every other member of the family. Do not commiserate; this only confirms the child in her illness. She knows you love her.

4. Do not be afraid to have the child separated from you, either at school or in separate housing, if it becomes obvious that her continued presence is undermining the emotional health of the family. The final separation is death; don't allow her to intimidate the family with threats of suicide.

5. Do not put down the child by comparing her to her more "successful" siblings or friends. Her self-esteem is a reflection of your esteem for her. Do not ask questions such as, "How are you feeling," or "How is your social life?" She already feels inadequate, and questions only aggravate the feeling.

DO

1. Love your child as you should love yourself. Love makes anyone feel worthwhile.

2. Trust your child to find her own values, ideals and standards, rather than insisting on yours. In any case, all ideals are just that . . . only ideals. In practice we fall short, too; our own behavior is adulterated with self-serving rewards.

3. Do everything to encourage her initiative, independence and autonomy. Be aware though, that anorexics tend to be perfectionists, so that they are never satisfied with themselves. Perfectionism justifies their dissatisfaction with themselves.

4. Be aware of the long-term nature of the illness. Anorexics do get better; many get completely well, very few die. But families must face months and sometimes years of treatment and anxiety. There are no counselors or psychiatrists with the same answer to every case. A support group such as a parents self-help group may make a significant difference to your family's survival; it helps you to *deal with yourself* in relation to your anorexic child. You must make the child understand that *your* life is as important as hers.

SOURCE: American Anorexia/Bulimia Association, Inc.

Table 6 Food-related Behaviors or Behavior Patterns

The following guidelines were published in *BASH Magazine,* April 1989, for identifying and monitoring the eating habits of eating-disordered patients:

A. Food Preferences (Anorexia)
1. Restrictive in fat and protein in all food selections.
2. Consumes most vegetables and specific fruits to control weight gain.
3. Observable increase in the amount of noncaloric condiments used to alter the flavor of food, possibly to make it less appealing (cinnamon, mustard, vinegar).
4. Increased desire for diet drinks, coffee and/or tea.

B. Food Preferences (Bulimia)
1. Polyphagic or carbohydrate specific during a binge; however, when not in a binge-purge cycle, specific "binge" foods, such as cereal, cakes, cookies, ice cream, bread, nuts, peanut butter, pasta, crackers and chips, are restricted.
2. Consumes easily purged foods to control weight gain, such as ice cream, cheese, eggs, vegetables, cereal, milk.
3. Craves foods that satisfy taste desires, usually for sweet or salty foods.
4. Increased desire for diet drinks, coffee and/or tea.
5. Consumes excess fluid to aid vomiting; attempts to suppress hunger and aid rehydration.

C. Physical Experience (Anorexia)
1. Cuts food into small pieces.
2. Arranges food on plate.
3. Eats slowly, with prolonged chewing time before swallowing.
4. Prefers small containers of food.
5. Throws away or hides food to avoid consumption.
6. Does not self-induce vomiting to control food intake. (The exception is the bulimic anorectic.)

D. Physical Experience (Bulimia)
1. Normal to large bites of food.
2. May mix foods together.
3. Eats rapidly with shortened chewing time before swallowing.
4. Prefers large containers of food.
5. Dislikes being responsible for food waste and will overeat or hoard food for an isolated binge experience.
6. Vomits to control food absorption by inducing vomiting, spontaneous rumination or regurgitation.

SOURCE: *BASH Magazine,* April 1989.

Table 7 Metropolitan Height and Weight Table for Women*
(Originally published 1959; revision 1983)

Height	Small Frame		Medium Frame		Large Frame	
	1959	1983	1959	1983	1959	1983
4' 9"	90–97	99–108	94–106	106–118	102–118	115–128
4'10"	92–100	100–110	97–109	108–120	105–121	117–131
4'11"	95–103	101–112	100–112	110–123	108–124	119–134
5' 0"	98–106	103–115	103–115	112–126	111–127	122–137
5' 1"	101–109	105–118	106–118	115–129	114–130	125–140
5' 2"	104–112	108–121	109–122	118–132	117–134	128–144
5' 3"	107–115	111–124	112–126	121–135	121–138	131–148
5' 4"	110–119	114–127	116–131	124–138	125–142	134–152
5' 5"	114–123	117–130	120–135	127–141	129–146	137–156
5' 6"	118–127	120–133	124–139	130–144	133–150	140–160
5' 7"	122–131	123–136	128–143	133–147	137–154	143–164
5' 8"	126–136	126–139	132–147	136–150	141–159	146–167
5' 9"	130–140	129–142	136–151	139–153	145–164	149–170
5'10"	134–144	132–145	140–155	142–156	149–169	152–173

*Height in feet and inches, without shoes. Weight in pounds, without clothes.
  Courtesy of Metropolitan Life Insurance Co.

Metropolitan Height and Weight Table for Men*

Height	Small Frame		Medium Frame		Large Frame	
	1959	1983	1959	1983	1959	1983
5' 1"	105–113	123–129	111–122	126–136	119–134	133–145
5' 2"	108–116	125–131	114–126	128–138	122–137	135–148
5' 3"	111–119	127–133	117–129	130–140	125–141	137–151
5' 4"	114–122	129–135	120–132	132–143	128–145	139–155
5' 5"	117–126	131–137	123–136	134–146	131–149	141–159
5' 6"	121–130	133–140	127–140	137–149	135–154	144–163
5' 7"	125–134	135–143	131–145	140–152	140–159	147–167
5' 8"	129–138	137–146	135–149	143–155	144–163	150–171
5' 9"	133–143	139–149	139–153	146–158	148–167	153–175
5'10"	137–147	141–152	143–158	149–161	152–172	156–179
5'11"	141–151	144–155	147–163	152–165	157–177	159–183
6' 0"	145–155	147–159	151–168	155–169	161–182	163–187
6' 1"	149–160	150–163	155–173	159–173	166–187	167–192
6' 2"	153–164	153–167	160–178	162–177	171–192	171–197
6' 3"	157–168	157–171	165–183	166–182	175–197	176–202

*Height in feet and inches, without shoes. Weight in pounds, without clothes.
  Courtesy of Metropolitan Life Insurance Co.

APPENDIX III

SOURCES OF INFORMATION

American Anorexia/Bulimia Association
(formerly the American Anorexia Nervosa
  Association)
418 E. 76th St.
New York, NY 10021
(212) 734-1114

American Anorexia/Bulimia Association of
  New Jersey
623 River Rd.
Fair Haven, NJ 07704
(908) 530-0387

American Anorexia/Bulimia Association of
  Philadelphia
Philadelphia Child Guidance Clinic
34th and Civic Center Blvd.
Philadelphia, PA 19104
(215) 387-1919

American Anorexia/Bulimia Association of
  Virginia, Inc.
PO Box 6644
Newport News, VA 23606
(804) 875-1307
Washington, DC information line: (202)
  362-3009

American Board of Medical Specialties
One Rotary Center, Suite 805
Evanston, IL 60201
(708) 491-9091

American Dietetic Association
216 W. Jackson Blvd., Suite 800
Chicago, IL 60606
(312) 899-0040

American Psychiatric Association
Division of Public Affairs

1400 K St. NW
Washington, DC 20005
(202) 682-6000

American Society for Bariatric Surgery
633 Post St. #639
San Francisco, CA 94109
(415) 753-6029

American Society of Bariatric Physicians
5600 S. Quebec, Suite 160D
Englewood, CO 80111
(303) 779-4833

American Society of Plastic and Reconstructive Surgeons
444 E. Algonquin Rd.
Arlington Heights, IL 60005
(708) 228-9900
(800) 635-0635

Anorexia Nervosa and Related Eating Disorders, Inc.
PO Box 5102
Eugene, OR 97405
(503) 344-1144

Center for Science in the Public Interest
1501 16th St. NW
Washington, DC 20036
(202) 332-9110

Council on Size and Weight Discrimina-
  tion, Inc.
PO Box 238
Columbia, MD 21045

Human Ecology Action League
PO Box 49126

Atlanta, GA 30359
(404) 248-1898

Maryland Association for Anorexia and
Bulimia, Inc. (MAANA)
Shettard Pratt Hospital
6501 N. Charles St.
Towson, MD 21204
(410) 323-1650

Mental Health Association of Broward
County
5546 W. Oakland Park Blvd.
Lauderhill, FL 33313
(305) 733-3994

National Anorexic Aid Society
1925 E. Dublin–Granville Rd.
Columbus, OH 43229
(614) 436-1112

National Association to Advance Fat Acceptance
(formerly the National Association to Aid
Fat Americans, Inc.)
PO Box 188620
Sacramento, CA 95818
(916) 443-0303

National Institute of Child Health and Human Development

NICHD NIH
Building 31, Room 2A32
9000 Rockville Pike
Bethesda, MD 20892
(301) 496-5133

National Institute of Mental Health Eating
Disorders Program
Building 10, Room 3S231
9000 Rockville Pike
Bethesda, MD 20892
(301) 496-1891

Overeaters Anonymous
4025 Spencer St. #203
Torrance, CA 90503
PO Box 92870
Los Angeles, CA 90009
(213) 542-8363

TOPS Club (Take Off Pounds Sensibly)
PO Box 07360
Milwaukee, WI 53207-0360
(414) 482-4620

Weight Watchers International
500 North Broadway
Jericho, NY 11753
(516) 939-0400

APPENDIX IV

OBESITY AND EATING DISORDER CENTERS
WEIGHT REDUCTION CAMPS FOR CHILDREN

OBESITY AND EATING DISORDER CENTERS

ALABAMA

UAB Nutrition Clinic
University of Alabama Hospital
222 Webb Building
1629 University Blvd.
UAB Station
Birmingham, AL 35294
(205) 934-5112

CALIFORNIA

Behavioral Medicine Clinic
Department of Psychiatry—Behavioral
  Medicine
Stanford University Medical Center
  Stanford, CA 94305
(415) 723-6811

Eating Disorders Clinic
Dept. of Psychiatry
Alta Bates/Herrick Hospital
2001 Swight Way
Berkeley, CA 94704
(510) 540-4444

Eating Disorders Resource and Referral
  Service
PO Box 34524
San Diego, CA 92103
(619) 236-0300

Oak Knoll Family Therapy Center
12307 Oak Knoll Road

Poway, CA 92064
(619) 748-4323

Physicians' Weight Reduction Centers
14104 Magnolia Blvd.
Sherman Oaks, CA 91423
(818) 501-3881

The Radar Institute
1663 Sawtelle Blvd., Third Floor
Los Angeles, CA 90025
(800) 255-1818

CONNECTICUT

ANAD of Connecticut Self-Help Group
Wheeler Clinic
91 Northwest Drive
Plainville, CT 06062
(203) 747-6801

Wilkins Center for Eating Disorders
#7 Riversville Road
Greenwich, CT 06831
(203) 531-1909

DISTRICT OF COLUMBIA

Department of Psychiatry
Children's National Medical Center
111 Michigan Ave. NW
Washington, DC 20010
(202) 745-5000

FLORIDA

Eating Disorders Unit
Bethesda Memorial Hospital
2815 South Seacrest Blvd.
Boynton Beach, FL 33435
(407) 737-7733

Eating Disorders Unit
Humana Hospital Sebastian
13695 N. U.S. Highway #1
Sebastian, FL 32958
(407) 589-3186

ERE Associates
8500 SW 92d St., Suite B102
Miami, FL 33156
(305) 279-3710

ERE Association
7325 SW 63d Ave., Suite 101
South Miami, FL 33143
(305) 284-1143

Glenbeigh Health Services
3102 East 138th Ave.
Tampa, FL 33613
(813) 971-5000

Willough at Naples
9001 Tamiami Trail East
Naples, FL 33962
(800) 722-0100
(800) 282-3508
(813) 775-4500

ILLINOIS

Control Over Nutrition
Forest Hospital
555 Wilson Lane
Des Plaines, IL 60016
(708) 635-4100

Eating Disorders Program
Northwestern Memorial Hospital
Superior St. & Fairbanks Ct.
Chicago, IL 60611
(312) 908-2000

MASSACHUSETTS

Adolescent Clinic
Children's Hospital Medical Center
300 Longwood Ave.
Boston, MA 02115
(617) 735-6000

Behavior Therapy Unit
McLean Hospital
115 Mill Street
Belmont, MA 02178
(617) 855-2000 ext. 2994

Eating Disorders Unit
Massachusetts General Hospital
55 Fruit Street
Boston, MA 02114
(617) 726-2000

MICHIGAN

Eating Disorders Support Group
Orchard Hills Psychiatric Center
42450 W. Twelve-Mile Rd. #305
Novi, MI 48377
(313) 349-7337

MINNESOTA

Department of Psychiatry
University of Minnesota Hospital and
   Clinic
Harvard St. at E. River Rd.
Minneapolis, MN 55455
(612) 626-6188

Psychiatry Department
Mayo Clinic
Baldwin Bldg., 4th Floor
200 First St. SW
Rochester, MN 55905
(507) 284-2933

MISSOURI

BASH Treatment and Research Center for
   Eating and Mood Disorders
Deaconess Hospital
6125 Clayton Ave., Suite 215

St. Louis, MO 63139
(314) 281-2904
(800) 227-4785

NEW JERSEY

Weight Watchers Center
210 Rte. 4 East
Paramus, NJ 07652
(201) 712-0266

NEW YORK

Adolescent Medicine
North Shore University Hospital
865 Northern Blvd.
Great Neck, NY 11020
(516) 773-7669

Center for the Study of Anorexia and
   Bulimia
1 West 91st St.
New York, NY 10024
(212) 595-3449

Dept. of Adolescent Medicine
Long Island Jewish–Hillside Medical
   Center
26901 76th Ave.
New Hyde Park, NY 11042
(718) 470-3000

Eating Disorders Group
St. Vincent's Hospital and Medical Center
203 W. 12th St.
New York, NY 10011
(212) 790-8273

Eating Disorders Research and Treatment
   Program
New York State Psychiatric Institute
Columbia-Presbyterian Medical Center
722 West 168th St.
New York, NY 10032
(212) 960-5754

Four Winds Hospital
800 Cross River Rd.

Katonah, NY 10536
(914) 763-8151

The Fredda Kray Weigh
   Wayside Cottage
1039 Post Rd.
Scarsdale, NY 10583
(914) 723-2997

Pediatrics Department
Mt. Sinai Medical Center
One Gustave L., Levy Pl.
New York, NY 10029
(212) 423-0900

Prader-Willi Association
Nassau County Medical Center
2201 Hempstead Turnpike
East Meadow, NY 11554
(516) 542-0123 Ext. 3391

Weight Watchers Center
117 Rockland Center
Nanuet, NY 10954
(914) 634-7809
(800) 221-2112

Weight Watchers Center
Cross Country Center
6M Upper Mall Walk
Yonkers, NY 10704
(914) 634-7809
(800) 221-2112

NORTH CAROLINA

Anorexia Nervosa Treatment Program
Box 3245
Duke University Medical Center
Durham, NC 27110
(919) 684-3073

OHIO

Eating Disorders Center
University of Cincinnati Medical Center
231 Bethesda Ave., ML 559
Cincinnati, OH 45267
(513) 558-1000

North Community Counseling—The Bridge
4897 Karl Road
Columbus, OH 43229
(614) 846-2588

Section of Child and Adolescent Psychiatry
Cleveland Clinic Hospital
9500 Euclid Ave.
Cleveland, OH 44195
(216) 444-2200

PENNSYLVANIA

AANA of Philadelphia
Philadelphia Child Guidance Clinic
34th and Civic Center Blvd.
Philadelphia, PA 19104
(215) 243-2600

Eating Disorder Unit (COPE)
Western Psychiatric Institute and Clinic
3811 O'Hara St.
Pittsburgh, PA 15213
(402) 624-5420

Juvenile Weight Control Program
Hahnemann University Hospital
Broad & Vine Sts.
Philadelphia, PA 19102
(215) 762-7000

Obesity Research Group
Hospital of the University of Pennsylvania
3600 Market St.
Philadelphia, PA 19104-2648
(215) 349-5220

Prader-Willi Clinic
Rehabilitation Institute of Pittsburgh
6301 Northumberland St.
Pittsburgh, PA 15217
(412) 521-9000

The Renfrew Center
475 Spring Lane
Philadelphia, PA 19128
(215) 482-5353

TEXAS

Department of Psychiatry
Baylor College of Medicine
Houston Medical Center
1200 Moursund Ave.
Houston, TX 77030
(713) 798-4856

WASHINGTON

Prader-Willi Clinic
Child Development and Mental Retardation
  Center
Mail Drop WJ-10
University of Washington
Seattle, WA 98195
(206) 685-1242

WISCONSIN

Eating Disorders Clinic
Department of Pediatrics
University of Wisconsin Hospital and
  Clinic
722 Hill St.
Madison, WI 53705
(608) 263-4760

Institute for Eating Disorders
330 South Whitney Way
Madison, WI 53705
(608) 223-7800

WEIGHT REDUCTION CAMPS FOR CHILDREN

CALIFORNIA

Camp Murietta for Girls
Camp Del Mar for Boys
6091 Charae St.
San Diego, CA 92122
(619) 450-3376
(800) 531-9186

MASSACHUSETTS

Kingsmont Camp
Box 100

West Stockbridge, MA 01266
(413) 232-8518

NEW YORK

Camp Camelot for Girls
949 Northfield Rd.

Woodmere, NY 11598
(516) 374-1366

Weight Watcher Camps
183 Madison Ave., Dept. 305
New York, NY 10016
(212) 889-9500

APPENDIX V

AUDIOVISUAL MATERIALS

"Anorexia & Bulimia," a 19-minute video that explains the dangerously addictive nature of anorexia and bulimia, and their possible effects on the cardiovascular and central nervous systems. A nutritionist demonstrates the extremes to which people with these eating disorders commonly go in their addiction. Available through Films for the Humanities & Sciences, Inc., Box 2053, Princeton, NJ 08543; (800) 257-5126.

"Bulimia." a 12-minute film that examines the dangers of bulimia and its effects on victims and their families through interviews with experts in eating disorders and with recovered bulimics and their parents (1983). Available through the CRM Educational Films, 2215 Faraday Ave., Carlsbad, CA 92008; (619) 431-9800.

"Bulimia: Out-of-Control Eating," a 23-minute video. Available through AIMS Media, 9710 DeSoto Ave., Chatsworth, CA 91311-4409; (818) 773-4300 or (800) 367-2467.

"Cathy Rigby on Eating Disorders" (originally titled "Faces of Recovery: Overcoming the Tragedy of Eating Disorders"), a 35-minute video tape narrated by Cathy Rigby McCoy, former Olympic gymnast, herself a former bulimic, now a successful actress. Offers insight into some of the successful techniques used in treating eating disorders as well as hope for eventual recovery. Through interviews with actual patients who have suffered from eating disorders for over 20 years, this video addresses some of the questions asked most often by patients and family members (1988). Available

through Increase Video, 6860 Canby Ave., Suite 118, Reseda CA 91335; (800) 233-2880.

"Eating Disorders," a 20-minute video (1987). Available through United Learning, 6633 W. Howard St., Niles, IL 60714; (800) 424-0362.

"Fight for Life," a 30-minute video tape that examines various eating and mood disorders, using members of real BASH families, with brief explanatory and informative passages by BASH staffers (1990). Available through BASH Treatment and Research Center, 6125 Clayton Ave., Suite 215, St. Louis, MO 63139; (314) 567-4080.

"Food Labeling: Understanding What You Eat," a video. Discusses nutrition and how to eat to solve a weight problem. Available through Altschul Group, 1560 Sherman Ave., Suite 100, Evanston, IL 60201; (708) 328-6700.

"The Food Platform," a 16mm film and video tape. Hundreds of young students assume the roles of body cells and meet to elect a diet for the body. Available through American Educational Films, PO Box 70188, Nashville, TN 37207; (615) 868-2040 or (800) 822-5678.

"How to Lose Weight," a 15-minute film and video tape. Discusses how much you should lose, how fast and traps to avoid. Available through Walter J. Klein Co., PO Box 472087, Charlotte, NC 28247-2087; (704) 542-1403.

"Learning about Eating Disorders: Bulimia," a 15-minute video (1987). Available through Churchill Media, 12210 Nebraska

Ave., Los Angeles, CA 90025; (310) 207-6600.

"Nutrition, Eating to Live or Living to Eat," a 60-minute video (1988). Available through PBS Video, 1320 Braddock Pl., Alexandria, VA 22314; (703) 739-5000.

BIBLIOGRAPHY

ARTICLES IN JOURNALS, NEWSPAPERS, AND PERIODICALS

Agras, W. Stewart; Schneider, John; Arnow, Bruce; Raeburn, Susan; and Telch, Christy. "Cognitive-Behavioral and Response-Prevention Treatments for Bulimia Nervosa." *Journal of Consulting and Clinical Psychology* 57 (April 1989).

Allinder, Rose M. "The Personality Differences between Women Diagnosed with Anorexia Nervosa versus Bulimia." *Dissertation Abstracts International* Vol. 48, No. 3 (1987).

Andersen, Arnold E. "Anorexic Behavior Isn't Quite the Same in Males." *BASH Magazine,* July 1989.

Andersen, Arnold E., and Mickalide, Angela D. "Anorexia Nervosa in the Male, an Underdiagnosed Disorder." *Psychosomatics* Vol. 24, No. 12 (December 1983).

"Anorexic Bone: Lost but Not Found." *Science News* 133.

Appelo, Tim. "Young Women Wasting Away." *Savvy,* May 1988.

Arbetter, Sandra R. "Emotional Food Fights." *Current Health* 2 (March 1989).

Arisimuno, G. G.; Foster, T. A.; Voors, A. W.; Srinivasan, S. R.; and Berenson, G. S. "Influence of Persistent Obesity in Children on Cardiovascular Risk Factors: The Bogalusa Heart Study." *Circulation* Vol. 70 (May 1984).

Aronson, H.; Fredman, Marla; and Gabriel, Marsha. "Personality Correlates of Eating Attitudes in a Nonclinical Sample." *International Journal of Eating Disorders* Vol. 9, No. 1 (January 1990).

"Assessing Dietary Fiber vis-a-vis Obesity and Diabetes." *BASH Magazine,* November 1989.

Atkinson, R. L. "Low and Very Low Calorie Diets." *Medical Clinics of North America* 73 (1) (January 1989).

Baldessarini, R. J. "Current Status of Antidepressants: Clinical Pharmacology and Therapy." *Journal of Clinical Psychiatry* 50 (4) (April 1989).

Bandini, L. G.; Schoeller, D. A.; Edwards, J.; Young, V. R.; Oh, S. H.; and Dietz, W. H. "Energy Expenditure during Carbohydrate Overfeeding in Obese and Nonobese Adolescents." *American Journal of Physiology* 256 (3 Pt 1) (March 1989).

Basilisco, G.; Camboni, G.; Bozzani, A.; Vita, P.; Doldi, S.; and Bianchi, P. A. "Orocecal Transit Delay in Obese Patients." *Digestive Diseases and Sciences* 34 (4) (April 1989).

Bassiouny, M. A., and Pollack, R. L. "Esthetic Management of Perimolysis with Porcelain Laminate Veneers." *Journal of the American Dental Association* Vol. 115, No. 3 (September 1987).

Bauer, Barbara, and Anderson, Wayne. "Bulimic Beliefs: Food for Thought." *Journal of Counseling and Development* 67 (7) (March 1989).

Bayer, A. E., and Baker, D. H. "Adolescent Eating Disorders: Anorexia and Bulimia." Virginia Polytechnic Institute and State University, Virginia Cooperative Extension Service, Publication No. 352–004, November 1983.

Bearn, J.; Treasure, J.; Murphy, M.; and Franey, C. "A Study of Sulphatoxymelatonin Excretion and Gonadotrophin." *British Journal of Psychiatry* Vol. 152 (March 1988).

Bennett, William, and Gurin, Joel. "NIH Obesity Report Is a Fatheaded Fright." *Cleveland Plain Dealer,* March 19, 1985.

Ben-Tovim, David I. "DSM-III, Draft DSM-III-R, and the Diagnosis and Prevalence of Bulimia in Australia." *American Journal of Psychiatry* Vol. 145, No. 8 (August 1988).

Ben-Tovim, David I.; Walker, M. K.; Murray, H.; and Chin, G. Body Size Estimates: Body Image or Body Attitude Measures?" *International Journal of Eating Disorders* Vol. 9, No. 1 (January 1990).

Berenstein, Frederick. "Dieting and Anorexia." *1,001 Home Ideas,* July 1989.

Beumont, Peter J. V. "Diet Guidance for Bulimics." *BASH Magazine,* June 1989.

———. "Trying to Make Sense of Body Image Distortion." *BASH Magazine,* June 1989.

Biller, Beverly M. K.; Saxe, Velia; Herzog, David B.; Rosenthal, Daniel I.; Holzman, Susan; and Klibanski, Anne. "Mechanisms of Osteoporosis in Adult and Adolescent Women with Anorexia Nervosa." *Journal of Clinical Endocrinology and Metabolism* 68 (1989).

Birk, Randi. "Eating Disorders and Diabetes." *Diabetes Self-Management* (September/October 1988).

Bjorkman, David J.; Alexander, James R.; and Simons, Margaret A. "Perforated Duodenal Ulcer after Gastric Bypass Surgery."*American Journal of Gastroenterology* 2 (February 1989).

Black, John L., and Bruce, Barbara K. "Behavior Therapy: A Clinical Update." *Hospital and Community Therapy* 40, No.11 (1989).

Blair, A. J.; Booth, D. A.; Lewis, V. J.; and Wainwright, C. J. "The Relative Success of Official and Informal Weight Reduction Techniques: Retrospective Correlational Evidence." *Psychology and Health* (in press).

Blinder, Barton J., and John, Jean Densmore. "Food-related Behaviors in Anorexia Nervosa and Bulimia Specificity and Differentiation." *BASH Magazine,* April 1989.

Bluestone, Mimi. "Fighting Depression with One of the Brain's Own Drugs." *Business Week,* February 22, 1988.

Blundell, John, and Hill, Andrew J. "Serotoninergic Modulation of the Pattern of Eating and the Profile of Hunger-Satiety in Humans." *International Journal of Obesity,* supplement, 1987.

"The Body Prison." *Life,* February 1988.

Bonavoglia, Angela. "I Am a Compulsive Overeater." *Cosmopolitan,* April 1991.

Boon, A. P.; Thompson, H.; and Baddeley, R. M. "Use of Histological Examination to Assess Ultrastructure of Liver in Patients with Long Standing Jejunoileal Bypass for Morbid Obesity." *Journal of Clinical Pathology* Vol. 41, No. 12 (December 1988).

Booth, D. A. "Holding Weight Down: Physiological and Psychological Considerations." *Medicographia* 7, No. 3 (1985).

———. "Mechanisms from Models—Actual Effects from Real Life: The Zero-Calorie Drink-Break Option." *Appetite,* (1988) 11, Supplement.

——. "Culturally Corralled into Food Abuse: The Eating Disorders as Physiologically Reinforced Excessive Appetites." In *Conditioned Binges*.

Botyanski, Nancy C. "Level of Object Representation and Psychic Structure Deficit in Obese Persons." *Psychological Reports*.

Bouchard, C. "Genetic Factors in Obesity." *Medical Clinics of North America* 73(1) (January 1989).

Bougneres, Pierre-Francois; Aravia-Loria, Ephrain; Henry, Sixtine; Basdevant, Arnaud; and Castano, Luis. "Increased Basal Glucose Production and Utilization in Children with Recent Obesity versus Adults with Long-Term Obesity." *Diabetes* 38 (April 1989).

Bray, George A. "Nutrient Balance and Obesity: An Approach to Control of Food Intake in Humans." *Medical Clinics of North America* 73(1) (January 1989).

——. Nutritional Aspects of Obesity." In *Nutrition and Medical Practice,* edited by Lewis A. Barness. Westport, Conn.: Avi, 1981.

Bringle, Mary Louise. "Confessions of a Glutton." *Christian Century,* October 25, 1989.

Brody, Jane E. "Personal Health." *New York Times,* March 18, 1987.

——. "Research Lifts Blame from Many Obese." *New York Times,* March 24, 1987.

Brody, Robert. "Update on Anorexia/Bulimia." *Cosmopolitan,* January 1991.

Brolin, Robert E.; Kenler, Hallis A.; Gorman, Robert C.; and Cody, Ronald P. "The Dilemma of Outcome Assessment after Operations for Morbid Obesity." *Surgery* 105 (3) (March 1989).

Brotleit, Ziona. "Moving Forward." *Renfrew Perspective,* Summer 1989.

Brotman, A. W.; Herzog, D. B.; and Hamburg, P. "Long-Term Course in Fourteen Bulimic Patients Treated with Psychotherapy." *Journal of Clinical Psychiatry* 49 (4) (April 1988).

Brouwers, Mariette. "Treatment of Body Image Dissatisfaction among Women with Bulimia Nervosa." *Journal of Counseling and Development* 69 (2) (November 1990).

Brownell, Kelly D. "Behavioral Managment of Obesity." *Medical Clinics of North America* Vol. 73, No. 1 (January 1989).

——. "When and How to Diet." *Psychology Today,* 23 (6) June 1989.

Buckholtz, N. S.; George, D. T.; Davies, A. O.; Jimerson, D. C.; and Potter, W. Z. "Lymphocyte Beta-adrenergic Receptor Modification in Bulimia." *Archives of Gerneral Psychiatry* 45 (5) (May 1988).

Burns, Diane Hubbard. "Diet Mania Obsesses Children." *Fort Lauderdale Sun-Sentinel,* March 29, 1988.

Burns, Trudy L.; Moll, Patricia P.; and Lauer, Ronald M. "The Relation between Ponderosity and Coronary Risk Factors in Children and Their Relatives." *American Journal of Epidemiology* 129 (5) (May 1989).

Calobrisi, A. "Eating Disorders." *Practical Diabetology* Vol. 4, No. 5 (September/October 1985).

Carlson, Eugene. " A Small Business Thrives on Oversize Clothes for Kids." *Wall Street Journal,* 1989.

Carmichael, Kim A. "How Self-starvation Damages Bone Structure." *BASH Magazine,* January 1990.

Cattanach, L.; Malley, R.; and Rodin, J. "Psychologic and Physiologic Reactivity to Stressors in Eating Disordered Individuals." *Psychosomatic Medicine* Vol. 50, No. 6 (November-December 1988).

Chapman, B. J.; Farquahar, D. L.; Galloway, S. McL.; Simpson, G. K.; and Munro, J. F. "The Effects of a New Beta-Adrenoceptor Agonist BRL 26830A in Obesity." *International Jounal of Obesity* 12 (2) (April 1988).

Chase, Marilyn. "Pigs May Provide Hints for Humans on Not Being Hogs." *Wall Street Journal,* December 8, 1988.

Chinnici, Madeline. "Picking the Perfect Diet." *Walking Magazine,* May/June 1989.

Claysos, Dennis E., and Klassen, Michael L. "Perception of Attractiveness by Obesity and Hair Color." *Perceptual and Motor Skills* Vol. 68, No. 1 (February 1989).

Clifton, P. G.; Barnfield, A. M. C.; and Philcox, L. "A Behavioral Profile of Fluoxetine-induced Anorexia." *Psychopharmacology* 97 (1989).

Cline, Carolyn. "Is Liposuction for You?" *Shape,* April 1988.

Coble, Sister Carrol. "Communication and the Family Process." *BASH Newsletter,* 1987.

Collins, M. Elizabeth. "Education for Healthy Body Weight: Helping Adolescents Balance the Cultural Pressure for Thinness." *Journal of School Health* 58 (6) (August 1988).

"Compulsive Eaters, Compulsive Exercisers." *Executive Fitness,* February 1988.

Cook, Lynn Crawford. "The Ideal Body: Gay vs. Straight." *Psychology Today,* July/August 1989.

Cooper, Stewart E. "Chemical Dependency and Eating Disorders: Are They Really So Different?" *Journal of Counseling and Development* 68 (1) (September 1989).

Copeland, Paul M., and Herzog, David B. "Hypoglycemia and Death in Anorexia Nervosa." *Psychotherapy and Psychosomatics* 48 (1987).

Corcoran, George B.; Salazar, Daniel E.; and Chan, Hannah H. "Obesity as a Risk Factor in Drug-induced Organ Injury." *Toxicology and Applied Pharmacology* 15 (March 15, 1989).

Cordido, Fernando; Casanueva, Felipe F.; and Dieguez, Carlos. "Cholinergic Receptor Activation by Pyridostigmine Restores Growth Hormone (GH) Responsiveness to GH-Releasing Hormone Administration in Obese Subjects: Evidence for Hypothalamic Somatostatinergic Participation in the Blunted GH Release of Obesity." *Journal of Clinical Endocrinology and Metabolism* 68 (February 1989).

Cowley, Geoffrey; Springen, Karen; Leonard, Elizabeth Ann; Robins, Kate; and Gordon, Jeanne. "The Promise of Prozac." *Newsweek,* March 26, 1990.

Cox, Gerald L., and Merkel, William T. "A Qualitative Review of Psychosocial Treatments for Bulimia." *Journal of Nervous and Mental Disorders* 177 (February 1989).

Craighead, Linda Wilcoxon. "Supervised Exercise in Behavioral Treatment for Moderate Obesity." *Behavior Therapy* 20 (1989).

Cuellar, R. E.; Kaye, W. H.; Hsu, L. K.; and Van Thiel, D. H. "Upper Gastrointestinal Tract Dysfunction in Bulimia." *Digestive Diseases and Sciences* Vol. 33, No. 12 (December 1988).

"Cut Fat Cravings and Lose Weight." *Executive Fitness,* September 1988.

Cytryn, Eileen S. "Comparative Psychological Assessment of Patients with Anorexia Nervosa and Their Siblings." *Dissertation Abstracts International* (October 1986).

"Dancing to Your Heart's Content." *University of California, Berkeley Wellness Letter,* February 1990.

Davis, Ron; Olmsted, Marion; and Rockert, Wendi. "Brief Group Psychoeducation for Bulimia Nervosa: Assessing the Clinical Significance of Change." *Journal of Consulting and Clinical Psychology* Vol. 58, No. 6 (December 1990).

Dawson, Marie. "Why Women Get Addicted to Food." *Ladies' Home Journal,* September 1990.

Dee, Sandra. "Learning to Live Again." *People Weekly,* March 18, 1991.

Depres, Jean-Pierre; Nadeau, Andre; Tremblay, Angelo; Ferland, Mario; Moorjani, Sital; Lupien, Paul J.; Theriault, Germain; Pinault, Sylvie; and Bouchard, Claude. "Role of Deep Abdominal Fat in the Association between Regional Adipose Tissue Distribution and Glucose Tolerance in Obese Women." *Diabetes* (March 1989).

Deutsch, J. Anthony. "Signals Determining Meal Size." In *Eating Habits,* edited by R. A. Boakes, D. A. Popplewell and M. J. Burton, John Wiley & Sons, 1987.

Devlin, Michael J.; Walsh, B. Timothy; Katz, Jack L.; Roose, Steven P.; Linkie, Daniel M.; Wright, Louise; Vande Wiele, Raymond; and Glassman, Alexander H. "Hypthalamic-Pituitary-Gonadal Function in Anoresia Nervosa and Bulimia." *Psychiatric Research* 28 (1989).

Dietzen, Mary Ann. "The Mother-Daughter Relationship, Locus of Control, and Personality Traits of Women with Eating Disorders." *Dissertation Abstracts International* 47, No. 6 (1986).

DiNicola, M. Phil. "Children Too Have Eating and Mood Disorders." *BASH Magazine,* June 1989.

Dolan, Bridget M.; Evans, Chris; and Lacey, J. Hubert. "Family Composition and Social Class in Bulimia: A Catchment Area Study of a Clinical and a Comparison Group." *Journal of Nervous and Mental Disease* 177, No. 5 (1989).

Dorsa, Daniel; Bernstein, Ilene; Broberg, Darla. "Nausea in Bulimic Women in Response to a Palatable Food." *Journal of Abnormal Psychology* 99 (2) (May 1990).

Dove, Jody. "Facts about Anorexia Nervosa." Office of Research Reporting at the National Institute of Child Health and Human Development, National Institutes of Health.

Downs, John; Downs, Anna; Rosethal, Ted. L.; Deal, Nancy; and Akiskal, Hagop S. "Increased Plasma Tricyclic Antidepressant Concentrations in Two Patients Concurrently Treated with Fluoxetine." *Journal of Clinical Psychiatry* 50 (1989).

Drake, Mary Anne. "Symptoms of Anorexia Nervosa in Female University Dietetic Majors." *Journal of the American Dietetic Association* 89 (1) (January 1989).

Dranoc, Paula. "The Fat of the Land." *Savvy Woman,* July 1989.

Drewnowski, A.; Hopkins, S. A.; and Kessler, R. C. "The Prevalence of Bulimia Nervosa in the U.S. College Student Population." *American Journal of Public Health* 78 (10) (October 1988).

Drewnowski, A.; Yee, D. K.; and Krahn, D. D. "Bulimia in College Women: Incidence and Recovery Rates." *American Journal of Psychiatry* 145 (6) (June 1988).

Duchmann, Erich G.; Williamson, Donald A.; and Stricker, Patricia M. "Bulimia, Dietary Restraint, and Concern for Dieting." *Journal of Psychopathology and Behavioral Assessment* 2, No. 1 (1989).

Dulloo, A. G.; Geissler, C. A.; Horton, T.; Collins, A.; and Miller, D. S. "Normal Caffeine Consumption: Influence on Thermogenesis and Daily Energy Expenditure in Lean and Postobese Human Volunteers." *American Journal of Clinical Nutrition* 49 (1) (January 1989).

Dura, Jason R., and Bornstein, R. A. "Differences between IQ and School Achievement in Anorexia Nervosa." *Journal of Clinical Psychology* 45 (3) (May 1989).

Earle, K. E.; Archer, A. G.; and Baillie, J. E. "Circulating and Excreted Levels of Chromium after an Oral Glucose Challenge: Influence of Body Mass Index, Hypoglycemic Drugs, and Presence and Absence of Diabetes Mellitus." *American Journal of Clinical Nutrition* 49(4) (April 1989).

"Eating and Hormones: Diet like a Pig." *Economist,* May 13, 1989.

Eckel, Robert H. "Lipoprotein Lipase: A Multifunctional Enzyme Relevant to Common Metabolic Diseases." *New England Journal of Medicine* 320(16) (April 20, 1989).

Eldridge, Kathleen; Wilson, G. Terence; and Whaley, Arthur. "Failure, Self-evaluation and Feeling Fat in Women." *International Journal of Eating Disorders* Vol. 9, No. 1 (January 1990).

Elliott, D. L.; Goldberg, L.; Kuehl, K. S.; and Bennett, W. M. "Sustained Depression of the Resting Metabolic Rate after Massive Weight Loss." *American Journal of Clinical Nutrition* Vol. 49 (January 1989).

Enright, Amy Baker, and Sansone, Randy. "An Overview of Eating Disorders." National Anorexic Aid Society, Inc., 1984.

Epstein, Leonard H.; Kuller, Lewis H.; Wing, Rena R.; Valoski, Alice; and McCurley, James. "The Effect of Weight Control on Lipid Changes in Obese Children." *American Journal of Diseases of Children* 143(4) (April 1989).

Epstein, Leonard, H.; Wing, Rena R.; Cluss, Patricia; Fernstrom, Madelyn H.; Penner, Barbara; Perkins, Kenneth A.; Nudelman, Sheila; Marks, Bonita; and Valoski, Alice. "Resting Metabolic Rate in Lean and Obese Children: Relationship to Child and Parent Weight and Percent-Overweight Change." *American Journal of Clinical Nutrition* 49(2) (February 1989).

Ernsberger, Paul. "Information about the Gastric Bubble ("Balloon") Procedure." *NAAFA Newsletter,* February 1986.

———. "Is Obesity Hazardous? The Case Against." *Debates in Medicine,* Vol. 2, 1989.

———. "Report on Weight-Loss Surgery." *NAAFA Newsletter,* 1984.

———. "The Rise, Fall and Rebirth of Intestinal Bypass." *NAAFA Newsletter* 10, No. 6 (1985).

Ernsberger, Paul, and Hirsch, Jules. "NIH Consensus Conference on Obesity: By Whom and for What? *Journal of Nutrition* 117(6) (June 1987).

Ernsberger, Paul, and Van Itallie, Theodore B. "Does Obesity Kill?" *Physician's Weekly,* October 6, 1986.

Ernsberger, Paul, and Nelson, Douglas O. "The Effects of Fasting and Refeeding on Blood Pressure Are Determined by Nutritional State, not by Body Weight Change." *American Journal of Hypertension.*

Ernsberger, Paul, and Nelson, Douglas O. "Refeeding Hypertension in Dietary Obesity." *American Journal of Physiology* 254 (1988).

Evans, D. J.; Barth, J. H.; and Burke, C. W. "Body Fat Topography in Women with Androgen Excess." *International Journal of Obesity* 12(2) (April 1988).

Fagher, Birger; Monti, Mario; and Theander, Sten. "Microcalorimetric Study of Muscle and Platelet Thermogenesis in Anorexia Nervosa and Bulimia." *American Journal of Clinical Nutrition* 49 (1989).

Fairburn, Christopher, and Beglin, Sarah. "Studies of the Epidemiology of Bulimia Nervosa." *American Journal of Psychiatry* 147(4) (April 1990).

Fanelli, Marie T.; Kuczmarski, Robert J.; and Hirsch, Margaret. "Estimation of Body Fat from Ultrasound Measures of Subcutaneous Fat and Circumferences in Obese Women." *International Journal of Obesity* 12(2) (April 1988).

Farley, Dixie. "Eating Disorders." *FDA Consumer,* May 1986.

Feibleman, Peter. "Confessions of a Food Addict." *Lear's,* April 1989.

Feingold, M.; Kaminer, Y.; Lyona, K.; Chaudhury, A. K.; et al. "Bulimia Nervosa in Pregnancy: A Case Report." *Obstetrics and Gynecology* 71(6) (June 1988).

Feldman, W.; Feldman, E.; and Goodman, J. T. "Culture versus Biology: Children's Attitudes toward Thinness and Fatness." *Pediatrics* 81(2) (February 1988).

Fernstrom, John D. "Food-induced Changes in Brain Serotonin Synthesis: Is There a Relationship to Appetite for Specific Macronutrients?" *Appetite* 8(3) (August 1987).

Ferretti, Fred. "Eating Disorders: New Treatments." *New York Times,* September 2, 1985.

Fieldsend, B. "Anorexia Nervosa and Turner's Syndrome." *British Journal of Psychiatry* Vol. 152 (February 1988).

Filstead, W. J.; Parrella, D. P.; and Ebbitt, J. "High-Risk Situations for Engaging in Substance Abuse and Binge-eating Behaviors." *Journal of Studies on Alcohol* 49(2) (March 1988).

Fisher, Martin, and Fornari, Victor. "Gynecomastia as a Precipitant of Eating Disorders in Adolescent Males." *International Journal of Eating Disorders* Vol. 9, No. 1 (January 1990).

Fitzgerald, B. A.; Wright, J. H.; Atala, K. D. "Bulimia Nervosa: Uncovering a Secret Disorder." *Postgraduate Medicine* 84(2) (August 1988).

Fletcher, J. M., and McKenzie, N. "The Effects of Dietary Fat Content on the Growth and Body Composition of Lean and Genetically Obese Zucker Rats Adrenalectomized before Weaning." *British Journal of Nutrition* Vol. 60, No. 3 (November 1988).

"Formula Diets for Obesity." *Medical Letter on Drugs and Therapeutics,* March 1989.

Franco, Kathleen S. N.; Tamburrino, Marijo B.; Carroll, Brendan T.; and Bernal, Guillermo A. A. "Eating Attitudes in College Males." *International Journal of Eating Disorders* Vol. 7, No. 2 (March 1988).

Frank, Emily. "Shame and Guilt in Eating Disorders." *American Journal of Orthopsychiatry* 61(2) (April 1991).

Freeman, C. P.; Barry, F.; Dunkeld-Turnbull, J.; and Henderson, A. "Controlled Trial of Psychotherapy for Bulimia Nervosa." *British Medical Journal* Vol. 296 (February 20, 1988).

Friedlander, Myrna, and Siegel, Sherri. "Separation-Individuation Difficulties and Cognitive-Behavioral Indicators of Eating Disorders among College Women." *Journal of Counseling Psychology* Vol. 37, No. 1 (January 1990).

Friedman, Enrique J. "Death from Ipecac Intoxification in a Patient with Anorexia Nervosa." *American Journal of Psychiatry* 141, No. 5 (1984).

Fry, Richard, and Crisp, Arthur H. "Adoption and Identity: A Case of Anorexia Nervosa." *British Journal of Medical Psychology* Vol. 62 (June 1989).

Galler, Janina R., and Ramsey, Frank. "A Follow-up Study of the Influence of Early Malnutrition on Development: Behavior at Home and at School." *Journal of the American Academy of Child Psychiatry* 28, No. 2 (1989).

Ganley, Richard M. "Eating Disorders Are Family Affairs." *Renfrew Perspective*, Spring 1988.

Gant, Thomas. "The Nuts and Bolts of Liposuction." *Shape*, April 1988.

Gardner, Rick M.; Urrutia, Russell; Morrell, James; Espinoza, Tracy; and Gallegos, Venice. "Physiological Arousal of Obese Persons to Food Stimuli." *Perceptual and Motor Skills* Vol. 67, No. 3 (December 1988).

Garner, David M.; Olmsted, Marion P.; Davis, Ron; Rockert, Wendi; Goldbloom, David; and Eagle, Morris. "The Association between Bulimic Symptoms and Reported Psychopathology." *International Journal of Eating Disorders* Vol. 9, No. 1 (January 1990).

Gartner, Alison; Marcus, Ronald; Halmi, Katherine; and Loranger, Armand. "DSM-III-R Personality Disorders in Patients with Eating Disorders." *American Journal of Psychiatry* 146(12) (December 1989).

Geracioti, Thomas D., Jr., and Liddle, Rodger, A. "Impaired Cholecystokinin Secretion in Bulimia Nervosa." *New England Journal of Medicine* 319(11) (September 15, 1988).

Giannini, A. James; Collins, James L.; and Lewis, Denise. "Anorexia Nervosa in the Elderly—Case Studies." *BASH Magazine*, May 1989.

"Girls, at Seven, Think Thin, Study Finds." *New York Times*, February 11, 1988.

Gold, P. W.; Gwirtsman, H.; Avgerinos, P. C.; and Nieman, L. K. "Abnormal Hypothalamic-Pituitary-Adrenal Function in Anorexia Nervosa." *New England Journal of Medicine* 314(21) (May 1986).

Gomez, Evaristo. "Promising Results of Fluoxetine When Tried on Depressed Bulimics." *BASH Magazine*, June 1989.

Goodner, Sherry. "Group Therapy for Eating Disorders." *BASH Newsletter*, 1987.

Grayson, Richard, and Grayson, June. "Dangers of Liposuction." *Sunday Times*, October 11, 1987.

"Grazing and Weight Loss." *University of California, Berkeley Wellness Letter*, February 1990.

Green, Bonnie L.; Wehling, Christina; and Talsky, Gerald J. "Group Art Therapy as an Adjunct to Treatment for Chronic Outpatient." *Hospital and Community Psychiatry* Vol. 38, No. 9 (September 1987).

Green, Tom. "In the Fight, She's Gained Self-respect." *USA Today*, Lifestyle section, November 27, 1989.

Greene, Geoffrey; Achterberg, Cheryl; Crumbaugh, Jeffrey; and Soper, Jan. "Dietary Intake and Dieting Practices of Bulimic and Non-bulimic Female College Students." *Journal of the American Dietetic Association* 90(4) (April 1990).

Gren, J., and Woolf, A. "Hypermagnesemia Associated with Catharsis in a Salicylate-intoxicated Patient with Anorexia Nervosa." *Annals of Emergency Medicine* 18(2) (February 1989).

Grilo, Carlos; Shiffman, Saul; and Wing, Rena. "Relapse Crises and Coping among Dieters." *Journal of Consulting and Clinical Psychology* 57(4) (August 1989).

Gurin, Joel. "Leaner, not Lighter." *Psychology Today,* June 1989.

Gwirtsman, H. E.; George, David T.; Carosella, Nicholas W.; Greene, Ronald C.; and Jimerson, David C. "Hyperamylasemia and Its Relationship to Binge-Purge Episodes: Development of a Clinically Relevant Laboratory Test." *Journal of Clinical Psychiatry* 50(6) (1989).

Gwirtsman, H. E.; George, D. T.; and Jimerson, D. C. "Central and Peripheral ACTH and Cortisol Levels in Anorexia Nervosa and Bulimia." *Archives of General Psychiatry* 46(1) (January 1989).

Gwirtsman, H. E.; Kaye, W. H.; Curtis, S. R.; and Lyter, L. M. "Energy Intake and Dietary Macronutrient Content in Women with Anorexia Nervosa and Volunteers." *Journal of the American Dietetic Association* 89(1) (January 1989).

Gwirtsman, H. E.; Obarzanek, E.; and George, D. T. "Decreased Caloric Intake in Normal-Weight Patients with Bulimia: Comparison with Female Volunteers." *American Journal of Clinical Nutrition* 49(1) (January 1989).

Haas, Carol. "Program Hears Victims' Inner Cries for Help." *Atlanta Constitution,* March 8, 1990.

Habermas, Tilmann, "The Psychiatric History of Anorexia and Bulimia: Weight Fears and Bulimic Symptoms in Early Cases." *International Journal of Eating Disorders* 8 No. 3 (1989).

Hacinli, Cynthia. "Why You Can—or Can't—Eat Another Bite." *Mademoiselle,* July 1989.

Haffner, Steven M.; Diehl, Andrew K.; Stern, Michael P.; and Hazuda, Helen P. "Central Adiposity and Gallbladder Disease in Mexican Americans." *American Journal of Epidemiology* 129(3) (March 1989).

Hahn, Cindy. "Why Eating Disorders Pervade Women's Tennis." *Tennis,* December 1990.

Haimes, Amy Lesser, and Katz, Jack L. "Sexual and Social Maturity versus Social Conformity in Restricting Anorectic, Bulimic, and Borderline Women." *International Journal of Eating Disorders* Vol. 7 (May 1988).

Hall, Alyson, and Crisp, Arthur H. "Brief Psychotherapy in the Treatment of Anorexia Nervosa: Outcome at One Year." *British Journal of Psychiatry* Vol. 151 (August 1987).

Hallgren, Per; Sjostrom, Lars; Hedlund, Henrik; Lundell, Lars; and Olbe, Lars. "Influence of Age, Fat Cell Weight, and Obesity on O2 Consumption of Human Adipose Tissue." *American Journal of Physiology* 256(4 Pt 1) (April 1989).

Hamilton, Linda H.; Brooks-Gunn, J.; Warren, Michelle P.; and Hamilton, William G. "The Role of Selectivity in the Pathogenesis of Eating Problems in Ballet Dancers." *Medicine and Science in Sports and Medicine* Vol. 20, No. 6 (December 1988).

Hammer, R. L.; Barrier, C. A.; Roundy, E. S.; Bradford, J. M.; and Fisher, A. G. "Calorie-restricted Low-Fat Diet and Exercise in Obese Women." *American Journal of Clinical Nutrition* 49(1) (January 1989).

"The Healthy Eater's Guide to Sugar." *University of California, Berkeley Wellness Letter,* December 1989.

Heber, David. "What Liposuction Can and Can't Do for You." *Shape,* April 1968.

Herzog, David B., and Copeland, Paul M. "Bulimia Nervosa—Psyche and Satiety." *New England Journal of Medicine* 319(11) (September 15, 1988).

———. "Eating Disorders." *New England Journal of Medicine* 313(5) (August 1, 1985).

Higgins, Linda. "Amylase Test May Provide Indication of Active Bulimia." *Medical World News,* August 28, 1989.

Higgs, J. F.; Goodyer, I. M.; and Birch, J. "Anorexia Nervosa and Food Avoidance Emotional Disorder." *Archives of Disease in Childhood* 64(3) (March 1989).

Hills, Andrew P., and Parker, Anthony W. "Obesity and Management via Diet and Exercise Intervention." *Child: Care, Health and Development* 14 (1988).

Hirsch, J.; Fried, S. K.; Edens, N. K.; and Leibel, R. L. "The Fat Cell." *Medical Clinics of North America* 73(1) (January 1989).

Holden, N. L., and Robinson, P. H. "Anorexia Nervosa and Bulimia Nervosa in British Blacks." *British Journal of Psychiatry* Vol. 152 (April 1988).

Horne, R. L.; Ferguson, J. M.; Pope, H. G., Jr., and Hudson, J. I. "Treatment of Bulimia with Bupropion: a Multicenter Controlled Trial." *Journal of Clinical Psychiatry* 49(7) (July 1988).

Horne, R. L.; Van Vactor, John; and Emerson, Shirley. "Disturbed Body Image in Patients with Eating Disorders." *American Journal of Psychiatry* 148(2) (February 1991).

Howat, Paula; Varner, Lisa; Hegsted, Maren; Brewer, Maria; and Mills, George. "The Effect of Bulimia upon Diet, Body Fat, Bone Density, and Blood Components." *Journal of the American Dietetic Association* 89(7) (July 1989).

Howat, Paula, Varner, L.; and Wampold, Richard. "The Effectiveness of a Dental/Dietitian Team in the Assessment of Bulimic Dental Health." *Journal of the American Dietetic Association* 90(8) (August 1990).

Howley, Kathleen. "Turning Teens' Lives Around." *Boston Globe,* March 31, 1991.

Hsu, L. K. George, and Zimmer, Ben. "Eating Disorders in Old Age." *International Journal of Eating Disorders* Vol. 7 (January 1988).

Hudson, James I., and Pope, Harrison G., Jr. "Affective Spectrum Disorder." *American Journal of Psychiatry* 147(5) (May 1990).

Hudson, J.I.; Pope, H.G., Jr.; Wurtman, J.; and Yurgelum-Todd, D. "Bulimia in Obese Individuals: Relationship to Normal-Weight Bulimia." *Journal of Nervous and Mental Disorders* 176(3) (March 1988).

Humphrey, Laura Lynn. "Observed Family Interactions among Subtypes of Eating Disorders Using Structural Analysis of Social Behavior." *Journal of Consulting and Clinical Psychology* 52(2) (April 1989).

Ince, Susan. "Indulgence and Denial." *Self,* March 1989.

Ishida, Yasuo. "Acupuncture Today." *Southern Medical Journal* 81(7) (July 1988).

Jenish, D. Arcy. "A Tragic Obsession." *Maclean's,* October 9, 1989.

Jensen, Michael D.; Haymond, Morey W.; Rizza, Robert A.; Cryer, Philip E.; and Miles, John M. "Influence of Body Fat Distribution on Free Fatty Acid Metabolism in Obesity." *Journal of Clinical Investigation* 83(4) (April 1989).

Jewell, Regina. "Affective, Eating Disorders: Their Common Ground." *BASH Magazine,* November 1989.

———. "Clinician Looks Hopefully to Fluoxetine for Results in Eating-Disorder Patients." *BASH Magazine,* August 1989.

———. "Computer Probe of the Eating-Disorder Personality." *BASH Magazine,* August 1989.

———. "Fantasies and Fat: The Cultural History of Dieting In America." *BASH Magazine*, February 1989.

———. "Self-mutilation and Its Kinship to Eating Disorders." *BASH Magazine*, November 1989.

Jirik-Babb, Pauline, and Katz, Jack L. "Impairment of Taste Perception in Anorexia Nervosa and Bulimia." *International Journal of Eating Disorders* Vol. 7 (May 1988).

Kaminer, Y.; Feingold, M.; and Lyons, K. "Bulimia in a Pair of Monozygotic Twins." *Journal of Nervous and Mental Disorders* 176(4) (April 1988).

Kapoor, S. "Treatment for Significant Others of Bulimic Patients May Be Beneficial." *Journal of the American Dietetic Association* 88(3) (March 1988).

Karnieli, E.; Moscona, R.; Rafaeloff, R.; Illouz, Y. G.; and Armoni, M. "Discrepancy between Glucose Transport and Transporters in Human Femoral Adipocytes." *American Journal of Physiology* 256(1 Pt 1) (January 1989).

Karpell, Merrily. "The Fear of Stepping Out of Line." *Renfrew Perspective*, Fall 1988.

Karpen, Maxine. "Quick Fixes." *effenelle* premier issue (1990).

Kassett, J. A.; Gwirtsman, H. E.; Aye, W. H.; Brandt, H. A.; and Jimerson, D. C. "Pattern of Onset of Bulimic Symptoms in Anorexia Nervosa." *American Journal of Psychiatry* 145(10) (October 1988).

Katahn, M. "Your Body Blueprint—Born to Be Fat?" *Mademoiselle*, September 1987.

Katz, Rebecca, L.; Keen, Carl L.; Litt, Iris F.; Hurley, Lucille S.; Kellams-Harrison, Kathleen M.; and Glader, Laurie J. "Zinc Deficiency in Anorexia Nervosa." *Journal of Adolescent Health Care* Vol. 8 (1987).

Keller, Martin B.; Herzog, David B.; Lavori, Philip W.; Ott, Ingrid L.; Bradburn, Isabel S.; and Mahoney, Elizabeth M. "High Rates of Chronicity and Rapidity of Relapse in Patients with Bulimia Nervosa and Depression." *Archives of General Psychiatry* 46(5) (1989).

Kennedy, S. H.; Garfinkel, P. E.; Parienti, V.; Costa, D.; and Brown, G. M. "Changes in Melatonin Levels but Not Cortisol Levels Are Associated with Depression in Patients with Eating Disorders." *Archives of General Psychiatry* 46(1) (January 1989).

Kent, J. S., and Clopton, J. R. "Bulimia: A Comparison of Psychological Adjustment and Familial Characteristics in a Nonclinical Sample." *Journal of Clinical Psychology* 44(6) (November 1988).

Killen, Joel D.; Taylor, C. Barr; Telch, Michael J.; Sayler, Keith E.; Maron, David J.; and Robinson, Thomas N. "Self-induced Vomiting and Laxatives and Diuretic Use among Teenagers." *JAMA*, 255(11) (March 21, 1986).

King, Pamela. "Turning Around Bulimia with Therapy." *Psychology Today*, September 1989.

Kiriike, Nobuo; Nagata, Toshihiko; Tanaka, Misono; Nishiwaki, Shinichi; Takakeuchi, Nobue; and Kawakita, Yukio. "Prevalence of Binge-eating and Bulimia among Adolescent Women in Japan." *Psychiatric Research* 26 (1988).

Kiyohara, K.; Tamai, H.; Kobayashi, N.; and Nakagawa, T. "Hypothalamic-Pituitary-Thyroidal Axis Alterations in Bulimic Patients." *American Journal of Clinical Nutrition* 47(5) (May 1988).

Klemchuk, Helen; Hutchinson, Cheryl; and Frank, Rochelle. "Body Dissatisfaction and Eating-related Problems on the College Campus: Usefulness of the Eating Disorder Inventory with a Nonclinical Population." *Journal of Counseling Psychology* 37(3) (July 1990).

Knapp, Caroline. "My Story." *New Woman,* March 1990.

Knobbe, Ann, and Kickham, Nancy. "The Role of Recreational Therapy and Music Therapy." *BASH Magazine,* January 1989.

Kobayashi, N.; Tamai, H.; Uehata, S.; Komaki, G.; et al. "Pancreatic Abnormalities in Patients with Eating Disorders." *Psychosomatic Medicine* (November-December 1988).

Koontz, Katy. "Women Who Love Food Too Much." *Health,* February 1988.

Kopeski, Lynne. "Diabetes and Bulimia—A Deadly Duo."

"Kral, J. G. "Surgical Treatment of Obesity." *Medical Clinics of North America* 73(1) (January 1989).

Kramer, F. M.; Stunkard, A. J.; Spiegel, T. A.; Deren, J. J.; et al. "Limited Weight Losses with a Gastric Balloon." *Archives of Internal Medicine* 149(2) (February 1989).

Krch, Frantisek D. "Growing Czech Awareness of Eating Disorders." *BASH Magazine,* November 1989.

Kreipe, R. E.; Strauss, J.; Hodgman, C. H.; Ryan, R. M. "Menstrual Cycle Abnormalities and Subclinical Eating Disorders: A Preliminary Report." *Psychosomatic Medicine* 51(1) (January-February 1989).

Kurtzman, F. D.; Yager, J.; Landsverk, J.; Wiesmeier, E.; and Bodurka, D. C. "Eating Disorders among Selected Female Student Populations at UCLA." *Journal of the American Dietetic Associatio.* 9(1) (January 1989).

Lacey, J. H., and Dolan, B. M. "Bulimia in British Blacks and Asians: A Catchment Area Study." *British Journal of Psychiatry* Vol. 152 (January 1988).

Lachenmeyer, J. R., and Muni-Brander, P. Eating Disorders in a Nonclinical Adolescent Population: Implications for Treatment." *Adolescence* 23(90) (Summer 1988).

Laessle, R. G.; Kittl, S.; Fichter, M. M.; Wittchen, H. U.; and Pirke, K. M. "Major Affective Disorder in Anorexia Nervosa and Bulimia: A Descriptive Diagnostic Study." *British Journal of Psychiatry* Vol. 151 (December 1987).

Laessle, Reinhold; Tuschl, Reinhard; Waadt, Sabine; and Pirke, Karl. "The Specific Psychology of Bulimia Nervosa: A Comparison with Restrained and Unrestrained (Normal) Eaters." *Journal of Consulting and Clinical Psychology* Vol. 57 (December 1989).

Langone, John. "Girth of a Nation." *Discover* magazine, February 1981.

Larocca, Félix E. F. "Concurrence of Turner's Syndrome, Anorexia Nervosa, and Mood Disorders: Case Report." *Journal of Clinical Psychiatry* 46(7) (July 1985).

———. "Gilles de la Tourette's (the Movement Disorder): The Association with a Case of Anorexia Nervosa in a Boy." *International Journal of Eating Disorders* Vol. 3 (Spring 1984).

———. "The Relevance of Self-help in the Management of Anorexia and Bulimia." *Res Medica* Vol. 1 (June 1983).

———. "The Treatment of Eating Disorders." *Journal of Chiropractic* (September 1987).

Larocca, Félix, E. F., and Della-Fera, Mary Anne. "Rumination: Its Significance in Adults with Bulimia Nervosa." *Journal of the Academy of Psychosomatic Medicine* (March 1986).

Larocca, Félix, E. F., and Goodner, Sherry A. "Eating Disorders in the Elderly: Transgenerational Psychiatry." *BASH Magazine.*

Larocca, Félix E. F. and Kolodny, Nancy J. "Treating Depression in Adolescence: The Psychiatric and Social Work Connection." *Therapeutic Potential of Mood Disorders Clinics* (September 1984).

Larocca, Félix, E. F., and Stern, John H. "Eating Disorders: Self-help and Treatment in Missouri." *Missouri Medicine* 81(12) (December 1984).

Lavallee, Patricia-Anne. "Religiosity, Rituals and Patterns in Anorexic and Bulimic Families." *Dissertation Abstracts International* 47, No. 11 (1987).

Lawrence, Jennifer; Liesse, Julie; and Dagnoli, Judann. "Appetite Grows for 'Light' Treats." *Advertising Age,* February 5, 1990.

Lee, Sing; Chiu, Helen F. K.; and Chen, Char-nie. "Anorexia Nervosa in Hong Kong: Why Not More in China? *British Journal of Psychiatry* 154 (1989).

Lehman, Adam, and Rodin, Judith. "Styles of Self-nurturance and Disordered Eating." *Journal of Consulting and Clinical Psychology* Vol. 57 (February 1989).

Lehman, Betsy A. "Obesity and Genetics." *Fort Lauderdale Sun-Sentinel* and *Boston Globe,* March 29, 1988.

Lehrman, K. "Anorexia and Bulimia: Causes and Cures." *Consumers' Research Magazine,* September 1987.

Leitenberg, Harold; Rosen, James; Agras, W. Stewart; Schneider, John; and Arnow, Bruce. "Cognitive-Behavioral Therapy with and without Exposure plus Response Prevention in Treatment of Bulimia Nervosa: Comment and Reply." *Journal of Consulting and Clinical Psychology* Vol. 57 (December 1989).

Lesem, Michael D.; George, David T.; Kaye, Walter H.; Goldstein, David S.; and Jimerson, David C. "State-related Changes in Norepinephrine Regulation in Anorexia Nervosa." *Biological Psychiatry* 25 (1989).

Levin, Barry E.; Hogan, Sue; and Sullivan, Ann C. "Initiation and Perpetuation of Obesity and Obesity Resistance in Rats." *American Journal of Physiology* 256(3 Pt 2) (March 1989).

Levitt, John L. "Treating Adults with Eating Disorders by Using an Inpatient Approach." *Health and Social Work* 11(2) (Spring 1986).

Levy, Alan B.; Dixon, Katharine N.; and Stern, Stephen L. "How Are Depression and Bulimia Related?" *American Journal of Psychiatry* 146(2) (February 1989).

Lewith, George. "Acupuncture." *Practitioner* Vol. 230 (December 1986).

Licinio-Paixao, J. "Hyperinsulinemia, a Mediator of Decreased Food Intake and Weight Loss in Anorexia Nervosa and Major Depression." *Medical Hypotheses* 28 (1989).

Linford, Patricia F., and Katsantonis, George P. "Food Allergies Exist but You Probably Don't Have One." *BASH Magazine,* December 1989.

Lissner, Lauren; Habicht, Jean-Pierre; Strupp, Barbara J.; Levistsky, David A.; Haas, Jere D.; and Roe, Daphne A. "Body Composition and Energy Intake: Do Overweight Women Overeat and Underreport?" *American Journal of Clinical Nutrition* 49(2) (February 1989).

Lloyd, G. G.; Steel, J. M.; and Young, R. J. "Eating Disorders and Psychiatric Morbidity in Patients with Diabetes Mellitus." *Psychotherapy and Psychosomatics* 48 (1987).

Logue, Alexandra. "Food Likes and Dislikes of the Eating-disordered." *BASH Magazine,* November 1989.

Lucas, Alexander R. "Self-starvation as an Adaptive Mechanism." *BASH Magazine,* February 1989.

Lundholm, J. K., and Littrell, J. M. "Desire for Thinness among High School Cheerleaders: Relationship to Disordered Eating and Weight Control Behaviors." *Adolescence* Vol. 21, No. 86 (Fall 1986).

McCann, J. P.; Bergman, E. N.; and Reimers, T. J. "Effects of Obesity and Ovarian Steroids on Insulin Secretion and Removal in Sheep." *American Journal of Physiology* 256(1 Pt 1) (January 1989).

McCann, Una, and Agras, W. Stewart. "Successful Treatment of Nonpurging Bulimia Nervosa with Desipramine." *American Journal of Psychiatry* 147 (November 1990).

McCarthy, Paul. "Bigger Plates, Smaller Portions." (May 1989).

McCrea, C.; Neil, W. J.; Flanigan, J. W.; and Summerfield, A. B. "Variable-Image Video Confrontation as a Method of Assessing Body Image: A Technical Report and Comparison with Similar Techniques." *Perceptual and Motor Skills* Vol. 67 (August 1988).

McGlynn, T. J., and Tinker, D. E. "Anorexia Nervosa in Adulthood." *American Family Physician* 39(1) (January 1989).

Mandel, Debra Lorraine. "Bulimia: Sex-Role Concepts and Self-esteem." *Dissertation Abstracts International* 48, No. 6 (1987).

Marcus, Marsha D.; Wing, Rena R.; Ewing, Linda; Kern, Edward; Gooding, Williams; and McDermott, Michael. "A Double-Blind, Placebo-controlled trial of Fluoxetine plus Behavior Modification in the Treatment of Obese Binge-eaters and Non–Binge Eaters." *American Journal of Psychiatry* 147(7) (July 1990).

———. "Psychiatric Disorders among Obese Binge Eaters." *International Journal of Eating Disorders* Vol. 9 (January 1990).

Marks, Jane. "We Have a Problem." *Parents,* April 1989.

Martin, Sue; Housley, Kathleen; and McCoy, Harriett. "Self-esteem of Adolescent Girls as Related to Weight." *Perceptual and Motor Skills* Vol. 67 (December 1988).

Matsubayashi, S.; Tamai, H.; Uehata, S.; and Kobayashi, N. "Anorexia Nervosa with Elevated Serum." *Psychosomatic Medicine* Vol. 50 (November-December 1988).

Mayo-Smith, W.; Hayes, C. W.; Biller, B. M.; Klibanski, A.; et al. "Body Fat Distribution Measured with CT: Correlations in Healthy Subjects, Patients with Anorexia Nervosa, and Patients with Cushing Syndrome." *Radiology* 170(2) (February 1989).

Mercer, Joy E. "In Philadelphia, a Place Where Women Can Overcome Eating Disorders." *Philadelphia Inquirer,* August 22, 1985.

Miller, Caroline Adams. "Dying to Be Thin." *New Woman,* May 1988.

Mitchell, James E.; Pomeroy, Claire; and Huber, Marguerite. "A Clinician's Guide to the Eating Disorders Medicine Cabinet." *International Journal of Eating Disorders* Vol. 7 (March 1988).

Mitchell, James E.; Pomeroy, Claire; Seppala, Marvin; and Huber, Marguerite. "Diuretic Use as a Marker for Eating Problems and Affective Disorders among Women." *Journal of Clinical Psychiatry* 49(7) (July 1988).

———. "Pseudo–Bartter's Syndrome, Diuretic Abuse, Idiopathic Edema, and Eating Disorders." *International Journal of Eating Disorders* Vol. 7 (March 1988).

Mitchell, James E.; Soll, Elizabeth; Eckert, Elke, O.; Pyle, Richard L.; and Hatsukami, Dorothy. "The Changing Population of Bulimia Nervosa Patients in an Eating Disorders Program." *Hospital and Community Psychiatry* Vol. 40 (November 1989).

Mole, Paul A.; Stern, Judith S.; Schultz, Cynthia L.; Bernauer, Edmund M.; and Holcomb, Bryan J. "Exercise Reverses Depressed Metabolic Rate Produced by Severe Caloric Restriction." *Medicine and Science in Sports and Exercise* 21(1) (February 1989).

Montgomery, Sy. "Vacuuming the Fat Away." *Working Woman,* May 1988.

Moore, Beth O., and Deutsch, J. A. "An Antiemetic Is Antidotal to the Satiety Effects of Cholecystokinin." *Nature* 315(6017) (May 1985).

Morgan, Carolyn; Affleck, Marilyn; and Solloway, Orin. "Gender Role Attitudes, Religiosity, and Food Behavior: Dieting and Bulimia in College Women." Social Science Quarterly (March 1990).

Morgan, H. G., and Hayward, A. E. "Clinical Assessment of Anorexia Nervosa: The Morgan-Russell Outcome Assessment Schedule." *British Journal of Psychiatry* Vol. 152 (March 1988).

Morrison, Beckie. "Learning to Overcome Addictions." *Renfrew Perspective,* Winter 1989.

Mortola, J. F.; Rasmussen, D. D.; and Yen, S. S. "Alterations of the Adrenocorticotropin-Cortisol Axis in Normal Weight Bulimic Women: Evidence for a Central Mechanism." *Journal of Clinical Endocrinology* 68(3) (March 1989).

Moses, Nancy; Banilivy, Mansour-Max; and Lifshitz, Fime. "Fear of Obesity among Adolescent Girls." *Pediatrics* 83(13) (March 1989).

"New Studies Link Fatness, Metabolism and Heredity." *NAAFA Newsletter,* March 1988.

Norring, C., and Sohlberg, S. "Eating Disorder Inventory in Sweden." *Acta Psychiatrica Scandinavica* 78 (1988).

North, Gail. "Exercise: Bulimia." *Cosmopolitan,* March 1989.

"Obesity and Dieting Linked to Gallstones." Insight, October 2, 1989.

O'Brien, G.; Hassanyeh, F.; Leake, A.; Schapira, K; et al. "The Dexamethasone Suppression Test in Bulimia Nervosa." *British Journal of Psychiatry* Vol. 152 (May 1988).

Orsulak, P. J. and Waller, D. "Antidepressant Drugs: Additional Clinical Uses." *Journal of Family Practice* 28(2) (February 1989).

Oberby, K. J., and Litt, I. F. "Mediastinal Emphysema in an Adolescent with Anorexia Nervosa and Self-induced Emesis." *Pediatrics* 81(1) (January 1988).

Owen, E. R. T. C.; Abraham, R.; and Kark, A. E. "Gastroplasty for Morbid Obesity: Technique, Complications and Results in Sixty Cases." *British Journal of Surgery* 76(2) (February 1989).

Palla, B. and Litt, I. F. "Medical Complications of Eating Disorders in Adolescents." *Pediatrics* 81(5) (May 1988).

Patton, George. "The Course of Anorexia Nervosa." *British Medical Journal* 299(6692) (July 15, 1989.)

Penner, Louis A.; Thompson, J. Kevin; and Coovert, Dale. "Size Overestimation among Anorexics: Much Ado about Very Little?" *Journal of Abnormal Psychology* 100(1) (February 1991).

Perez, E. L.; Blouin, J.; and Blouin, A. "The Dexamethasone Suppression Test in Bulimia: Nonsuppression Associated with Depression and Suboptimal Weight." *Journal of Clinical Psychiatry* 49(3) (March 1988).

Perrone, Vinnie. "Pound for Pound, a Most Dangerous Sport." *Washington Post,* April 28, 1991.

Poldinger, W., and Krambeck, K. "The Relevance of Creativity for Psychiatric Therapy and Rehabilitation." *Comprehensive Psychiatry* Vol. 13, No. 10 (October 1987).

Polivy, Janet. "Dangers of Dieting." *NAAS Newsletter,* January-March 1988.

———. "Is Dieting Itself an Eating Disorder?" *BASH Magazine,* July 1989.

Pomeroy, Claire; Mitchell, James E.; Seim, Harold C.; and Seppala, Marvin. "Prescription Diuretic Abuse in Patients with Bulimia Nervosa." *Journal of Family Practice* (November 1988).

Potter, J. F.; Schafer, D. F.; and Bohi, R. L. "In-hospital Mortality as a Function of Body Mass Index: An Age-dependent Variable." *Journal of Gerontology* 43(3) (May 1988).

Potts, N. L. "Eating Disorders: The Secret Pattern of Binge/Purge." *American Journal of Nursing* 84(1) (January 1984).

Powers, Mary A., and Pappas, Theodore N. "Physiologic Approaches to the Control of Obesity." *Annals of Surgery* 209(3) (March 1989).

Powers, Pauline S.; Coovert, Dale Lee; Brightwell, Dennis R.; and Stevens, Beth A. "Other Psychiatric Disorders among Bulimic Patients." *Comprehensive Psychiatry* Vol. 14 (September/October 1988).

Prendergast, Alan. "Hooked on Perfection." *Special Report,* November 1989.

Pressman, Deborah. "Somatic Complaints Intensified by Psychotherapy." *Renfrew Perspective,* Winter 1989.

Price, W. A. "Pharmacologic Management of Eating Disorders." *American Family Physician* 37(5) (May 1988).

Prince, Isolde. "Pica and Geophagia in Cross-cultural Perspective." *Transcultural Psychiatric Research Review* 26 (1989).

Provenzale, J. M. "Anorexia Nervosa—Thinness as Illness." *Postgraduate Medicine* (October 1983).

Pyle, Richard L. "Bulimia Nervosa: An Ominous Variant of Anorexia Nervosa." *Journal of Clinical Psychiatry* Vol. 42 (February 1981).

Pyle, Richard L., and Mitchell, James E. "The Subtle, Puzzling Affinity of Drugs and Bulimia." *BASH Magazine,* September 1989.

Radke-Sharpe, Norean; Whitney-Saltiel, Deborah; and Rodin, Judith. "Fat Distribution as a Risk Factor for Weight and Eating Concerns." *International Journal of Eating Disorders* 9 (January 1990).

Raynes, Ellen; Auerbach, Carl; and Botyanski, Nancy C. "Level of Object Representation and Psychic Structure Deficit in Obese Persons." *Psychological Reports* 64(1) (1989).

Reeve, T.; Jackson, B.; Scott-Conner, C.; and Sledge, C. "Near-Total Gastric Necrosis Caused by Acute Gastric Dilatation." *Southern Medical Journal* 81(4) (April 1988).

Rigotti, N. A. "Osteoporosis in Women with Anorexia Nervosa." *New England Journal of Medicine* Vol. 311 (December 20, 1984).

Roberts, M. W. and Li, S. H. "Oral Findings in Anorexia Nervosa and Bulimia Nervosa: A Study of Forty-Seven Cases." *Journal of the American Dental Association* 115(3) (September 1987).

Robinson, P. H.; Clarke, M.; and Barrett, J. "Determinants of Delayed Gastric Emptying in Anorexia Nervosa and Bulimia Nervosa." *Gut* 29(4) (April 1988).

Rodin, J.; Schank, D.; and Striegel-Moore, R. "Psychological Features of Obesity." *Medical Clinics of North America* 73(1) (January 1989).

Rogers, Fred B. "Mandala Symbolism and Creative Arts Therapy." *Pennsylvania Medicine* Vol. 90 (November 1987).

Rohlfing, Carla. "The Healthy Family—CCK: The Hormone That Makes You Thin." *Family Circle,* February 20, 1990.

Rohner-Jeanrenaud, F.; Walker, C. D.; Greco-Perotto, R.; and Jeanrenaud, B. "Central Corticotropin-releasing Factor Administration Prevents the Excessive Body Weight Gain of Genetically Obese Rats." *Endocrinology* 124(2) (February 1989).

Rookus, Maartje A.; Burema, Jan; and Frijters, Jan E. R. "Changes in Body Mass Index in Young Adults in Relation to Number of Life Events Experienced." *International Journal of Obesity* 12(1) (February 1988).

Roper, Pamela, and Biggs, Thomas. "Consider the Facts First." *Shape,* April 1988.

Rosen, James C.; Tacy, Barbara; and Howell, David. "Life Stress, Psychological Symptoms and Weight Reducing Behavior in Adolescent Girls: A Prospective Analysis." *International Journal of Eating Disorders* Vol. 9 (January 1990).

Rosenfeld, Anne. "New Treatment for Bulimia." *Psychology Today,* March 1989.

Rossiter, Elise M.; Agras, W. Stewart; Losch, Martha, and Telch, Christy F. "Dietary Restraint of Bulimic Subjects Following Cognitive-Behavioral or Pharmacological Treatment." *Behavior Research and Therapy* 26(6) (1988).

Rucinski, Ann. "Relationship of Body Image and Dietary Intake of Competitive Ice Skaters." *Journal of the American Dietetic Association* 89(1) (January 1989).

Sanger, E., and Cassino, T. "Eating Disorders: Avoiding the Power Struggle." *American Journal of Nursing* 84(1) (January 1984).

Schlesier-Carter, Barbara; Hamilton, Sharon; O'Neil, Patrick; Lydiard, R. Bruce; and Malcolm, Robert. "Depression and Bulimia: The Link between Depression and Bulimic Cognitions." *Journal of Abnormal Psychology* 98(3) (August 1989).

Schmolling, Paul. "Eating Attitudes Test Scores in Relation to Weight, Socioeconomic Status, and Family Stability." *Psychological Reports* Vol. 64 (August 1988).

Schnitt, Diana. "Psychological Issues in Dancers—An Overview." *Journal of Physical Education, Recreation and Dance* 61(9) (November 1990).

Schocken, D. D.; Holloway, J. D.; and Powers, P. S. "Weight Loss and the Heart: Effects of Anorexia Nervosa and Starvation." *Archives of Internal Medicine* 14(9 Pt 4) (April 1989).

Schotte, David E.; McNally, Richard J.; and Turner, Mary L. "A Dichotic Listening Analysis of Body Weight Concern in Bulimia Nervosa." *International Journal of Eating Disorders* Vol. 9 (January 1990).

Schotte, David E., and Stunkard, Albert J. "Bulimia vs Bulimic Behaviors on a College Campus." *JAMA: Journal of the American Medical Association* Vol. 257 (September 4, 1987).

Scott, R. L., and Baroffio, J. R. "An MMPI Analysis of Similarities and Differences in Three Classifications of Eating Disorders: Anorexia Nervosa, Bulimia, and Morbid Obesity." *Journal of Clinical Psychology* Vol. 42 (September 1986).

Sedlet, Kathy L., and Ireton-Jones, Carol S. "Energy Expenditure and the Abnormal Eating Pattern of a Bulimic: A Case Report." *Journal of the American Dietetic Association* 39(1) (January 1989).

Segal, K. R., and Pi-Sunyer, F. X. "Exercise and Obesity." *Medical Clinics of North America* 73(1) (January 1989).

Shapiro, S. "Bulimia: An Entity in Search of Definition." *Journal of Clinical Psychology* 44(4) (July 1988).

Shimokata, H.; Tobin, J. D.; Muller, D. C.; and Elahi, D. "Studies in the Distribution of Body Fat: Effects of Age, Sex, and Obesity." *Journal of Gerontology* 44(2) (March 1989).

Shisslak, Catherine M.; Pazda, Susan; and Crago, Marjorie. "Body Weight and Bulimia as Discriminators of Psychological Characteristics among Anorexics, Bulimic, and Obese Women." *Journal of Abnormal Psychology* (November 1990).

Shisslak, Catherine M.; Schnaps, Laura. S.; and Crago, Marjorie. "Eating Disorders and Substance Abuse in Women: A Comparative Study of MMPI Patterns." *Journal of Substance Abuse* Vol. 1 (January 1989).

Shur, E.; Alloway, R.; Obrecht, R.; and Russell, G. F. "Physical Complications in Anorexia Nervosa: Hematological and Neuromuscular Changes in Twelve Patients." *British Journal of Psychiatry* (July 1988).

Shure, Jane. "Sexual Abuse Linked to Eating Disorders." *Renfrew Perspective,* Summer 1989.

Siegel, D. M. "Bulimia, Tricyclic Antidepressants, and Mania." *Clinical Pediatrics* 28(3) (March 1989).

Simon, Cheryl. "The Triumphant Dieter." *Psychology Today,* June 1989.

Sims, E. A. "Storage and Expenditure of Energy in Obesity and Their Implications for Management." *Medical Clinics of North America* 73(1) (January 1989).

Skaggs, Judy. "The Use of Self-help in Family Support." *BASH Newsletter,* May 1986.

Slade, Peter D. "The Misery That Neurotic Perfectionism Can Create." *BASH Magazine,* July 1989.

Sohlberg, Staffan; Rosmark, Borje; Norring, Claes; and Holmgren, Sven. "Impulsivity and Long-Term Prognosis of Psychiatric Patients with Anorexia Nervosa/Bulimia Nervosa." *Journal of Nervous and Mental Disease* 177(5) (May 1989).

————. "Two Year Outcome in Anorexia Nervosa/Bulimia: A Controlled Study of an Eating Control Program Combined with Psychoanalytically Oriented Psychotherapy." *International Journal of Eating Disorders* (March 1987).

Sorensen, Thorkild; Price, R. Arlen; Stunkard, Albert J.; and Schulsinger, Fini. "Genetics of Obesity in Adult Adoptees and Their Biological Siblings." *British Medical Journal* Vol. 297 (January 14, 1989).

Spiegelman, B. M.; Lowell, B.; Napolitano, A.; Dubuc, P.; et al. "Adrenal Glucocorticoids Regulate Adipsin Gene Expression in Genetically Obese Mice." *Journal of Biological Chemistry* 264(3) (January 1989).

Steel, J. M.; Young, R. J.; Lloyd, G. G.; and Clarke B. F. "Clinically Apparent Eating Disorders in Young Diabetic Women: Associations with Painful Neuropathy and Other Complications." *British Medical Journal* (Clinical Research Ed.) 294(6576) (April 1987).

Steiger, H.; Fraenkel, L.; and Leichner, P. P. "Relationship of Body-Image Distortion to Sex-Role Identification, Irrational Cognitions, and Body Weight in Eating-disordered Females." *Journal of Clinical Psychology* Vol. 45 (January 1989).

Stein, David M., and Laakso, William. "Bulimia: A Historical Perspective." *International Journal of Eating Disorders* Vol. 7 (March 1988).

Steinberg, Stacey; Tobin, David; and Johnson, Craig. "The Role of Bulimic Behaviors in Affect Regulation: Different Functions for Different Patient Subgroups." *International Journal of Eating Disorders* Vol. 9 (January 1990).

Stern, Loraine. "Your Child's Health: Early Signs of Serious Problems." *Woman's Day,* April 18, 1989.

Stirling, Mack C., and Orringer, Mark B. "Continued Assessment of the Combined Collis-Nissen Operation." *Annals of Thoracic Surgery* 47(2) (February 1989).

Stunkard, Albert J. "A Description of Eating Disorders in 1932." *American Journal of Psychiatry* Vol. 147 (March 1990).

———. "Obesity: Risk Factors, Consequences and Control." *Medical Journal of Australia* Vol. 148 (February 1, 1988).

"Substitute Fat May Mean Slim Gains." *U.S. News & World Report,* March 5, 1990.

Szmukler, G. I. "Premature Loss of Bone in Chronic Anorexia Nervosa." *British Medical Journal* 290(6461) (January 5, 1985).

Szymanski, Ludwik S., and Biederman, Joseph. "Depression and Anorexia Nervosa of Persons with Down's Syndrome." *American Journal of Mental Deficiency* 89(3) (November 1984).

Telch, Christy; Agras, W. Stewart; and Rossiter, Elise M. "Binge Eating Increases with Increasing Adiposity." *International Journal of Eating Disorders* Vol. 7 (January 1988).

———. "Group Cognitive-Behavioral Treatment for the Nonpurging Bulimic: An Initial Evaluation." *Journal of Consulting and Clinical Psychology* Vol. 58 (October 1990).

Thelen, Mark; Farmer, Janet; Mann, Laura McLaughlin; and Pruitt, Julie. "Bulimia and Interpersonal Relationships: A Longitudinal Study." *Journal of Counseling Psychology* Vol. 37 (January 1990).

Thornton, Lisa, and DeBlassie, Richard. "Treating Bulimia." *Adolescence* Vol. 24 (Fall 1989).

Tisdale, M. J., and Brennan, R. A. "A Comparison of Long-Chain Triglycerides and Medium-Chain Triglycerides on Weight Loss and Tumour Size in a Cachexia Model." *British Journal of Cancer* Vol. 58 (November 1988).

Tobin, David, and Johnson, Craig. "Multifactorial Assessment of Bulimia Nervosa." *Journal of Abnormal Psychology* Vol. 100 (February 1991).

Toner, Brenda B.; Garfinkel, Paul E.; and Garner, David M. "Affective and Anxiety Disorders in the Long-Term Follow-up of Anorexia Nervosa." *International Journal of Psychiatry in Medicine* Vol. 18, No. 4 (1988).

Treasure, J. L.; Wheeler, M.; King, E. A.; Gordon, P. A. L.; and Russell, G. F. M. "Weight Gain and Reproductive Function: Ultrasonographic and Endocrine Features in Anorexia Nervosa." *Clinical Endocrinology* 29 (1988).

Tucker, Larry A., and Friedman, Glenn M. "Television Viewing and Obesity in Adult Males." *American Journal of Public Health* 79(4) (April 1989).

Vaisman, Nachum; Corey, M.; Rossi, Miriam F.; Goldberg, Eudice; and Pencharz, Paul B. "Changes in Body Composition during Refeeding of Patients with Anorexia Nervosa." *Journal of Pediatrics* 113(5) (November 1988).

Vaisman, Nachum; Rossi, Miriam F.; Goldberg, Eudice; Dibden, Lionel J.; Wykes, Linda J.; and Pencharz, Paul B. "Energy Expenditure and Body Composition in Patients with Anorexia Nervosa." *Journal of Pediatrics* 113 (1988).

van Binsbergen, C. J. M.; Odink, J.; van den Berg, H.; Koppeschaar, H.; and Binnink, H. J. T. Coelingh. "Nutritional Status in Anorexia Nervosa: Clinical Chemistry, Vitamins, Iron and Zinc." *European Journal of Clinical Nutrition* 42 (1988).

van Dale, Djoeke, and Saris, Wim H. M. "Repetitive Weight Loss and Weight Regain: Effects on Weight Reduction, Resting Metabolic Rate, and Lipolytic Activity before and after Exercise and/or Diet Treatment." *American Journal of Clinical Nutrition* Vol. 50 (March 1989).

Vanderbroucke, J. P.; Mauritz, B. J.; de Bruin, A.; Verheesen, J. H.; et al. "Weight, Smoking, and Mortality." *JAMA: Journal of the American Medical Association* Vol. 252 (November 23–30, 1984).

Vandereycken, Walter. "The Addiction Model in Eating Disorders: Some Critical Remarks and a Selected Bibliography." *International Journal of Eating Disorders* Vol. 9 (January 1990).

Vanderlinden, Johan, and Vandereycken, Walter. "Family Therapy in Bulimia Nervosa." *BASH Newsletter.*

———. "Perception of Changes in Eating Disorder Patients during Group Treatment." *Psychotherapy and Psychosomatics* 49 (1988).

Van Deth, Ron, and Vandereycken, Walter. "Reflections on the History of Self-starvation." *BASH Magazine,* April 1984.

Van Pelt, Dina. "Laser in Liposuction a Disputed Addiction." *Insight,* February 5, 1990.

———. "Metabolism May Offer Eating Disorder Clues." *Insight,* November 27, 1989.

Vansant, Greet; Den Besten, Cathaline; Weststrate, Jan; and Deurenberg, Paul. "Body Fat Distribution and the Prognosis for Weight Reduction: Preliminary Observations." *International Journal of Obesity* 12(2) (April 1988).

Van Vreckem, Ellie, and Vandereycken, Walter. "Therapeutic Significance in the Sibling Relationship." *BASH Magazine,* July 1989.

"Very Low Calorie Diets." *Perspectives on Weight Management,* Ross Laboratories, Vol. 2, No. 4 (1989).

Vincent, C. A., and Richardson, P. H. "Acupuncture for Some Common Disorders: A Review of Evaluative Research." *Journal of the Royal College of General Practitioners* Vol. 37 (February 1987).

Walsh, B. Timothy. "Antidepressants and Bulimia: Where Are We?" *International Journal of Eating Disorders* Vol. 7 (May 1988).

———. "Phenelzine vs Placebo in Fifty Patients with Bulimia." *Archives of General Psychiatry* 45(5) (May 1988).

Walsh, B. Timothy; Kissileff, Harry R.; Cassidy, Susan M.; and Dantzic, Sondra. "Eating Behavior of Women with Bulimia." *Archives of General Psychiatry* 46(1) (January 1989).

Wamboldt, F. S.; Kaslow, N. J.; Swift, W. J.; and Ritholz, M. "Short-Term Course of Depressive Symptoms in Patients with Eating Disorders." *American Journal of Psychiatry* 144(3) (March 1987).

Warshaw, Hope S. "Liquid Protein Diets." *Diabetes Self-Management,* July/August 1989.

Weiner, Herbert. "Psychoendocrinology of Anorexia Nervosa." *Psychiatric Clinics of North America* 12(1) (March 1989).

Weingarten, H. P.; Hendler, R.; and Rodin, J. "Metabolism and Endocrine Secretion in Response to a Test Meal in Normal-Weight Bulimic Women." *Psychosomatic Medicine* 50(3) (May-June 1988).

Weintraub, M., and Bray, George A. "Drug Treatment of Obesity." *Medical Clinics of North America* Vol. 73 (January 1989).

Welch, Garry; Hall, Anne; and Norring, Claes. "The Factor Structure of the Eating Disorder Inventory in a Patient Setting." *International Journal of Eating Disorders* Vol. 9 (January 1990).

Willi, Jurg; Giacometti, Graziella; and Limacher, Bernhar. "Update on the Epidemiology of Anorexia Nervosa in a Defined Region of Switzerland." *American Journal of Psychiatry* Vol. 147 (November 1990).

Williamson, Donald; Davis, C. J.; Goreczny, Anthony; and Blouin, David. "Body-Image Disturbances in Bulimia Nervosa: Influences of Actual Body Size." *Journal of Abnormal Psychology* 98(1) (February 1989).

Willis, D. C., and Rand, G. S. "Pregnancy in Bulimic Women." *Obstetrics and Gynecology* 71(5) (May 1988).

Willis, Judith Levine. "How to Take Weight Off (and Keep It Off) without Getting Ripped Off." *FDA Consumer*, DHHS Publication No. (FDA) 89-1116.

Wolf, Naomi. "Fear of Eating: How U.S. Women Lock Themselves into Hunger Camps." *Los Angeles Times*, May 12, 1991.

———. "Hunger Artists." *Village Voice*, December 12, 1989.

Wonderlich, Stephen, and Swift, William. "Perceptions of Parental Relationships in the Eating Disorders: The Relevance of Depressed Mood." *Journal of Abnormal Psychology* 99(4) (November 1990).

Wooley, O. Wayne, and Wooley, Susan C. "An Indictment of Dieting." *NAAFA Newsletter*, January-February 1980.

Wright, Peter. "Hunger, Satiety and Feeding Behavior in Early Infancy." In *Eating Habits*, edited by R. A. Boakes, David A. Popplewell and Michael J. Burton, New York: Wiley, 1987.

———. "Mothers' Assessment of Hunger in Relation to Meal Size in Breastfed Infants." *Journal of Reproductive and Infant Psychology* 5 (1987).

———. "The Psychology of Eating and Eating Disorders." In *Psychology Survey No. 6*, edited by H. Beloff and A. Coleman. British Psychological Society, 1987.

Wu, Joseph; Hagman, Jennifer; Buchsbaum, Monte; Blinder, Barton; and Derrfler, Melissa. "Greater Left Cerebral Hemispheric Metabolism in Bulimia." *American Journal of Psychiatry* 147(3) (March 1990).

Yager, Joel. "The Treatment of Eating Disorders." *Journal of Clinical Psychiatry* 49 Suppl:18–25 (September 1988).

Yager, J.; Kurtzman, F.; Landsverk, J.; and Wiesmeier, E. "Behaviors and Attitudes Related to Eating Disorders in Homosexual Male College Students." *American Journal of Psychiatry* Vol. 145 (April 1988).

Yager, Joel; Landsverk, John; and Edelstein, Carole K. "A Twenty-Month Follow-up Study of 628 Women with Eating Disorders." *American Journal of Psychiatry* 144(9) (September 1987).

Yager, J.; Landsverk, J.; Edelstein, C. K.; and Hyler, Steven E. "Screening for Axis II Personality Disorders in Women with Bulimic Eating Disorders." *Psychosomatics* 30(3) (Summer 1989).

Yale, Jean-Francois; Leiter, Lawrence A.; and Marliss, Errol B. "Metabolic Responses to Intense Exercise in Lean and Obese Subjects." *Journal of Clinical Endocrinology and Metabolism* 68(2) (February 1989).

Yates, William R.; Sieleni, Bruce; Reich, James; and Brass, Clint. "Comorbidity of Bulimia Nervosa and Personality Disorder." *Journal of Clinical Psychiatry* 50 (1989).

Yost, Trudy J., and Eckel, Robert H. "Hypocaloric Feeding in Obese Women: Metabolic Effects of Medium-Chain Triglyceride Substitution." *American Journal of Clinical Nutrition* 49(2) (February 1989).

Zaslow, Jeffrey. "Fourth Grade Girls These Days Ponder Weighty Matters." *Wall Street Journal*, February 11, 1986.

Zellner, Debra; Harner, Debra; and Adler, Robbie. "Effects of Eating Abnormalities and Gender on Perception of Desirable Body Shape." *Journal of Abnormal Psychology* 98(1) (February 1989).

BOOKS AND REPORTS

B., Bill. *Compulsive Overeater*. Minneapolis, Minn.: CompCare Publications, 1981.

Bauer, Barbara G.; Anderson, Wayne P.; and Hyatt, Robert A. *Bulimia: Book for Therapist and Client*. Muncie, Ind.: Accelerated Development, 1986.

Bayrd, Edwin. *The Thin Game*. New York: Newsweek, 1978.

Beaulieu, Michael S. *Obesity: A Disease of the Mind*. New Haven, Conn: Prometheus Bound, 1985.

Beller, Anne Scott. *Fat & Thin: A Natural History of Obesity*. New York: McGraw-Hill, 1977.

Bemporad, J. R., and Herzog, D. B., eds. *Psychoanalysis & Eating Disorders*. New York: Gilford Press, 1989.

Bennett, William, and Gurin, Joel. *The Dieter's Dilemma*. New York: Basic Books, 1982.

Berland, Theodore. *Rating the Diets*. New York: Beekman House, 1980.

Blinder, B. J., et al., eds. *Modern Concepts of the Eating Disorders*. 1988.

Boakes, Robert A., ed. *Eating Habits: Food, Physiology and Learned Behavior*. London: John Wiley & Sons, 1987.

Boskind-White, Marlene, and White, William C. *Bulimarexia*. New York: W. W. Norton, 1983.

Brownell, K. D., Foreyt, J. P., eds. *Handbook of Eating Disorders: Physiology, Psychology, and Treatment of Obesity, Anorexia, and Bulimia*. New York: Basic Books, 1986.

Bruch, Hilde. *Eating Disorders: Obesity, Anorexia Nervosa, and the Person Within*. New York: Basic Books, 1973.

———. *The Golden Cage: The Enigma of Anorexia Nervosa*. Cambridge: Harvard University Press, 1978.

Brumberg, Joan Jacobs. *Fasting Girls*. Cambridge: Harvard University Press, 1988.

Byrne, Katherine. *A Parent's Guide to Anorexia and Bulimia.* New York: Schocken, 1987.

Cauwels, Janice M. *Bulimia.* Garden City, N.Y.: Doubleday, 1983.

Christian, Shannon, with Margaret Johnson. *The Very Private Matter of Anorexia Nervosa.* Grand Rapids, Mich.: Zondervan, 1986.

Collipp, Platon J., ed. *Childhood Obesity.* New York: Warner, 1986.

Cooper, Kenneth H. *The New Aerobics.* New York: Bantam, 1970.

Crisp, Arthur H. *Anorexia Nervosa: Let Me Be.* London: Academic Press, 1980.

Donovan, Dennis M., and Marlatt, G. Alan. *Assessment of Addictive Behaviors.* New York: Guilford Press, 1988.

Ernsberger, Paul, and Haskew, Paul. *Rethinking Obesity: An Alternative View of Its Health Implications.* New York: Human Sciences Press, 1987.

Friedman, Abraham. *Fat Can Be Beautiful.* New York: G. P. Putnam's Sons, 1974.

Furst, Lillian R., and Graham, Peter W., eds. *Disorderly Eaters: Texts in Self-empowerment.* University Park, Pa., 1992.

Garfinkel, Paul E., and Garner, David M. *Anorexia Nervosa.* New York: Brunner/Mazel, 1982.

――――, eds. *The Role of Drug Treatments for Eating Disorders.* New York: Brunner/Mazel, 1987.

Haskew, Paul, and Adams, Cynthia H. *When Food Is a Four-Letter Word.* Englewood Cliffs, N.J.: Prentice-Hall, 1984.

Hirschmann, Jane R., and Munter, Carol H. *Overcoming Overeating.* Reading, Mass: Addison-Wesley, 1988.

Hollis, Judi. *Fat Is a Family Affair.* San Francisco: Harper & Row, 1985.

Hornyak, L. M., and Baker, E. K., eds. *Experiential Therapies for Eating Disorders.* New York: Guilford Press, 1989.

Hunt, Douglas. *No More Cravings.* New York: Warner, 1987.

Huon, G. F., and Brown, L. B. *Fighting with Food: Overcoming Bulimia Nervosa.* Australia: New South Wales Press.

Johnston, F. E., ed. *Nutritional Anthropology.* New York: Alan R. Liss, 1987.

Larocca, Félix E. F., ed. in chief. *Eating Disorders: Effective Care and Treatment.* St. Louis: Ishiyaku EuroAmerica, 1986.

――――. guest ed. *The Psychiatric Clinics of North America,* Vol. 7, No. 2: *Symposium on Eating Disorders.* Philadelphia: W. B. Saunders, 1984.

Larocca, Félix E. F., with Nancy J. Kolodny. *Facilitator's Training Manual.* St. Louis: Midwest Medical Publications, 1983.

Lawrence, Marilyn. *The Anorexic Experience.* London: Women's Press, 1984.

――――, ed. *Fed Up and Hungry.* New York: Peter Bedrick, 1987.

Levenkron, Steven. *Treating and Overcoming Anorexia Nervosa.* New York: Warner, 1982.

McCurdy, John A., Jr. *Sculpturing Your Body: Diet, Exercise and Lipo (Fat) Suction.* Hollywood, Fla.: Frederick Fell Publishers, 1987.

MacLeod, Sheila. *The Art of Starvation.* New York: Schocken, 1982.

Miller, Caroline Adams. *My Name is Caroline.* New York: Doubleday, 1988.

Mitchell, James E., ed. *Anorexia Nervosa & Bulimia—Diagnosis and Treatment.* Minneapolis: University of Minnesota Press, 1985.

Muslin, H. D., and Val, E. R. *The Psychotherapy of the Self.* New York: Brunner/Mazel, 1987.

Neuman, Patricia A., and Halvorson, Patricia A. *Anorexia Nervosa and Bulimia: A Handbook for Counselors and Therapists.* New York: Van Nostrand Reinhold, 1983.

Orbach, Susie. *Fat Is a Feminist Issue.* New York: Berkley, 1978.

Palmer, R. L. *Anorexia Nervosa.* New York: Penguin, 1980.

Pope, Harrison G., and Hudson, James I. *New Hope for Binge Eaters.* New York: Harper & Row, 1984.

Romeo, Felicia. *Understanding Anorexia Nervosa.* Springfield, Ill.: Charles C. Thomas, 1986.

Root, Maria P. P.; Fallon, Patricia; and Friedrich, William N. *Bulimia: A Systems Approach to Treatment.* New York: W. W. Norton, 1986.

Rumney, Avis. *Dying to Please.* Jefferson, N.C.: McFarland, 1983.

Sacker, Ira M., and Zimmer, Marc. A. *Dying to Be Thin.* New York: Warner, 1987.

Schemmel, Rachel, ed. *Nutrition, Physiology, and Obesity.* Boca Raton, Fla.: CRC Press, 1980.

Schwartz, Hillel. *Never Satisfied: A Cultural History of Diets, Fantasies, and Fat.* New York: Free Press, 1986.

Siegel, Michele; Brisman, Judith; and Weinshel, Margot. *Surviving an Eating Disorder.* New York: Harper & Row, 1988.

Slochower, Joyce Anne. *Excessive Eating.* New York: Human Sciences Press, 1983.

Stierlin, Helm, and Weber, Gunthard. *Unlocking the Family Door: A Systemic Approach to the Understanding and Treatment of Anorexia Nervosa.* New York: Brunner/ Mazel, 1989.

Stoltz, Sandra Gordon. *The Food Fix.* Englewood Cliffs, N.J.: Prentice-Hall, 1983.

Toguchi, Masaru, and Warren, Frank Z. *Complete Guide to Acupuncture and Acupressure.* New York: Gramercy, 1985.

Tupin, J. P., and Shader, R. I., eds. *Handbook of Clinical Psychopharmacology.* Northvale, N.J.: Jason Aronson, 1988.

Useful Information on Anorexia Nervosa and Bulimia, (ADM) 87-1514. Superintendent of Documents, U.S. Government Printing Office, PO Box 371954, Pittsburgh, PA 15250-7954. GPO No. 017-024-01322-6, $17.00 per 50 copies.

Vandereycken, W.; Kog, E.; and Vanderlinden, J., eds. *The Family Approach to Eating Disorders: Assessment and Treatment of Anorexia Nervosa and Bulimia.* New York: PMA, 1989.

Walsh, B. Timothy, ed. *Eating Behavior in Eating Disorders.* Washington, D.C.: American Psychiatric Press, 1988.

Webb, Linda J. ed. *Diagnostic and Statistical Manual of Mental Disorders* (DSM III and DSM III-R). Washington, D.C.: American Psychiatric Press, 1980/1987.

Wise, Jonathan, and Wise, Susan Kierr. *The Overeaters.* New York: Human Sciences Press, 1979.

Yalom, I. D. *Love's Executioner and Other Tales of Psychotherapy.* New York: Basic Books, 1989.

PERIODICALS

International Journal of Eating Disorders, John Wiley & Sons, PO Box 7247-8491, Philadelphia, PA 19170-8491.

Light Delight, 12505 W. Jefferson Blvd. #-305, Los Angeles, CA 90066.

Obesity and Health, Route 2, Box 905, Hettinger, ND 58639.

INDEX

Main essays are indicated by **bold** page numbers.
Tables are indicated by *"t"*